Autism Spectrum Disorders in Infants and Toddlers

Diagnosis, Assessment, and Treatment

Edited by

KATARZYNA CHAWARSKA
AMI KLIN
FRED R. VOLKMAR

Foreword by Michael D. Powers

THE GUILFORD PRESS
New York   London

Printed in the United States of America

This book is printed on acid-free paper.

Last digit is print number: 9 8 7 6 5 4 3 2

Library of Congress Cataloging-in-Publication Data

Autism spectrum disorders in infants and toddlers : diagnosis, assessment, and treatment / edited by Katarzyna Chawarska, Ami Klin, Fred R. Volkmar ; foreword by Michael D. Powers.
    p. ; cm.
Includes bibliographical references and index.
ISBN 978-1-59385-649-6 (hardcover : alk. paper)
    1. Autism in children. 2. Infants—Mental health. 3. Toddlers—Mental health.
I. Chawarska, Katarzyna. II. Klin, Ami. III. Volkmar, Fred R.
    [DNLM: 1. Autistic Disorder—diagnosis. 2. Autistic Disorder—therapy.
3. Child. 4. Infant. WM 203.5 A93849 2008]
    RJ506.A9A92393 2008
    618.92′85882—dc22

                                                                2007044633

To Marek, Szymon, and Julek;
Siomara, Ian, Liana, and Daniel;
Lisa, Lucy, and Emily

About the Editors

Katarzyna Chawarska, PhD, is Assistant Professor and Director of the Developmental Disabilities Clinic for Infants and Toddlers at the Child Study Center at Yale University School of Medicine. Dr. Chawarska received her graduate degree in developmental psychology at Yale University and completed her clinical training at the Yale Child Study Center. Dr. Chawarska is a principal investigator on several research grants focused on early mechanisms of social development and sponsored by the National Institute of Child Health and Human Development, National Institute of Mental Health, as well as private foundations, including Autism Speaks and the National Alliance for Autism Research. Her research is focused on the early expression of autism spectrum disorders and on experimental studies of face and gaze processing in infants and toddlers.

Ami Klin, PhD, is the Harris Associate Professor of Child Psychology and Psychiatry at the Child Study Center at Yale University School of Medicine. Dr. Klin is Director of the Autism Program at Yale, which has been named one of the National Institutes of Health's Autism Centers of Excellence. Dr. Klin's primary research activities focus on the social mind and the social brain, and on various aspects of autism from infancy through adulthood. He is the editor or coeditor of several books and special issues of professional journals, including *Asperger Syndrome* and the *Handbook of Autism and Pervasive Developmental Disorders*.

Fred R. Volkmar, MD, is the Irving B. Harris Professor of Child Psychiatry, Pediatrics, and Psychology and Director of the Child Study Center at

Yale University School of Medicine. He is also the Chief of Child Psychiatry at Yale–New Haven Hospital and serves as Director of Autism Research at Yale. Dr. Volkmar was the primary author of the American Psychiatric Association's DSM-IV autism and Pervasive Developmental Disorders section, and is the author, coauthor, or coeditor of several hundred scientific papers and chapters and a number of books, including *Asperger Syndrome, Healthcare for Children on the Autism Spectrum*, and the *Handbook of Autism and Pervasive Developmental Disorders*. He has served as an associate editor of the *Journal of Child Psychology and Psychiatry* and the *American Journal of Psychiatry*, and is editor-in-chief of the *Journal of Autism and Developmental Disorders*. He has served as co-chairperson of the autism/intellectual disabilities committee of the American Academy of Child and Adolescent Psychiatry. Dr. Volkmar is the principal investigator of three program project grants, including a CPEA (Collaborative Program of Excellence in Autism) grant from the National Institute of Child Health and Human Development and a STAART (Studies to Advance Autism Research and Treatment) Autism Center Grant from the National Institute of Mental Health.

Contributors

Karyn Bailey, LCSW, MSW, Yale Child Study Center, New Haven, Connecticut

Grace T. Baranek, PhD, OTR/L, FAOTA, Department of Allied Health Sciences, University of North Carolina at Chapel Hill, Chapel Hill, North Carolina

Karen Bearss, PhD, Yale Child Study Center, New Haven, Connecticut

Somer L. Bishop, PhD, University of Michigan Autism and Communication Disorders Center, Ann Arbor, Michigan

Katarzyna Chawarska, PhD, Yale Child Study Center, New Haven, Connecticut

Fabian J. David, MS, PT, Department of Movement Sciences and Nutrition, University of Illinois at Chicago, Chicago, Illinois

Rosy M. Fredeen, PhD, Koegel Autism Center, University of California, Santa Barbara, Santa Barbara, California

Grace W. Gengoux, MA, Department of Counseling, Clinical, and School Psychology, University of California, Santa Barbara, Santa Barbara, California

Abha R. Gupta, MD, PhD, Yale Child Study Center, New Haven, Connecticut

Ami Klin, PhD, Yale Child Study Center, New Haven, Connecticut

Lynn Kern Koegel, PhD, Koegel Autism Center, University of California, Santa Barbara, Santa Barbara, California

Robert L. Koegel, PhD, Department of Counseling, Clinical, and School Psychology, and Koegel Autism Center, University of California, Santa Barbara, Santa Barbara, California

Catherine Lord, PhD, University of Michigan Autism and Communication Disorders Center, Ann Arbor, Michigan

Rhiannon Luyster, PhD, University of Michigan Autism and Communication Disorders Center, Ann Arbor, Michigan

Rhea Paul, PhD, CCC-SLP, Department of Communication Disorders, Southern Connecticut State University, and Yale Child Study Center, New Haven, Connecticut

Jennifer Richler, PhD, University of Michigan Autism and Communication Disorders Center, Ann Arbor, Michigan

Celine Saulnier, PhD, Yale Child Study Center, New Haven, Connecticut

Tristram Smith, PhD, Strong Center for Developmental Disabilities, University of Rochester Medical Center, Rochester, New York

Fred R. Volkmar, MD, Yale Child Study Center, New Haven, Connecticut

Linn Wakeford, MS, OTR/L, Department of Allied Health Sciences, University of North Carolina at Chapel Hill, Chapel Hill, North Carolina

Alexander Westphal, MD, Yale Child Study Center, New Haven, Connecticut

Amy M. Wetherby, PhD, CCC-SLP, Department of Communication Disorders, Florida State University, Tallahassee, Florida

Jennifer Wick, MA, Strong Center for Developmental Disabilities, University of Rochester Medical Center, Rochester, New York

Lisa Wiesner, MD, private practice, Orange, Connecticut

Juliann Woods, PhD, CCC-SLP, Department of Communication Disorders, Florida State University, Tallahassee, Florida

Foreword

The poet William Blake (1757–1827) once suggested that we can "see a world in a grain of sand." In studying the details of life, we better understand more complex mechanisms as they evolve developmentally into adaptive patterns of learning, behavior, and cognition. The task of synthesizing complexity is not a small one, particularly where the changing landscape of early childhood development is involved. That we must synthesize and collaborate across disciplines is now widely accepted; to do less is myopic at best, malfeasance or malpractice at worst. Undertaking the task of integrating the science and clinical practice of various disciplines was the intent of Katarzyna Chawarska, Ami Klin, and Fred R. Volkmar in creating this book, and they have succeeded with remarkable clarity. Because *Autism Spectrum Disorders in Infants and Toddlers* captures at once the breadth of the disorders, the most current research and applications, and the questions yet unanswered, it will quickly become the essential guide to this fascinating, complex universe of understanding and helping these children and their families.

A knowing smile. The exuberance and excitement of a shared observation. The drama between the instance of fear and the moment of comfort. Events so commonplace in the life of a toddler as to be taken for granted, unless they fail to occur. So expected and seemingly natural are these behaviors that when discrepant, or worse yet, absent, we often attribute the errors to external events. It comes as little surprise, then, that as we have begun to better understand the automatic and effortless process of social and communication development in young children, we have also come to appreciate the pervasive effects on a young child of the failure to understand the social world. As any parent readily understands, those pervasive developmental failures have a rippling and compounding impact not only on the child, but on the life of everyone touched by that child. If, as some have stated, autism is the prototypical developmental disorder, then rigorous investigation holds tremendous promise for those so affected and for other children as well. In their groundbreaking work, the editors have brought together a group of eminent researchers from many disciplines who are also remarkable clinicians. These authors review the expanding fields of basic and applied research on very young children with or suspected with autism spectrum disorders (ASD) in a manner both comprehensive and accessible. As important, however, applications to the child in need today are articulated with precision. Throughout, the emphasis on practice derived from exceptional science is evident, whether establishing diagnostic parameters, developing social or communication repertoires, understanding and addressing sensory and motor problems, or helping families make sense of it all.

Although it is exciting to read what is known, and in its comprehensiveness *Autism Spectrum Disorders in Infants and Toddlers* provides just that, it is also humbling to consider what is not. As we come to understand the basic mechanisms of social thinking and social communication, and of the genetic and neurobiological differences whose confluence we call autism, we appreciate the power of science, of knowledge, and of the ability to affirmatively alter the developmental course of a child with a severe developmental disability. But the responsibility that comes with this power and knowledge—to reach the 1 in 150 children with a diagnosis of ASD in impoverished, geographically remote, or other vastly underserved regions—is even greater, and unmet. Chawarska, Klin, and Volkmar, together with their contributors, empower us with this extensive knowledge, but also simultaneously task us to apply it.

In Chapter 1, Volkmar, Chawarska, and Klin quickly establish the mandate for this volume. Beginning with a description of diagnostic conceptualizations from Kanner through DSM-IV-TR and ICD-10, they move seamlessly into clinical presentation of autistic symptomatology in the first, second, and third years of life. Their formulation provides essential context for understanding the subsequent chapters on diagnosis, assessment, and treatment.

The chapters on diagnostic, cognitive, adaptive, communication, and sensory–motor assessment provide the foundation for the basic and applied research discussed throughout the rest of the book. Bishop, Luyster, Richler, and Lord summarize social, play, and communication behavior in typically developing children, with more extensive discussion of screening and diagnostic instruments used to detect ASD. Their thoughtful observations on differential diagnosis of children under 24 months suspected of ASD are particularly valuable. Chawarska and Bearss highlight the importance of developmental, cognitive, and adaptive assessment from a dynamic, interdisciplinary framework. They review in detail the most commonly used measures in these domains, incorporating astute clinical observations and specific strategies that make direct assessment more fruitful. By providing a review of long-term follow-up on some of these measures, the authors underscore the very developmental discontinuity that is emblematic of ASD while simultaneously providing sound advice on interpreting and reporting findings.

Given that a child's discrepancies in communicating in social contexts is often the first concern noted by parents about their toddler, Paul's chapter outlining the development of typical preverbal and spoken language and the very specific deviant patterns observed in infants and toddlers with ASD is especially welcome. Even more valuable are the discussions of normative and criterion-referenced assessment methods and strategies. Through detailed clinical descriptions supported and expanded by a comprehensive review of relevant research, Paul provides a solid grounding for understanding and evaluating communication deficits from the earliest months.

Irregularities in interpreting, regulating, and responding to the sensory world are much discussed (often with some controversy) in the autism literature. For this reason, Baranek, Wakeford, and David's chapter is particularly relevant and welcome. They provide an exceptional review of the literature on infants and toddlers, establishing a framework for comprehensive review of assessment procedures used to evaluate sensory–motor functions. Their discussion of intervention strategies appropriately begins with review of theoretical models and launches into a more detailed discussion of traditional and controversial approaches. The strength of this chapter is its emphasis on evidence-based practice derived from studies of efficacy of treatment procedures. Numerous case examples throughout the chapter bring clarity to the concepts presented.

The detailed presentation of case studies of three children first identified with ASD between 15 and 20 months, and subsequently followed through age 4, is a virtuoso clinic on the content and process of early identification. Although important discrepancies of clinical presentation are evident in these children, this chapter by Klin, Saulnier, Chawarska, and Volkmar provides a clinically sophisticated and detailed background against which to apply the diagnostic and assessment practices of the previous five chapters as context to the subsequent three on treatment. At once thorough and scholarly, these case presentations ultimately capture the developing, dynamic child with clarity, precision, and humanity.

The chapters devoted to treatment methods thoughtfully explore the relationship between developmental and behavioral models of intervention with infants and toddlers with ASD as well as medical considerations for this group. Wetherby and Woods review the primary social communication deficits of young children with ASD, identify basic principles guiding developmental treatment models, and describe those core elements of developmental models that enjoy a firmer empirical footing. In the process they also provide a thoughtful comparison of the similarities and differences between developmental and behavioral models of intervention. For their part, Koegel, Koegel, Fredeen, and Gengoux cogently describe what may be termed the "third wave" of behavioral treatment in autism. By clearly articulating the importance of naturalistic language and social teaching paradigms while simultaneously underscoring the essential ingredient of empirical validation of both treatment procedures and learning outcomes, these authors may well provide the foundation for systematic investigation—and possible synthesis—of behavioral and developmental models of treatment that is needed in the field.

Smith and Wick bring this entire discussion of treatment (and possible mistreatment) into clear focus with their thought-provoking and well-documented review of popular but controversial treatments in autism. With the demand that the treatment interventions offered must stand up to the dual tests of empirical validation and replicability, the authors provide ample support for the expanding calls for evidence-based practice in recent federal legislation, including the Individuals with Disabilities Education Act and the No Child Left Behind Act. Further, and perhaps most important, they help to operationalize the concept that intervention cannot be merely "appropriate"; it must be "effective" in delivering predicted learning outcomes. Effectiveness is an empirical question that can be measured even in a single child. The rubric for empirical validation common to the behavioral sciences is thus offered as a consideration for other disciplines and methodologies.

Genetic and proposed environmental causes of autism, as well as components of a comprehensive medical evaluation of children with autism, are discussed by Volkmar, Westphal, Gupta, and Wiesner. Providing a clear and well-documented review of the genetics of autism is one of the exceptional features of this chapter, rivaled by the thorough discussion of associated conditions that may be seen by primary care providers and how to address them in the office or clinic. Equally important, however, is the excellent review of scientific evidence that refutes the autism–measles–mumps–rubella (MMR) vaccine link. Although the authors acknowledge the persistence of this belief in the absence of empirical support, they also collectively provide the reader with a means of understanding the controversy and its implications.

Like a pebble thrown into a lake, the rippling effects of a diagnosis of ASD in a child impact the immediate and extended family, kinship networks, the community, and a family's perception of its role and function. Bailey carefully and sensitively outlines the emotional terrain families confront before and after diagnosis, providing an excellent introduction to the educational, social, and advocacy networks in which they now must become expert. If a sense of self-efficacy and personal hardiness in the face of a diagnosis of ASD matters (and research has shown that it indeed does), then Bailey provides the guidance that can support hope, optimism, and confidence—and ultimately better outcomes—for the child with ASD and his or her family.

Like bookends, the first and last chapters frame our understanding of what is known, and must become known. In Chapter 1, Volkmar, Chawarska, and Klin introduced the work that is possible now, and the exemplary manner in which evaluation and treatment must be accomplished in order to effect the best outcomes for infants and toddlers with ASD. In closing this volume, they direct us to those issues and questions that will engender future possibilities. By emphasizing the extension of current research findings, the authors explicitly underscore the necessity of interdisciplinary collaboration. Investigation of the complexity of ASD as we now understand it will—if we are lucky—create better questions and answers about those most basic impairments observed, and even more exciting opportunities for translating research into effective clinical practice.

At once scholarly and practical, Chawarska, Klin, and Volkmar have created the interdisciplinary standard by which other work in autism will be judged for years to come. By weaving seamlessly the weft of developmental, neurobiological, and family considerations against the warp of rigorous science and evidence-based clinical practice, they have unified seemingly disparate parts into a complex whole, rendering the detail of basic research findings as thoughtfully as the elegance of the developing child as a person. In so doing, they remind us—even demand—that we see and know the infant and toddler with autism first and foremost as a child of promise, to be understood. But more than this, as a teacher who will surely continue to give up his or her secrets if only we ask our questions with equal measures of scientific rigor and awe.

MICHAEL D. POWERS, PsyD
Director, The Center for Children with Special Needs,
Glastonbury, Connecticut, and
Yale Child Study Center,
Yale University School of Medicine,
New Haven, Connecticut

Preface

Although the first symptoms of autism spectrum disorders (ASD) appear in the first or second year of life, most children affected by the disorder are not diagnosed and appropriately treated until preschool or early school age. This disparity between onset of symptoms and diagnosis is discouraging for both clinical and research reasons. Fortunately, over the past decade, advances in research on diagnosis and treatment have been made. It is clear that the early diagnosis is relatively stable and that timely initiation of treatment leads to improved outcomes in terms of cognition, social interactions, communication, and adaptive functioning. In addition to the importance of early identification for improving the quality of life of individuals with ASD, it also provides the opportunity for studying pathogenesis of the disorder when confounding effects of treatment, compensatory strategies, and comorbid disorders have not yet had an impact on syndrome expression.

This volume reflects our attempt to synthesize state-of-the-art knowledge regarding early expression of the syndrome while nonetheless highlighting the areas of research and clinical practice that still remain to be addressed and elucidated. It contains a critical review of current issues related to classification, diagnosis, assessment, and treatment of ASD in infants and toddlers. Experts in the field share their clinical insights as well as empirical findings that can be readily translated into practice. The book is addressed to psychologists, psychiatrists, pediatricians, educators, early intervention providers, speech and language pathologists, social workers, as well as parents.

We thank our colleagues who contributed to this volume as well as the staff at The Guilford Press, particularly Kitty Moore, who supported its development. Finally, we thank our young patients and their families who have taught us so much about the earliest manifestations of autism and the challenges they face.

Contents

CHAPTER 1

Autism Spectrum Disorders in Infants and Toddlers

An Introduction

FRED R. VOLKMAR
KATARZYNA CHAWARSKA
AMI KLIN

In his original report on the syndrome of early infantile autism, Leo Kanner (1943/1968) indicated that autism was a congenital disorder. Although a minority of children seem to develop autism after some months of normal development, most of the subsequent work on autism has generally supported his contention (see Volkmar, Chawarska, & Klin, 2005, for a review). This observation would also be highly consistent with the large body of work supporting a genetic basis for the condition (Rutter, 2005). Somewhat paradoxically, however, our knowledge of autism as it is expressed in the first year of life is quite limited.

Fortunately, within the last decade this situation has begun to change. A little more than a decade ago various factors acted to delay case detection and early diagnosis (Siegel, Pliner, Eschler, & Elliott, 1988), but now various programs specifically focused on early diagnosis of infants at risk for autism have been developed. Growing public awareness of the condition and an increasingly large body of work on the importance of early intervention and stability of early diagnosis (National Research Council, 2001) have increased interest in the early stages of autism. A growing body of research work focused on this age group has begun to

1

appear. In previous years most of this work was based on either parent report (Chawarska, Paul, et al., 2007; Cohen, Volkmar, & Paul, 1986) or review of videotapes or movies (e.g., Osterling & Dawson, 1994; Werner, Dawson, Osterling, & Dinno, 2000), with all the attendant problems associated with the lack of contemporaneous methods. The first prospective longitudinal studies of young children (Lord, 1995; Lord et al., 2006) and the recognition of the importance of early intervention have stimulated the National Institute of Mental Health to set the ambitious goal of reducing the number of children with autism through early diagnosis and intervention. In this chapter we are concerned with issues of the clinical expression of autism in infants. Although our major focus is on infancy and early childhood, some of the work on preschool children is highly relevant and is touched upon as well. We attempt to highlight areas critical for future research on this important topic.

AUTISM AS A DIAGNOSTIC CONCEPT

Kanner's Original Report

Kanner's (1943/1968) original report contrasted the lack of social interest (autism) with the normative marked predisposition to engage with others in reciprocal interactions; he carefully framed his observation developmentally by citing the work of Gesell on the early emergence of social interest in the first weeks of life. We now are aware that this interest is present from birth in the typically developing infant. Since Kanner's first description, the diagnostic concept has undergone modification based on research and clinical work. At the same time, the diagnostic conceptualization retains important historical and conceptual continuities with Kanner's first description. Kanner emphasized the centrality of the social difficulties, as well as the presence of a set of unusual behaviors he subsumed under the term "insistence of sameness" or "resistance to change." These unusual behaviors included unusual movements and mannerisms as well as problems in dealing with change and novelty. Of the first 11 patients described in his report, only one was below age 3 years when Kanner first examined him, and three children were between the ages of 3 and 4 years.

Although Kanner emphasized the uniqueness of the condition and its apparent difference from schizophrenia, other clinicians tended to assume some form of continuity of the two conditions. This issue was clarified over the next several decades as longitudinal and other data made it clear that autism formed a distinct diagnostic category. As a result, however, Kanner's early focus on "early infantile autism" was lost and most research focused on school-age or adolescent children.

DSM-I and DSM-II:
Confusion with Childhood Schizophrenia

In the first two editions of the *Diagnostic and Statistical Manual of Mental Disorders* (DSM) only the term *childhood schizophrenia* was officially available to describe autism. This situation was very unfortunate. Subsequently, the work of Kolvin (1971) and Rutter (1972) made it clear that autism was distinctive and could not simply be considered an early form of schizophrenia (Volkmar & Klin, 2005). Furthermore, available research suggested that autism was a brain-based disorder and not a result of deviant parent–child interaction. In parallel with attempts to provide better definitions of adult psychiatric disorders for research (Spitzer, Endicott, & Robins, 1978), similar attempts were made of childhood-onset disorders like autism. Among the investigators of this time, Rutter (1978) provided an important and influential synthesis of Kanner's original report with subsequent research. Rutter suggested the importance of four essential features: (1) early onset, (2) distinctively impaired social development, (3) distinctively impaired communication, and (4) unusual behaviors of the type suggested in Kanner's concept of "insistence on sameness" (resistance to change, idiosyncratic responses to the environment, motor mannerisms and stereotypies, etc.). Rutter was clear that the social and communication difficulties were not just a function of associated intellectual disability. These various issues were considered as autism was first included in the landmark, third edition of DSM (DSM-III; American Psychiatric Association, 1980).

DSM-III and DSM-III-R

DSM-III (American Psychiatric Association, 1980) represented a marked change from its two predecessors. The taxonomy proposed was based on research findings and emphasized the importance of an atheoretical and empirically based set of criteria. Autism was included in a newly designated class of childhood-onset disorders, Pervasive Developmental Disorders (PDD). A "subthreshold" condition was included as well, *atypical PDD*; this term had considerable (if unintended) overlap with earlier terms such as *atypical personality development* (Volkmar & Klin, 2005). The definition included in DSM-III was heavily dependent on Rutter's earlier conceptualization and provided for a clear differentiation of autism from schizophrenia. Interestingly, the original DSM-III approach lacked a developmental orientation and, if anything, the criteria proposed were much more appropriate to very young children with autism, that is, consistent with the term *infantile autism*. Although the use of a multiaxial approach was a clear benefit for child psychiatry, some aspects of the organization of this system were confusing—for example, autism and related disorders were placed on a different axis than other developmental disorders. A much more developmental orientation was introduced in DSM-III-R (American Psychiatric Association, 1987), which was greatly influenced by the work of Lorna Wing (Wing & Gould, 1979). Although the now familiar three major areas of dysfunction were still included, the new criteria were much more detailed and included a range of examples (with the goal of producing an approach applicable to the broad range of age and developmental levels). The use of a polythetic approach was also adopted, and the requirement for early onset was dropped (although onset before or after age 3 could still be specified). The official name of the condition was changed from *infantile autism* to *Autistic Disorder* in reflection of these changes. Although many aspects of the DSM-III-R approach were improvements, it quickly became apparent that the system tended to "overdiagnose" autism, particularly in the cases of more intellectually challenged children (Rutter & Schopler, 1992). This observation led to the potential for major difficulties in the comparison of studies using different diagnostic criteria and also posed problems for pending revision in the International Classification of Diseases—tenth edition (ICD-10; World Health Organization, 1990). The ICD and DSM approaches are fundamentally related and share many aspects of diagnostic coding, although there are also important differences.

ICD-10 and DSM-IV

Extensive revision of both the ICD and DSM systems was undertaken early in 1994. As part of the DSM-IV revision process (American Psychiatric Association, 1994), attempts were made to identify areas of both consensus and controversy such as clinical utility, reliability, and descriptive validity of categories and criteria. Coordination with the pending ICD revision was also a consideration. Literature reviews and data reanalyses were also undertaken for specific issues, such as those relative to the concept of Childhood Disintegrative Disorder—a concept included in previous versions of ICD but not DSM. Data reanalyses suggested that the DSM-III-R approach was overbroad, and a decision was made to undertake a large multinational field trial (Volkmar et al., 1994). This field trial was conducted in coordination with the ICD-10 revision effort and included more than 100 raters working at more than 20 sites around the world. The final sample included information on nearly 1,000 cases seen by one (or sometimes more than one) rater. In the nearly 1,000 cases, more than 300 children were less than 5 years of age (although most were between ages 3 and 5 and no child younger than 2 was seen). A standard coding system was used to provide basic information on a case and rater and on a number of diagnostic criteria.

The overall results of the field trial (see Table 1.1) confirmed that DSM-III-R had a higher sensitivity but lower specificity, whereas the ICD-10 draft definition, designed to be a research diagnostic system, had, as expected, higher specificity. A series of analyses were undertaken, including reliability of criteria and diagnosis, factor analyses, signal detection analysis, and so forth (Volkmar et al., 1994, Klin, Lang, Cicchetti, & Volkmar, 2000). As expected, social criteria were, as individual diagnostic items, generally the most potent single diagnostic predictors, and a decision was made to weight them more heavily in the final DSM-IV definition. Possible modifications in the ICD-10 system were examined, the goal being to have convergent definitions in the DSM and ICD. The final diagnostic approach provided reasonable coverage over the range of syndrome expression in autism as reflected in the field trial sample and was applicable from early childhood (i.e., at about age 3) through adulthood.

It must be emphasized that the DSM-IV and ICD-10 approach did consider developmental aspects of syndrome change, but, not surprisingly at that time, the focus was *not* on infants and very young children; that is, it appeared that the approach derived worked satisfactorily starting at about age 3. Interestingly, examination of some of the DSM-IV field trial data (children under age 5) reveals a few items with stronger developmental correlates. In general, such items were discarded because they would not be applicable to the entire range of syndrome expression. For example, attachment to unusual objects has low sensitivity (.50) but high specificity (.90), so that when it is observed, it has high predictive power for autism but only in this younger age group.

Interest in the earliest development of children with problems included in the autism spectrum was also fueled by inclusion of additional

TABLE 1.1. Sensitivity/Specificity by IQ Level

	n	DSM-III[a]		DSM-III-R		ICD-10[b]	
		Se	Sp	Se	Sp	Se	Sp
Overall	940	.82	.80	.86	.83	.79	.89
By IQ level							
< 25	64	.90	.76	.84	.39	.74	.88
25–39	148	.88	.76	.90	.60	.88	.92
40–54	191	.79	.76	.93	.74	.84	.83
55–69	167	.86	.78	.84	.77	.78	.89
70–85	152	.79	.81	.88	.81	.74	.96
> 85	218	.78	.83	.78	.78	.78	.91

Note. Se, sensitivity; Sp, specificity.
[a]"Lifetime" diagnosis (current infantile autism or "residual" infantile autism).
[b]Original ICD-10 criteria and scoring table adapted from Volkmar et al. (1994). Copyright 1994 by the American Psychiatric Association. Adapted by permission.

disorders within the revised PDD section of DSM-IV (e.g., Asperger's Disorder, Rett's Disorder, and Childhood Disintegrative Disorder). A need to differentiate these disorders highlighted the importance of understanding developmental history and early clinical presentations.

At the time that DSM-IV appeared (1994), there was little concern with the manifestation of autism in infants and very young children. For children by about age 3, the DSM system appeared to generally work well with reasonable stability of diagnosis (Lord & Risi, 2000). However, with the growing interest in genetic mechanisms, screening of at-risk populations such as siblings, and the marked increase in research in the earliest manifestations of autism, there has been progressively more concern about autism as it is manifested in infancy. We consider these issues before returning to the problem of early diagnosis.

CLINICAL PHENOMENOLOGY

Onset of the Condition

As noted, Kanner (1943/1968) emphasized the apparently congenital nature of autism in his original report. Direct evidence regarding the actual onset of the symptoms is still lacking, and a vast majority of the current reports rely on parental recollection regarding the age of onset and type of first abnormalities. Although these reports have their obvious limitations and the onset of parental concerns is likely to follow the actual time when the symptoms of autism spectrum disorder (ASD) (equivalent to the term PDD) begin to manifest, they also offer some insight into the nature of the first concerns that are likely to motivate parents to seek professional advice, which in turn may lead to an earlier initiation of treatment. Raising parental awareness of the first signs of various developmental disorders, including ASD, has become one of the priorities of a number of parent organizations, such as Autism Speaks (*www.autismspeaks. org*) and the Centers for Disease Control and Prevention (*www.cdc.gov/ ncbddd/autism/actearly/*), as one of the factors that are likely to contribute to early identification and treatment of infants with developmental disabilities.

A number of studies have suggested that the vast majority of parents of children with ASD first notice abnormalities during the course of the first 2 years of life (Baghdadli, Picot, Pascal, Pry, & Aussilloux, 2003; Chawarska, Paul, et al., 2007; De Giacomo & Fombonne, 1998; Rogers & DiLalla, 1990; Tolbert, Brown, Fowler, & Parsons, 2001; Volkmar, Stier, & Cohen, 1985). The first concerns arise, on average, in the second year, usually at about 14 months (Chawarska, Paul, et al., 2007), 17 months (Baghdadli et al., 2003), or 19 months (De Giacomo & Fombonne, 1998). These ages are likely to be sensitive to several factors, such as the time elapsing between the onset of parental concerns and the time when the information was collected. With a shorter lag, reports of earlier ages of onset are to be expected; otherwise a "forward-telescoping" effect seems to apply (Cooper, Kim, Taylor, & Lord, 2001), that is, a shift of the estimate regarding the age when the child began manifesting first symptoms to later ages.

The time when parents begin to notice the first abnormities varies, such that 30–50% of parents report concerns in the first year of the child's life and 80–90% by the second birthday (Baghdadli et al., 2003; Chawarska, Paul, et al., 2007; De Giacomo & Fombonne, 1998; Volkmar et al., 1985). There are relatively few studies reporting on the association between clinical outcome and the onset of parental concerns. Most of the studies were conducted retrospectively and produced very mixed results. A recent study examined prospectively the link between the onset of parental concerns, measured when the toddlers were between 18 and 36 months, and clinical diagnosis at the age of 4 (Chawarska, Paul, et al., 2007). Children who were identified by their parents as having problems between birth and 10 months were four times more likely to be later diagnosed with autism than with Pervasive Developmental Disorder-Not Otherwise Specified (PDD-NOS). However, those identified by parents as having difficulties between 11 and 18 months were equally likely to receive a diagnosis of autism or PDD-NOS at 4 years. Finally, all children in the group with concerns arising at or after 18 months received a diagnosis of autism at the age of 4. This finding suggests a strong and nonlinear relationship between the age of parental recognition (and presumably the onset of symptoms) and clinical diagnosis assigned 2–3 years later and raises a question of possible variants that manifest differently in the onset of symptoms.

Among the most common and often first noted concerns are delays in speech and language development, followed by an abnormal social responsivity level, medical problems, and nonspecific difficulties related to sleeping, eating, and attention (Chawarska, Paul, et al., 2007; De Giacomo & Fombonne 1998). Notably, in young children, the appearance of stereotyped behaviors, motor mannerisms, and unusual interests rarely trigger parental concerns, most likely because of their relatively mild manifestations in infancy or a later onset. Although concerns regarding the development of speech and the level of social engagement are frequent for toddlers with autism and PDD-NOS, the nonspecific concerns related to feeding, eating, and sleep appear to be more frequent for toddlers with PDD-NOS (Chawarska, Paul, et al., 2007).

Although the presence of specific delays constitutes a strong basis for parental concerns, such concerns may also emerge in response to unusual variations in the rate of progress, such as an apparent slowing of development (e.g., if babbling is not followed by the emergence of the first words) or a loss of previously acquired skills (regression) (Siperstein & Volkmar, 2004). Regression is usually reported in 20–35% of cases (Chawarska, Paul, et al., 2007; Goldberg et al., 2003; Luyster et al., 2005; Rapin & Katzman, 1998; Rogers, 2004; Werner & Dawson, 2005) and can involve the loss of words, vocalizations, nonverbal communication skills (e.g., eye contact, gestures), social dyadic interaction skills, imitation, or pretend play (Davidovitch, Glick, Holtzman, Tirosh, & Safir, 2000; Goldberg et al., 2003; Luyster et al., 2005). The perception of regression appears to be specific, though clearly not universal, to ASD (Luyster et al., 2005; Siperstein & Volkmar, 2004). Parental reports of regression do not necessarily indicate normal development prior to the perceived loss of skills, nor do early abnormalities preclude regression (Lord, Shulman, & DiLavore, 2004; Siperstein & Volkmar, 2004; Werner & Dawson, 2005; Wilson, Djukie, Shinnar, Dharmani, & Rapin, 2003). In fact, unequivocal loss of skills following normal developmental milestones is relatively uncommon (Siperstein & Volkmar, 2004; see Figure 1.1). An analysis of developmental history in a large sample of children with autism suggested that in most instances of reported loss, the development seemed to reach a plateau and then stagnate rather than undergo a true loss of skills. In other instances, parents reported a loss in a child who was already experiencing developmental delays (Siperstein & Volkmar, 2004). However, it is clear that in some cases a marked regression does occur—such regression has been documented in very young children with ASD through analysis of video recordings in the first year of life (Werner & Dawson, 2005). Werner and Dawson (2005) used home videotapes of the first and second birthday parties of children with ASD and of typically developing con-

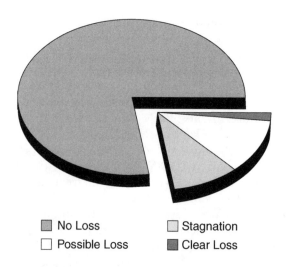

FIGURE 1.1. Loss of developmental skills.

trols. Raters blind to diagnosis and history of regression confirmed regression, as defined by a decline in frequency of joint attention acts and word/babble use in a subset of the ASD sample.

It is clear that skill loss after a prolonged period of normal development (e.g., to 3 or 4 years) is relatively uncommon. A specific diagnostic term, *Childhood Disintegrative Disorder*, exists for this category of cases, and the outcome appears to be worse than that in autism, with little or no recovery of previously exhibited abilities (Volkmar, Koenig, & State, 2005). Given the complexities of understanding the role of regression in autism, it remains unclear as to what relationship exists between this less common later-onset condition and reported early regression in autism.

Among the factors that precipitate the onset of parental concerns are concurrent cognitive delays, delays in motor development, and the presence of medical problems (De Giacomo & Fombonne, 1998). The presence of perinatal complications and sensory deficits has also been associated with earlier recognition (Baghdadli et al., 2003). A more recent study suggests that in the first year, late onset of social smile, delays in responsivity to speech and language understanding, and late onset of independent walking are possible factors precipitating parental concerns (Chawarska, Paul, et al., 2007). Factors that have not been found to influence the age of recognition include birth order, social class, and gender (De Giacomo & Fombonne, 1998). More recently, the growing appreciation of the genetic factors in autism and increased risk for ASD in younger siblings of the affected children may sensitize parents to early signs of vulnerability and contribute to earlier recognition of developmental problems (Klin et al., 2004; Zwaigenbaum et al., 2007).

Clinical Presentation in the First Year of Life

Kanner's original report emphasized the central role of social difficulties in autism. It is a tribute to his powers of observation that most subsequent research has supported this observation, albeit with considerable refinement (Carter, Davis, Klin, & Volkmar, 2005; see also Chawarska & Volkmar, 2005, for a review). Although early reports on symptoms of autism in the first year of life relied heavily on parental report (e.g., Dahlgren & Gillberg, 1989; Klin, Volkmar, & Sparrow, 1992) and single case studies (Dawson, Osterling, Meltzoff, & Kuhl, 2000), these reports were later supplemented by analytic studies of home video recordings depicting, for instance, a first birthday party or other family events (e.g., Baranek, 1999; Maestro et al., 2001; Osterling, Dawson, & Munson, 2002; Werner et al., 2000). Studies based on these approaches have contributed greatly to raising awareness, regardless of possible early symptoms of ASD. However, they suffer a number of important methodological limitations related, for instance, to parental ability to detect and report on the more subtle and contextualized symptoms of ASD (Chawarska, Klin, Paul,

& Volkmar, 2007; Stone, Hoffman, Lewis, & Ousley, 1994) as well as to the sensitivity and specificity of the identified deficits to ASD owing to issues with control groups or the representativeness of the source material (i.e., videotapes) (see also Zwaigenbaum et al., 2007, for a review).

More recently, however, the findings of increased genetic liability for ASD in younger children enabled researchers to study ASD *in statu nascendi* by following prospectively large cohorts of younger siblings at risk for developing the disorders (Zwiegenbaum et al., 2007). The sibling recurrence rate of autism has been estimated between 3 and 8% (Bailey et al., 1995; Bailey, Phillips, & Rutter, 1996; Ritvo et al., 1989). These numbers may underestimate the true recurrence rate for several reasons, including (1) increased prevalence rates related to the employment of more inclusive diagnostic criteria for autism and PDD-NOS since the advent of DSM-IV, and (2) the stoppage phenomenon exemplified by a high number of families avoiding further pregnancies once an offspring is diagnosed with autism (Jones & Szatmari, 1988; Slager, Faroud, Haghighi, Spence, & Hodge, 2001). Increased rates for nonautistic PDD in siblings (Asperger syndrome, PDD-NOS) have also been reported (Bailey et al., 1995; Le Couteur et al., 1996). Features of a broader autism phenotype (BAP) have been reported in 15–45% of family members (Bailey, Palferman, Heavey, & Le Couteur, 1998; Folstein et al., 1999), with higher rates of both narrow and broad autistic phenotype in male rather than female relatives of individuals with autism (Bolton et al., 1994; Pickles et al., 1995; Piven, Palmer, Jacobi, Childress, & Arndt, 1997). Preliminary findings from ongoing studies on high-risk siblings suggest that 20–25% of younger siblings of children with autism may exhibit developmental impairments in the first or second year of life (Zwaigenbaum et al., 2005), though studies examining the developmental trajectories of younger siblings are clearly needed and are slowly emerging (Landa & Garrett-Mayer, 2006; Yirmiya et al., 2006).

Analysis of videotapes suggests that as compared with typical controls, infants who were later diagnosed with ASD were less likely to look at and seek other people, and they were less likely to smile and vocalize at others in the first 6 months of life (Maestro et al., 2002). In the second half of the first year, infants later diagnosed with ASD might show difficulties in responding when their names were called and look at others less frequently, as compared with typically developing children or infants with developmental delays (Baranek, 1999; Osterling et al., 2002; Werner et al., 2000). However, as a recent prospective study of high-risk infants suggests, limited response to their names at 12 months, although quite specific to infants with ASD as well as high-risk siblings with developmental delays, is by no means universally present in all infants who are later diagnosed with the disorder (Nadig et al., 2007). Thus, failure to respond to his or her name may be an indicator that a 12-month-old child would benefit from further evaluation, but passing the "name-calling" test does not mean that the child is not at risk of developing ASD. Studies of the presence of unusual sensory behaviors and motor stereotypies in samples of children with ASD, as compared with children with developmental delays, yield mixed results. Although some suggest the presence of excessive mouthing and possibly aversion to social touch (Baranek, 1999; Loh et al., 2007; Osterling et al., 2002), others fail to detect similar effects. Furthermore, motor stereotypies have been reported in some samples (Loh et al., 2007; Osterling et al., 2002) but not in others (Baranek, 1999; Werner & Dawson, 2005).

Presently the vast majority of prospective baby sibling studies report on the expression of the broader autism phenotype that can be detected in infant siblings who are not affected with a full-blown ASD, rather than in children who were actually diagnosed with ASD later on (e.g., Toth, Dawson, Meltzoff, Greenson, & Fein, 2007; Cassel et al., 2007; Merin, Young, Ozonoff, & Rogers, 2007; Gamliel, Yirmiya, & Sigman, 2007). This current trend is related to the fact that owing to a relatively low recurrence rate among siblings, very large longitudinal samples need to accumulate for certain research questions to be addressed. Nonetheless, the first experimental studies reporting on the presentation of infants with ASD in the first year of life are beginning to emerge. Prospective studies of infant siblings, followed from 6 to 24 or 36 months and identified as having some form of ASD, suggest that robust behavioral features of ASD that could be captured through standard assessment instruments such the Autism Observation Scale for Infants (AOSI; Bryson, Zwaigenbaum, McDermott, Rombough, & Brian, 2007) and the Mullen Scales of Early Learning (MSEL; Mullen, 1995) may not emerge until some time after 6 months and before 12 months, with further intensification of their expression occurring between 12 and 24 months (Bryson, Zwaigenbaum, Brian, et al., 2007; Landa & Garrett-Mayer, 2006; Zwaigenbaum et al., 2005). Zwaigenbaum and colleagues (2005) identified several features at 12 months that are likely to differentiate siblings with ASD from those without social disability. Among the features were poor eye contact, limited social interest and smiling, limited use of gestures, poor response to name, poor imitation, and delays in receptive and expressive language. These infants also exhibited temperamental abnormalities, including initial passivity in early development followed by the emergence of a tendency for extreme distress reactions by 12 months. Difficulties in disengagement of visual attention were also noted. Studies such as these constitute the first step toward establishing clear diagnostic criteria for ASD in the first year of life, although extensive studies are needed to establish both sensitivity to and specificity of the identified abnormalities.

A complementary approach to identifying behavioral markers of ASD in infancy involves the employment of experimental designs targeting basic perceptual and cognitive processes involved in development of social interactions and communication. Among these are eye-tracking studies of perception of social and nonsocial stimuli (e.g., Chawarska & Shic, 2007; Klin & Jones, in press; Merin et al., 2007) and speech perception (Nadig et al., 2007). These studies are discussed in greater detail by Klin, Saulnier, Chawarska, and Volkmar (Chapter 6, this volume).

Symptoms of ASD in the Second and Third Years of Life

Several factors have contributed to a much larger body of data on autism as it manifests after the first birthday and before age 3. Recent advances in clinical research suggest that in 2- and 3-year-olds, symptoms of autism center on areas of social interaction and communication and are often accompanied by delays in multiple areas of functioning, including motor and nonverbal cognitive development (see Chawarska & Volkmar, 2005, for a review; see also Bishop, Luyster, Richler, & Lord, Chapter 2; Chawarska & Bearss, Chapter 3; and Paul, Chapter 4, this volume). In the social domain, the most frequently reported symptoms are diminished eye contact, limited interest in social games and turn-taking exchanges, low frequency of looking referentially at parents, and preference for being alone (Cox et al., 1999; Lord, 1995; Stone, Lee, et al., 1999). Vocal and motor imitation and symbolic play skills appear delayed as compared with the children's overall developmental levels (Baron-Cohen, Cox, Baird, Sweettenham, & Nightingale, 1996; Cox et al., 1999). Young children with autism direct their visual attention more frequently toward objects than toward people (Dawson et al., 2004; Swettenham et al., 1998). A limited range of facial expressions and infrequent instances of sharing affect (e.g., by smiling and looking at others) have been reported as well (Cox et al., 1999; Lord, 1995; Stone, Lee, et al., 1999). In the area of communication, the most striking differences relate to early emerging social communicative exchanges through nonverbal (e.g., use of gestures or gaze to communicate interest or joint attention) and vocal or verbal means. The child's responsivity to speech in general, and to his or her name in particular, continues to be limited (Baron-Cohen et al., 1996; Cox et al., 1999; DiLavore, Lord, & Rutter, 1995; Klin, 1991; Lord & Pickles, 1996; Paul, Chawarska, Klin, & Volkmar, 2007). Vocalizations may take on an abnormal quality (Sheinkopf, Mundy, Oller, & Steffens, 2000; Wetherby, Yonclas, & Bryan, 1989). Stereotypic and repetitive behaviors reach a clinical threshold in the second year in some children (Chawarska, Klin, et al., 2007), and in a vast majority of children by the age of 4 (e.g., Lord, 1995). Adaptive skills are usually delayed beyond what would be expected based on the developmental level (Klin et al., 1992; Stone, Ousley, Hepburn, Hogan, & Brown, 1999).

The relatively mild expression of the unusual repetitive behaviors (stereotyped movements and mannerisms) and the general category of "resistance to change" behaviors in this age group is of some interest (e.g., Chawarska, Klin, et al., 2007; Loh et al., 2007; Lord, 1995). The absence of clear-cut behaviors in this general category is one of the more general conceptual problems in the application of categorical (DSM-IV or ICD-10) diagnostic criteria. In Lord's longitudinal study the absence of such behaviors before age 3 was a frequent reason that a diagnosis of autism could not be made (Lord, 1995; Lord et al., 2006). Although clear precursors of such behaviors may potentially be used as alternatives for this age group, relatively few attempts have been made to identify such precursors (Loh et al., 2007) and to assess their specificity to ASD. However, difficulties in adapting to new situations, interest in visually repetitive phenomena (e.g., ceiling fans), and overattention to the nonsocial environment (focusing on alphabet letters on blocks or small details of play materials) are potential candidates. Furthermore, an increase in the second year, rather than the expected decrease, of some of the repetitive movements observed in the first year (Thelen, 1979) may be a sign of abnormal development in this area (Loh et al., 2007).

IMPLICATIONS FOR DIAGNOSIS AND SCREENING

Issues of diagnosis and screening are discussed in detail by Bishop et al. (Chapter 2, this volume) and are only briefly touched upon here. Clearly, by about age 3 (and often even before) the current DSM-IV/ICD-10 categorical approach can be used with little difficulty. Available work does highlight some limitations of their criteria for very young children (Stone, Lee, et al., 1999). An alternative categorical classification (National Center for Clinical Infant Programs [NCCIP], 1994) has been proposed, but its utilization in the clinical community has been limited, probably because its underlying conceptualization has been developed outside the body of nosological research in autism. Thus, there is little information on its concurrent validity with DSM-IV and related literature. Because the history of this system precedes the current wave of nosological efforts related to children under the age of 3 years, it would be critical for the NCCIP (now Zero to Three) system to be properly researched and its clinical and concurrent validity (relative to other systems), reliability, and other psychometric properties to be adequately assessed.

More generally, well-documented diagnostic instruments may work well after age 3–4 years or past a certain developmental level (often around 18 months), but their use is not clearly established for the first years of life. Dimensional assessment instruments have a number of potential advantages—for example, in their approach to developmental change and/or developmental level—and may be of particular use, given the greater potential for change in this age group. Similarly, screening approaches (see Bishop et al., Chapter 2, this volume) are particularly important in terms of identification of children in need of services but present their own issues in terms of design and evaluation. Unfortunately, what is critically needed, but not yet available, are methods that rely on biological markers or some other robust, readily measured indicator of risk. Given the lack of such markers, clinician-assigned diagnosis, as provided by experienced clinicians, remains the "gold standard" for diagnosis in infancy (Chawarska, Klin, et al., 2007; Cox et al., 1999; Gillberg et al., 1990; Lord, 1995; Stone, Lee, et al., 1999).

SUMMARY AND CONCLUSIONS: THE SIGNIFICANCE OF EARLY CASE DETECTION

The growing body of work on autism in infants is important for several reasons. Available data suggest that with earlier case detection the outcome of autism is gradually improving; for example, more and more individuals are able to live independently and fewer are likely to remain mute and to exhibit comorbid intellectual disability (Howlin, 2005). The recent National Research Council (2001) review of evidence on early treatment notes that, despite various limitations, a considerable body of work on the importance of early intervention now exists. In addition to its being important for treatment and long-term outcome, early detection is also important in clarifying the earliest developmental processes, which may be disrupted in autism.

Prospective research is critically needed to help us to more fully understand the basic mechanisms of psychopathology and to clarify how early difficulties become entrained in subsequent development. Somewhat paradoxically, those who work with both higher-functioning older individuals with autism and very young infants are impressed not only by the potential for significant developmental change, but also by the severity and continuity of difficulties across time and development—for example, in modulation of the human voice in prosody and in the use of eye contact to mediate social interaction (Paul, Augustyn, Klin, & Volkmar, 2005). The ability to observe these early processes without the accompanying overlay of subsequent development will be particularly important. Study of the range of early developmental skills in this population may also result in some clinical surprises; for example, there is now a suggestion that for a subgroup of infants, difficulties in affect regulation and temperament may be the more striking initial signs of autism rather than disturbances in social interaction (Bryson, Zwaigenbaum, Brian, et al., 2007).

Consistent with Kanner's (1943/1968) original description, it appears that in many cases infants are born with autism. It is also clear that in a variably reported, apparently small number of cases, the child develops reasonably normally for a time before autism appears. Although much work remains to be done, it is possible even now to begin to understand how some of the early manifestations of autism become entrained in subsequent development. Data from this age group may shed important light on perplexing clinical questions—for instance, the well-established differences in gender ratio and severity may be apparent before age 3 years (Carter et al., 2007). Careful follow-up studies also emphasize the potential difficulties of early diagnosis (Sutera et al., 2007), further underscoring the importance of biological markers and the study of specific biological and neuropsychological processes for better early diagnosis. To this end, the study of very specific social processes under highly controlled conditions may be particularly important (e.g., Chawarska, Klin, & Volkmar, 2003; Chawarska & Volkmar, 2005; Chawarska & Shic, 2007; Klin, 1992; Klin & Jones, in press; Klin, Jones, Schultz, Volkmar, & Cohen, 2002; Merin et al., 2007; Presmanes et al., 2007). As such processes are identified, siblings can also be studied to address potential contributions of these processes to the broader autism phenotype (Cassel et al., 2007; Presmanes, Walden, Stone, & Yoder, 2007; Toth et al., 2007; Gamliel et al., 2007).

ACKNOWLEDGMENTS

Preparation of this chapter was supported in part by grants from the National Alliance for Autism Research/Autism Speaks and the National Institute of Mental Health (Grant No. U54 MH676494) to Fred R. Volkmar, Katarzyna Chawarska, and Ami Klin.

REFERENCES

American Psychiatric Association. (1980). *Diagnostic and statistical manual of mental disorders* (3rd ed.). Washington, DC: Author.

American Psychiatric Association. (1987). *Diagnostic and statistical manual of mental disorders* (3rd ed., text rev.). Washington, DC: Author.

American Psychiatric Association. (1994). *Diagnostic and statistical manual of mental disorders* (4th ed.). Washington, DC: Author.

Baghdadli, A., Picot, M. C., Pascal, C., Pry, R., & Aussilloux, C. (2003). Relationship between age of recognition of first disturbances and severity in young children with autism. *European Child and Adolescent Psychiatry, 12*(3), 122–127.

Bailey, A., Le Couteur, A., Gottesman, I., Bolton, P., Simonoff, E., Yuzda, E., et al. (1995). Autism as a strongly genetic disorder: Evidence from a British twin study. *Psychological Medicine, 25*(1), 63–77.

Bailey, A., Palferman, S., Heavey, L., & Le Couteur, A. (1998). Autism: The phenotype in relatives. *Journal of Autism and Developmental Disorders, 28*(5), 369–392.

Bailey, A., Phillips, W., & Rutter, M. (1996). Autism: Towards an integration of clinical, genetic, neuropsychological, and neurobiological perspectives. *Journal of Child Psychology and Psychiatry and Allied Disciplines, 37*(1), 89–126.

Baranek, G. T. (1999). Autism during infancy: A retrospective video analysis of sensory-motor and social behaviors at 9–12 months of age. *Journal of Autism and Developmental Disorders, 29*(3), 213–224.

Baron-Cohen, S., Cox, A., Baird, G., Sweettenham, J., & Nightingale, N. (1996). Psychological markers in the detection of autism in infancy in a large population. *British Journal of Psychiatry, 168*(2), 158–163.

Bolton, P., Macdonald, H., Pickles, A., Rios, P., Goode, S., Crowson, M., et al. (1994). A case–control family history study of autism. *Journal of Child Psychology and Psychiatry and Allied Disciplines, 35*(5), 877–900.

Bryson, S. E., Zwaigenbaum, L., Brian, J., Roberts, W., Szatmari, P., Rombough, V., et al. (2007). A prospective case series of high-risk infants who developed autism. *Journal of Autism and Developmental Disorders, 37*(1), 12–24.

Bryson, S. E., Zwaigenbaum, L., McDermott, C., Rombough, V., & Brian, J. (2007). The Autism Observation Scale for Infants: Scale development and reliability data. *Journal of Autism and Developmental Disorders.* Retrieved from *www.springerlinks.com/content/104757*

Carter, A. S., Black, D. O., Tewani, S., Connolly, C. E., Kadlec, M. B., & Tager-Flusberg, H. (2007). Sex differences in toddlers with autism spectrum disorders. *Journal of Autism and Developmental Disorders, 37*(1), 86–97.

Carter, A. S., Davis, N. O., Klin, A., & Volkmar, F. R. (2005). Social development in autism. In F. R. Volkmar, A. Klin, R. Paul, & D. J. Cohen (Eds.), *Handbook of autism and pervasive developmental disorders* (3rd ed., Vol. 1, pp. 312–334). Hoboken, NJ: Wiley.

Cassel, T. D., Messinger, D. S., Ibanez, L. V., Haltigan, J. D., Acosta, S. I., & Buchman, A. C. (2007). Early social and emotional communication in the infant siblings of children with autism spectrum disorders: An examination of the broad phenotype. *Journal of Autism and Developmental Disorders, 37*(1), 122–132.

Chawarska, K., Klin, A., Paul, R., & Volkmar, F. (2007). Autism spectrum disorder in the second year: Stability and change in syndrome expression. *Journal of Child Psychology and Psychiatry, 48*(2), 128–138.

Chawarska, K., Klin, A., & Volkmar, F. (2003). Automatic attention cueing through eye movement in 2-year-old children with autism. *Child Development, 74*(4), 1108–1122.

Chawarska, K., Paul, R., Klin, A., Hannigen, S., Dichtel, L. E., & Volkmar, F. (2007). Parental recognition of developmental problems in toddlers with autism spectrum disorders. *Journal of Autism and Developmental Disorders, 37*(1), 62–73.

Chawarska, K., & Shic, F. (2007). *Visual scanning and recognition of static facial and non-facial stimuli in 2-year-olds*. Paper presented at the International Meeting for Autism Research, Seattle, WA.

Chawarska, K., & Volkmar, F. (2005). Autism in infancy and early childhood. In F. Volkmar, R. Paul, A. Klin, & D. J. Cohen (Eds.), *Handbook of autism and pervasive developmental disorders* (3rd ed., Vol. 1, pp. 223–246). Hoboken, NJ: Wiley.

Cohen, D. J., Volkmar, F. R., & Paul, R. (1986). Issues in the classification of pervasive developmental disorders: History and current status of nosology. *Journal of the American Academy of Child Psychiatry, 25*(2), 158–161.

Cooper, J., Kim P., Taylor, A., & Lord, C. (2001). *Early communication and social skills in children with autism spectrum disorders, with and without early word loss.* Paper presented at the International Meeting for Autism Research, San Diego, CA.

Cox, A., Klein, K., Charman, T., Baird, G., Baron-Cohen, S., Swettenham, J., et al. (1999). Autism spectrum disorders at 20 and 42 months of age: Stability of clinical and ADI-R diagnosis. *Journal of Child Psychology and Psychiatry and Allied Disciplines, 40*(5), 719–732.

Dahlgren, S. O., & Gillberg, C. (1989). Symptoms in the first two years of life: A preliminary population study of infantile autism. *European Archives of Psychiatry and Neurological Science, 238*(3), 169–174.

Davidovitch, M., Glick, L., Holtzman, G., Tirosh, E., & Safir, M. P. (2000). Developmental regression in autism: Maternal perception. *Journal of Autism and Developmental Disorders, 30*(2), 113–119.

Dawson, G., Osterling, J., Meltzoff, A. N., & Kuhl, P. (2000). Case study of the development of an infant with autism from birth to two years of age. *Journal of Applied Developmental Psychology, 21*(3), 299–313.

Dawson, G., Toth, K., Abbott, R., Osterling, J., Munson, J., Estes, A., et al. (2004). Early social attention impairments in autism: Social orienting, joint attention, and attention to distress. *Developmental Psychology, 40*(2), 271–283.

De Giacomo, A., & Fombonne, E. (1998). Parental recognition of developmental abnormalities in autism. *European Child and Adolescent Psychiatry, 7*(3), 131–136.

DiLavore, P. C., Lord, C., & Rutter, M. (1995). Pre-linguistic autism diagnostic observation schedule. *Journal of Autism and Developmental Disorders, 25*(4), 355–379.

Folstein, S. E., Santangelo, S. L., Gilman, S. E., Piven, J., Landa, R., Lainhart, J., et al. (1999). Predictors of cognitive test patterns in autism families. *Journal of Child Psychology and Psychiatry and Allied Disciplines, 40*(7), 1117–1128.

Gamliel, I., Yirmiya, N., & Sigman, M. (2007). The development of young siblings of children with autism from 4 to 54 months. *Journal of Autism and Developmental Disorders, 37*(1), 171–183.

Gillberg, C., Ehlers, S., Schaumann, H., Jakobsson, G., Dahlgren, S. O., Lindblom, R., et al. (1990). Autism under age 3 years: A clinical study of 28 cases referred for autistic symptoms in infancy [see comments]. *Journal of Child Psychology and Psychiatry, 31*(6), 921–934.

Goldberg, W. A., Osann, K., Filipek, P. A., Laulhere, T., Jarvis, K., Jodahl, C., et al. (2003). Language and other regression: Assessment and timing. *Journal of Autism and Developmental Disorders, 33*(6), 607–616.

Howlin, P. (2005). Outcomes in autism spectrum disorders. In F. R. Volkmar, R. Paul, A. Klin, & D. J. Cohen (Eds.), *Handbook of autism and pervasive developmental disorders* (3rd ed., Vol. 1, pp. 201–222). Hoboken, NJ: Wiley.

Jones, M., & Szatmari, P. (1988). Stoppage rules and genetic studies of autism. *Journal of Autism and Developmental Disorders, 18*(1), 31–40.

Kanner, L. (1968). Autistic disturbances of affective contact. *Acta Paedopsychiatrica, 35*(4), 100–136. (Original work published 1943)

Klin, A. (1991). Young autistic children's listening preferences in regard to speech: A possible characterization of the symptom of social withdrawal. *Journal of Autism and Developmental Disorders, 21*(1), 29–42.

Klin, A. (1992). Listening preferences in regard to speech in four children with developmental disabilities. *Journal of Child Psychology and Psychiatry, 33*(4), 763–769.

Klin, A., Chawarska, K., Paul, R., Rubin, E., Morgan, T., Wiesner, L., et al. (2004). Autism in a 15-month-old child. *American Journal of Psychiatry, 161*(11), 1981–1988.

Klin, A., & Jones, W. (in press). Altered face scanning and impaired recognition of biological motion in a 15-month-old infant with autism. *Developmental Science*.

Klin, A., Jones, W., Schultz, R., Volkmar, F., & Cohen, D. (2002). Visual fixation patterns during viewing of naturalistic social situations as predictors of social competence in individuals with autism. *Archives of General Psychiatry, 59*(9), 809–816.

Klin, A., Lang, J., Cicchetti, D. V., & Volkmar, F. R. (2000). Brief report: Interrater reliability of clinical diagnosis and DSM-IV criteria for autistic disorder: Results of the DSM-IV autism field trial. *Journal of Autism and Developmental Disorders, 30*(2), 163–167.

Klin, A., Volkmar, F. R., & Sparrow, S. (1992). Autistic social dysfunction: Some limitations of the theory of mind hypothesis. *Journal of Child Psychology and Psychiatry, 33*(5), 861–876.

Kolvin, I. (1971). Studies in the childhood psychoses. I. Diagnostic criteria and classification. *British Journal of Psychiatry, 118*(545), 381–384.

Landa, R., & Garrett-Mayer, E. (2006). Development in infants with autism spectrum disorders: A prospective study. *Journal of Child Psychology and Psychiatry, 47*(6), 629–638.

Le Couteur, A., Bailey, A., Goode, S., Pickles, A., Robertson, S., Gottesman, I., et al. (1996). A broader phenotype of autism: The clinical spectrum in twins. *Journal of Child Psychology and Psychiatry and Allied Disciplines, 37*(7), 785–801.

Loh, A., Soman, T., Brian, J., Bryson, S. E., Roberts, W., Szatmari, P., et al. (2007). Stereotyped motor behaviors associated with autism in high-risk infants: A pilot videotape analysis of a sibling sample. *Journal of Autism and Developmental Disorders, 37*(1), 25–36.

Lord, C. (1995). Follow-up of two-year-olds referred for possible autism. *Journal of Child Psychology and Psychiatry, 36*(8), 1365–1382.

Lord, C., & Pickles, A. (1996). Language level and nonverbal social-communicative behaviors in autistic and language-delayed children. *Journal of the American Academy of Child and Adolescent Psychiatry, 35*(11), 1542–1550.

Lord, C., & Risi, S. (2000). Diagnosis of autism spectrum disorders in young children. In A. M. Wetherby & B. M. Prizant (Eds.), *Autism spectrum disorders: A transactional developmental perspective* (pp. 11–30). Baltimore: Brookes.

Lord, C., Risi, S., DiLavore, P. S., Shulman, C., Thurm, A., & Pickles, A. (2006). Autism from 2 to 9 years of age. *Archives of General Psychiatry, 63*(6), 694–701.

Lord, C., Shulman, C., & DiLavore, P. (2004). Regression and word loss in autistic spectrum disorders. *Journal of Child Psychology and Psychiatry, 45*(5), 936–955.

Luyster, R., Richler, J., Risi, S., Hsu, W. L., Dawson, G., Bernier, R., et al. (2005). Early regression in social communication in autism spectrum disorders: A CPEA study. *Developmental Neuropsychology, 27*(3), 311–336.

Maestro, S., Muratori, F., Barbieri, F., Casella, C., Cattaneo, V., Cavallaro, M., et al. (2001). Early behavioral development in autistic children: The first 2 years of life through home movies. *Psychopathology, 34*(3), 147–152.

Maestro, S., Muratori, F., Cavallaro, M. C., Pei, F., Stern, D., Golse, B., et al. (2002). Attentional skills during the first 6 months of age in autism spectrum disorder. *Journal of the American Academy of Child and Adolescent Psychiatry, 41*(10), 1239–1245.

Merin, N., Young, G. S., Ozonoff, S., & Rogers, S. (2007). Visual fixation patterns during reciprocal social interaction distinguish a subgroup of 6-month-old infants at risk for autism from comparison infants. *Journal of Autism and Developmental Disorders, 37*(1), 108–121.

Mullen, E. (1995). *Mullen Scales of Early Learning (AGS ed.).* Circle Pines, MN: American Guidance Service.

Nadig, A. S., Ozonoff, S., Young, G. S., Rozqa, A., Sigman, M., & Rogers, S. J. (2007). A prospective study of response to name in infants at risk for autism. *Archives of Pediatric and Adolescent Medicine, 161*(4), 378–383.

National Center for Clinical Infant Programs. (1994). *Diagnostic classification of mental health and developmental disorders of infancy and early childhood.* Washington, DC: Author.

National Research Council. (2001). *Educating young children with autism.* Washington, DC: National Academy Press.

Osterling, J., & Dawson, G. (1994). Early recognition of children with autism: A study of first birthday home videotapes. *Journal of Autism and Developmental Disorders, 24*(3), 247–257.

Osterling, J. A., Dawson, G., & Munson, J. A. (2002). Early recognition of 1-year-old infants with autism spectrum disorder versus mental retardation. *Development and Psychopathology, 14*(2), 239–251.

Paul, R., Augustyn, A., Klin, A., & Volkmar, F. R. (2005). Perception and production of prosody by speakers with autism spectrum disorders. *Journal of Autism and Developmental Disorders, 35*(2), 205–220.

Paul, R., Chawarska, K., Klin, A., & Volkmar, F. (2007). Dissociations in the development of early communication in autism spectrum disorders. In R. Paul (Ed.), *Language disorders from a developmental perspective: Essays in honor of Robin S. Chapman* (pp. 163–194). Mahwah, NJ: Erlbaum.

Pickles, A., Bolton, P., Macdonald, H., Bailey, A., Le Couteur, A., Sim, C. H., et al. (1995). Latent-class analysis of recurrence risks for complex phenotypes with selection and measurement error: A twin and family history study of autism. *American Journal of Human Genetics, 57*(3), 717–726.

Piven, J., Palmer, P., Jacobi, D., Childress, D., & Arndt, S. (1997). Broader autism phenotype: Evidence from a family history study of multiple-incidence autism families. *American Journal of Psychiatry, 154*(2), 185–190.

Presmanes, A. G., Walden, T. A., Stone, W. L., & Yoder, P. J. (2007). Effects of different attentional cues on responding to joint attention in younger siblings of children with autism spectrum disorders. *Journal of Autism and Developmental Disorders, 37*(1), 133–144.

Rapin, I., & Katzman, R. (1998). Neurobiology of autism. *Annals of Neurology, 43*(1), 7–14.

Ritvo, E. R., Jorde, L. B., Mason-Brothers, A., Freeman, B. J., Pingree, C., Jones, M. B., et al. (1989). The UCLA–University of Utah epidemiologic survey of autism: Recurrence risk estimates and genetic counseling. *American Journal of Psychiatry, 146*(8), 1032–1036.

Rogers, S. J. (2004). Developmental regression in autism spectrum disorders. *Mental Retardation and Developmental Disabilities Research Reviews, 10*(2), 139–143.

Rogers, S. J., & DiLalla, D. L. (1990). Age of symptom onset in young children with pervasive developmental disorders. *Journal of the American Academy of Child and Adolescent Psychiatry, 29*(6), 863–872.

Rutter, M. (1972). Childhood schizophrenia reconsidered. *Journal of Autism and Childhood Schizophrenia, 2*(4), 315–337.

Rutter, M. (1978). Diagnosis and definition of childhood autism. *Journal of Autism and Childhood Schizophrenia, 8*(2), 139–161.

Rutter, M. (2005). Genetic influences and autism. In F. R. Volkmar, R. Paul, A. Klin, & D. J. Cohen (Eds.), *Handbook of autism and pervasive developmental disorders* (3rd ed., Vol. 1, pp. 425–452). Hoboken, NJ: Wiley.

Rutter, M., & Schopler, E. (1992). Classification of pervasive developmental disorders: Some concepts and practical considerations. *Journal of Autism and Developmental Disorders, 22*(4), 459–482.

Sheinkopf, S. J., Mundy, P., Oller, D., & Steffens, M. (2000). Vocal atypicalities of preverbal autistic children. *Journal of Autism and Developmental Disorders, 30*(4), 345–354.

Siegel, B., Pliner, C., Eschler, J., & Elliott, G. R. (1988). How children with autism are diagnosed: Difficulties in identification of children with multiple developmental delays. *Journal of Developmental and Behavioral Pediatrics, 9*(4), 199–204.

Siperstein, R., & Volkmar, F. (2004). Brief report: Parental reporting of regression in children with pervasive developmental disorders. *Journal of Autism and Developmental Disorders, 34*(6), 731–734.

Slager, S., Foroud, T., Haghighi, F., Spence, M. A., & Hodge, S. E. (2001). Stoppage: An issue for segregation analysis. *Genetic Epidemiology, 20*(3), 328–339.

Spitzer, R. L., Endicott, J. E., & Robins, E. (1978). Research diagnostic criteria. *Archives of General Psychiatry, 35*, 773–782.

Stone, W. L., Hoffman, E. L., Lewis, S. E., & Ousley, O. Y. (1994). Early recognition of autism: Parental reports vs. clinical observation. *Archives of Pediatrics and Adolescent Medicine, 148*(2), 174–179.

Stone, W. L., Lee, E. B., Ashford, L., Brissie, J., Hepburn, S. L., Coonrod, E. E., et al. (1999). Can autism be diagnosed accurately in children under 3 years? *Journal of Child Psychology and Psychiatry, 40*(2), 219–226.

Stone, W. L., Ousley, O. Y., Hepburn, S. L., Hogan, K. L., & Brown, C. S. (1999). Patterns of adaptive behavior in very young children with autism. *American Journal on Mental Retardation, 104*(2), 187–199.

Sutera, S., Pandey, J., Esser, E. L., Rosenthal, M. A., Wilson, L. B., Barton, M., et al. (2007). Predictors of optimal outcome in toddlers diagnosed with autism spectrum disorders. *Journal of Autism and Developmental Disorders, 37*(1), 98–107.

Swettenham, J., Baron-Cohen, S., Charman, T., Cox, A., Baird, G., Drew, A., et al. (1998). The frequency and distribution of spontaneous attention shifts between social and nonsocial stimuli in autistic, typically developing, and nonautistic developmentally delayed infants. *Journal of Child Psychology and Psychiatry and Allied Disciplines, 39*(5), 747–753.

Thelen, E. (1979). Rhythmical stereotypies in normal human infants. *Animal Behaviour, 27*, 699–715.

Tolbert, L., Brown, R., Fowler, P., & Parsons, D. (2001). Brief report: Lack of correlation between age of symptom onset and contemporaneous presentation. *Journal of Autism and Developmental Disorders, 31*(2), 241–245.

Toth, K., Dawson, G., Meltzoff, A. N., Greenson, J., & Fein, D. (2007). Early social, imitation, play and language abilities of young non-autistic siblings of children with autism. *Journal of Autism and Developmental Disorders, 37*(1), 158–170.

Wilson, S., Djukie, A., Shinnar, S., Dharmani, C., & Rapin, I. (2003). Clinical characteristics of language regression in children. *Developmental Medicine and Child Neurology, 45*, 508–514.

Volkmar, F. R., Chawarska, K., & Klin, A. (2005). Autism in infancy and early childhood. *Annual Review of Psychology, 56*, 315–336.

Volkmar, F. R., & Klin, A. (2005). Issues in the classification of autism and related conditions. In F. R. Volkmar, A. Klin, R. Paul, & D. J. Cohen (Eds.), *Handbook of autism and pervasive developmental disorders* (3rd ed., Vol. 1, pp. 5–41). Hoboken, NJ: Wiley.

Volkmar, F. R., Klin, A., Siegel, B., Szatmari, P., Lord, C., Campbell, M., et al. (1994). Field trial for autistic disorder in DSM-IV. *American Journal of Psychiatry, 151*(9), 1361–1367.

Volkmar, F. R., Koenig, K., & State, M. (2005). Childhood disintegrative disorder. In F. R. Volkmar, A. Klin, R. Paul, & D. J. Cohen (Eds.), *Handbook of autism and pervasive developmental disorders* (3rd ed., Vol. 1, pp. 70–78). Hoboken, NJ: Wiley.

Volkmar, F. R., Stier, D. M., & Cohen, D. J. (1985). Age of recognition of pervasive developmental disorder. *American Journal of Psychiatry, 142*(12), 1450–1452.

Werner, E., & Dawson, G. (2005). Validation of the phenomenon of autistic regression using home videotapes. *Archives of General Psychiatry, 62*(8), 889–895.

Werner, E., Dawson, G., Osterling, J., & Dinno, N. (2000). Brief report: Recognition of autism spectrum disorder before one year of age: A retrospective study based on home videotapes. *Journal of Autism and Developmental Disorders, 30*(2), 157–162.

Wetherby, A. M., Yonclas, D. G., & Bryan, A. A. (1989). Communicative profiles of preschool children with handicaps: Implications for early identification. *Journal of Speech and Hearing Disorders, 54*(2), 148–158.

Wing, L., & Gould, J. (1979). Severe impairments of social interaction and associated abnormalities. *Journal of Autism and Developmental Disorders, 9*(1), 11–29.

World Health Organization. (1990). *International classification of diseases (draft version: Diagnostic Criteria for Research)* (10th ed.). Geneva: Author.

Yirmiya, N., Gamliel, I., Pilowsky, T., Feldman, R., Baron-Cohen, S., & Sigman, M. (2006). The development of siblings of children with autism at 4 and 14 months: Social engagement, communication, and cognition. *Journal of Child Psychology and Psychiatry, 47*(5), 511–523.

Zwaigenbaum, L., Bryson, S., Rogers, T., Roberts, W., Brian, J., & Szatmari, P. (2005). Behavioral manifestations of autism in the first year of life. *International Journal of Developmental Neuroscience 23*(2–3), 143–152.

Zwaigenbaum, L., Thurm, A., Stone, W., Baranek, G., Bryson, S., Iverson, J., et al. (2007). Studying the emergence of autism spectrum disorders in high-risk infants: Methodological and practical issues. *Journal of Autism and Developmental Disorders, 37*(3), 466–480.

CHAPTER 2

Diagnostic Assessment

SOMER L. BISHOP
RHIANNON LUYSTER
JENNIFER RICHLER
CATHERINE LORD

Autism is a neurodevelopmental disorder characterized by deficits in social reciprocity and communication and by the presence of restricted and repetitive behaviors and/or interests. According to the criteria outlined in the *Diagnostic and Statistical Manual of Mental Disorders* (DSM-IV; American Psychiatric Association, 1994) and the *International Classification of Diseases* (ICD-10; World Health Organization, 1992), in order to receive a diagnosis of autism, a child must have shown abnormalities in social interaction, language as used in social communication, or symbolic/imaginative play before the age of 3 years. If a child does not meet all of the above criteria for autism, he or she may be given a diagnosis of Asperger syndrome (AS) or Pervasive Developmental Disorder-Not Otherwise Specified (PDD-NOS). We refer to these three diagnoses together as autism spectrum disorders (ASD).

Because there is not yet a biological marker for ASD, a diagnosis of ASD is made on the basis of a behavioral profile, which is characterized by both the absence of typical behaviors as well as the presence of atypical behaviors. Recently, researchers and clinicians have sought to identify ASD earlier and earlier, owing to findings that early intervention is associated with improved outcomes (Harris & Handleman, 2000). This is somewhat problematic, however, because whereas the behavioral features of ASD are well established for children in the preschool years and beyond, less is known about symptom presentation in the first 2 years of life

(Zwaigenbaum et al., 2005; Mitchell et al., 2006). Indeed, DSM-IV criteria were established based on the profile exhibited in early and middle childhood and do not necessarily apply to children under the age of 3. Therefore, professionals should exercise caution when making diagnoses in very young children. Furthermore, any assessment for possible ASD needs to be comprehensive and include a consideration of other disorders of early childhood. Because ASD is a developmental disorder and different symptoms are diagnostic at different points in development, understanding what is developmentally appropriate for children under 3 is an important first step in early identification of the disorder.

This chapter addresses issues in the assessment and diagnosis of ASD in infants and toddlers. The first section provides a brief summary of the development of social, communication, and play behaviors in typically developing young children. Next, we provide guidelines for assessment and differential diagnosis of children with ASD, including the importance of considering social, communication, and play behaviors in the context of a child's overall developmental functioning. Finally, we review the currently available screening instruments for identifying ASD in infants and toddlers, with special attention given to their appropriateness and limitations for use with children under 3 years of age.

EARLY TYPICAL DEVELOPMENT

The impairments that result from ASD are defined in relation to typical development. Reciprocal interaction and communication difficulties involve deficits in behaviors that emerge in typically developing children without explicit teaching and that are adaptive in their social contexts. In the area of restricted and repetitive behaviors and interests (RRBs), impairment refers to the presence of unusual, sometimes maladaptive behaviors that are, at least according to common wisdom, not usually seen in typically developing children. Thus, in order to determine if a child is showing signs of ASD, it is crucial to have a clear understanding of what constitutes typical behavior in a child of the same developmental level. As more and more children are being referred for a diagnosis of ASD at very young ages, it has become particularly important to have a comprehensive picture of social and communicative behavior in typically developing infants and toddlers. This understanding can help clinicians and researchers avoid overdiagnosing autism as well as wrongly dismissing real, appropriate concerns about behaviors associated with ASD.

A large body of evidence suggests that children come into the world already socially oriented and that their social understanding becomes richer and more sophisticated in a relatively short period of time. Newborns prefer looking at faces over nonface patterns (Valenza, Simion,

Cassia, & Umilta, 1996) and prefer listening to speech over nonspeech sounds (Vouloumanos & Werker, 2004). Meltzoff and Moore (1989) have shown that newborns can imitate simple human gestures, such as tongue protrusions and head movements, and by just 6 weeks of age they can engage in deferred imitation, emulating others' facial movements after a 24-hour delay (Meltzoff & Moore, 1994). Children as young as 6 months can distinguish between purposeful and nonpurposeful action (Woodward, 1999), and by 9 months of age they are able to follow and direct the attention of adults to outside entities, a capacity known as joint attention (Tomasello, 1995). At approximately 12 months of age, infants begin to engage in social referencing by using the emotional reactions of others to determine how to behave (Walden & Ogan, 1988). At approximately 18 months, toddlers can infer an adult's intended action by watching failed attempts (Meltzoff, 1995). By 24 months of age, children adjust the language they use in conversation based on their understanding of what the listener knows (Tomasello, Farrar, & Dines, 1984).

This progression shows an increasing understanding of others' intentions in the first 2 years of life. Tomasello (1995) has proposed a developmental trajectory for the understanding of others' intentions, whereby children progress from following and directing the attention of others without understanding their intentions, to understanding others as intentional agents, to learning that others' intentions may not always match the situation. This work has recently been expanded to suggest that these early developments culminate in the understanding of shared intentions with another individual, which is believed to be a defining feature of human social interaction (Tomasello, Carpenter, Call, Behne, & Moll, 2005). Understanding of others' intentions is also thought to underlie the ability to learn words. According to this view, early language acquisition represents a form of social cognition. In order for a child to learn the referent of a novel word, he or she must infer the referential intent of the speaker, using subtle cues such as the direction of the speaker's gaze and other contextual clues (Baldwin, 1993).

One of the most remarkable aspects of early development is its rapid pace. In a relatively short period of time, children's understanding of the social world becomes quite sophisticated. Yet it is important to remember that there is a great deal of variability in early trajectories of social and communication development. Fenson et al. (1994) emphasize the importance of going beyond descriptions of the "modal child" in order to understand the range of variability that can be expected in typically developing children.

For example, there is a great deal of variability in both early receptive language and expressive vocabulary development. As children get older, this variability increases, because children whose initial language is more advanced also show a higher rate of word acquisition. When considering variability in early social and communication development, then, it may be useful to examine not only differences in children's abilities at a given point in development, but also differences in the developmental trajectories of these abilities over time.

Marked individual differences have been found in other areas of communication, such as use of gestures, as well as in the development of social cognition. In a comprehensive study of children's social and communication development from 9 to 15 months of age, Carpenter, Nagell, Tomasello, Butterworth, and Moore (1998) found considerable variability in attention and gaze following, imitation, gesture production, and joint engagement, among other skills. Although the majority of the children in their sample displayed these skills by the age of 12 months, some children acquired these skills earlier than others (e.g., as young as 9 months) and some children had not acquired certain skills by 15 months.

Some researchers have argued that differences in child temperament might explain some of the variability in early social and communication development. Dixon and Smith (2000) found that temperament exhibited in early development was related to subsequent language skills, both receptive and expressive. In their sample, children who showed greater adaptability, more positive mood, and greater persistence at 13 months tended to have more productive language at 20 months, and children who had long durations of orientation, smiled and laughed frequently, or were easily soothed at 7 months tended to have advanced comprehension at 7 and 10 months of age.

Other studies have found similar relationships between children's early temperament and later language (Slomkowski, Nelson, Dunn, & Plomin, 1992). Dixon and Smith (2000) suggest that the relationship between temperament and language may be mediated by amount of joint engagement. That is, parents and others may be less likely to enter into a social exchange with a child who shows negative affect and poor adaptability than they would with a child who shows positive affect. The reduced amount of social interaction may in turn adversely affect the child's understanding and production of language. This model is partly supported by a finding in the study by Carpenter et al. (1998) that the amount of time mother–infant dyads spent in joint engagement was related to the child's early verbal and nonverbal communication skills.

The fact that there is a wide range of social and communication skills among typically developing young children presents a challenge to those trying to identify "markers" of ASD in children of this age. How does one decide if a toddler has a true impairment in reciprocal social interaction and/or communication that puts him at risk for a diagnosis of ASD, or whether he simply falls on the lower end of the continuum of typical development in these areas? Is a toddler who does not smile at others very often simply showing less positive affect than the "average" typical child of the same age because of her temperament, or does she have a more fundamental difficulty in interacting with others? It is also important to consider the role that cultural differences play in a child's social and communication behaviors (see Babad et al., 1983). The child's social environment, including culturally based parenting practices, is likely to influence some of the aspects of infant social communication behaviors.

Additional insight into this issue may come from considering "constellations" of deficits, rather than individual impairments. ASD is commonly thought of as involving deficits in several different areas (Siegel, Pliner, Eschler, & Elliott, 1988). It may be that, in order to be considered "at risk" for ASD, a child should be showing deficits in more than one of these areas. Therefore, when considering a particular social or communicative behavior in a young child, it may be important to consider whether the child is "below average" or "impaired" in a specific behavior, but also whether difficulties in that behavior occur in the context of other impairments. For example, a child who shows delays in using sounds and words but who shows positive affect, good eye contact, and use of early gestures would likely not elicit much concern as a child who, in addition to having delayed expressive language, shows impairments in other areas. Practitioners may also want to consider these issues when conducting evaluations of slightly older children. Despite the minimum onset requirement presented by DSM-IV—delay or abnormality in social interaction, *or* in language as used in social communication, *or* in imaginative play prior to age 3—practitioners may want to require that these types of early atypicalities occur in conjunction with one another in order to establish the onset of ASD.

Even with these distinctions in mind, it can be difficult for clinicians and researchers to determine whether a child who shows two or three developmental difficulties falls somewhere on the autism spectrum, is developmentally delayed but not on the spectrum, or is simply behind relative to the "average" typical child, but still within the range of typical development. PDD-NOS is usually diagnosed in young children who show some impairments characteristic of autism, but in such instances the number of impairments is fewer than that required for a diagnosis of autism, the impairments do not occur across all three areas specified (i.e., social, communication, RRBs), or the impairments are not as severe. This could explain why studies have found that early diagnoses of PDD-NOS are not as stable as diagnoses of autism (Chawarska, Klin, Paul, & Volkmar, 2007). A recent study found that the majority of children diagnosed with PDD-NOS at age 2 remained on the autism spectrum at age 9. Nevertheless, more than 10% of the children with PDD-NOS diagnoses at 2 years moved to a nonspectrum classification by 5 or 9 years (Lord et al., 2006). Given these criteria, it is possible to see how some young children thought to have "mild autism" might, at older ages, more clearly appear to have nonspectrum developmental delays or fall at the lower end of the continuum of typical development.

RRBs differ from most social and communication deficits required for a diagnosis of ASD, because they involve the presence of "atypical" behaviors rather than the absence of typical ones. Yet it is important to remember that some RRBs are actually seen in young children with typical development. Thelen (1979) reported motor stereotypies, such as kicking, waving, banging, rocking, and bouncing in normal infants in their first year of life, especially between the ages of 24 and 42 weeks. As toddlers and preschoolers, many typical young children display compulsive-like behaviors, such as insistence on sameness in their routines and/or environment, strong likes and dislikes, a rigid idea of how things should look, feel, taste, or smell, and a strict adherence to rituals during times of transition, such as at bedtime. Evans et al. (1997) found evidence for two kinds of compulsive-like behaviors in a substantial portion of young children: "just right" behaviors (e.g., lining objects up or insisting that they be arranged in a precise way) and repetitive behaviors/insistence on sameness (e.g., preferring to have the same schedule every day). It has also been argued that some repetition in object use or exploration (i.e., Piagetian secondary circular reactions) is important for developing cognitive skills, such as problem solving.

It is interesting to note the similarities between these behaviors and those considered to be "restricted and repetitive behaviors and interests" (American Psychiatric Association, 1994) in children with ASD. Many of the behaviors that constitute the category of RRBs are similar to those described in studies of typical children. Factor analyses of RRB scales in ASD have also found evidence for the two "subtypes" of RRBs described above (Cuccaro et al., 2003; Bishop, Richler, & Lord, 2006). Given these similarities, it is important to ask what is different about these behaviors in typically developing children as opposed to children on the autism spectrum, and why their presence at a young age is not necessarily an indicator of later impairment.

Part of the answer may lie in the developmental trajectories of these behaviors in typically developing children as compared to those of children with ASD. In the study by Evans et al. (1997), children between the ages of 24 and 36 months were found to exhibit the highest frequency and intensity of compulsive-like behaviors; after 36 months, scores tended to decrease steadily and then more steeply, so that mean scores between the ages of 48 and 72 months were significantly lower. This pattern suggests that most typically developing children tend to "grow out of" these behaviors, although this conclusion should be made with caution, given that the data in this study were cross-sectional. In contrast, longitudinal studies of RRBs in children with ASD have found that many of these behaviors tend to increase in prevalence and severity with time, at least up until the age of 5 and possible until older ages (Moore & Goodson, 2003; Charman et al., 2005). One of the main differences in these behaviors in typically developing children versus those with ASD could be that, for most typical children, the behaviors tend to be common only within a relatively narrow window of development, in contrast to children with ASD, who exhibit these behaviors for longer periods of time (Thelen, 1979).

This again highlights the importance of considering the differences in constellations of behaviors in young children with typical development as opposed to those with ASD. In the study by Evans et al. (1997), mean scores of typical children on the Childhood Routines Inventory (CRI) were very low relative to the maximum achievable score. Most children exhibited one or two of these behaviors, or if they did exhibit a few, the behaviors were relatively mild. In contrast, studies of RRBs in children with ASD indicate that the majority of children, even those at young ages, tend to exhibit more than two repetitive behaviors, and that these behaviors often interfere with the functioning of the child or the family (Richler, Bishop, Kleinke, & Lord, 2007). These findings suggest that it is important to consider whether a child who shows one particular compulsive-like behavior (e.g., lining up toy cars) also shows other similar behaviors (e.g., insisting that objects be placed in specific locations). Similarly, it is important to consider whether the presence of such behaviors occurs in concert with impairments in social interaction and communication.

Part of the reason that repetitive behaviors tend not to be as severe in typically developing children may be that these children do not have the added component of impairment in social interaction and communication to contend with. As a result, they are likely to spend more of their time interacting and communicating with others than engaging in repetitive activities. Even when they do engage in repetitive activities, they are likely to involve others in these activities, which makes the activities more social and flexible. In contrast, children with ASD often prefer to participate in repetitive activities rather than interact with others, which further deprives them of social stimulation (Rogers & Ozonoff, 2005).

Considering the early pictures of typical development and atypical development in social interaction and communication side by side, it is interesting to consider why the trajectories of typical development begin to diverge from those of the development of children with ASD. Some have argued that most children are born "hard-wired" to be oriented to the social world, responding to social input in their environment, and in turn, receiving more input (see Johnson et al., 2005). It has also been suggested that the early plasticity of the brain may provide an opportunity for experience to shape synaptic connections, eliminating those that are not needed and strengthening those that are crucial for higher-order functions, such as social cognition (Courchesne, Carper, & Akshoomoff,

2003). In contrast, some children may be born without the same predisposition to prioritize social input over nonsocial input (Dawson, Meltzoff, Osterling, Rinaldi, & Brown, 1998; Dawson et al., 2004) or may experience changes in trajectories of social and communication development, such as reaching a developmental plateau (Siperstein & Volkmar, 2004) or experiencing an actual worsening or regression in social and communication skills (Ozonoff, Williams, & Landa, 2005). Thus, for a number of reasons, children with ASD may not receive the same social input from the environment as typically developing children during this critical period of brain development (Mundy & Neal, 2001). Consequently, the parts of the brain normally involved in social cognition may not be selectively shaped for this role (Johnson et al., 2005). As typically developing children become more socially sophisticated in the first few years of life, the impairments of children with ASD may build on each other and become more apparent.

EARLY ASSESSMENT OF ASD

Because of the cumulative effects of early appearing deficits, such as those described above, detection of the symptoms of ASD tends to become easier as children get older. However, as we have come to understand more about early development of ASD, it has become increasingly possible to differentiate children with ASD from typically developing young children. Furthermore, whereas professionals have traditionally been hesitant to make diagnoses of ASD in children under the age of 3, recent literature suggests that when made by experienced clinicians, diagnoses of toddlers are relatively stable over time. Because different methods (i.e., clinical observation and parent report) provide different types of information, diagnoses are most accurate and stable when based on information obtained from multiple sources (e.g., Lord et al., 2006; Chawarska, Klin, et al., 2007).

Even for experienced clinicians, diagnosis can be difficult when trying to distinguish between ASD and other early childhood disorders. Psychological diagnoses, such as intellectual disability, expressive and receptive language disorders, anxiety disorders, and Attention-Deficit/ Hyperactivity Disorder (ADHD), as well as genetic disorders, such as fragile-X syndrome, share many features with ASD. Making diagnostic distinctions in very young children is therefore a difficult process.

Diagnosis of ASD is further complicated when a researcher or clinician is trying to determine whether a child meets the criteria for autism versus another spectrum condition (e.g., PDD-NOS, AS). Childhood Disintegrative Disorder (CDD) and Rett syndrome are quite rare and are less likely to be confused with autism, especially if a thorough medical history is obtained. On the other hand, clinicians often find themselves trying to distinguish between autism and AS or PDD-NOS, in part because of poor agreement about the diagnostic criteria of these disorders (Ozonoff, South, & Miller, 2000). DSM-IV provides guidelines for making diagnostic distinctions between these disorders, but these guidelines were written on the basis of studies of substantially older children (Volkmar et al., 1994; Chawarska & Volkmar, 2005).

Both CDD and Rett syndrome are characterized by a period of apparently normal development followed by a substantial regression. The onset of CDD must occur after 2 years of age, and the child must exhibit loss of previously acquired skills in at least two areas, such as language, social skills, adaptive behavior, play, toileting, or motor skills (American Psychiatric Association, 1994). After the regression, children with CDD must also exhibit impairments in at least two of the three domains in autism (i.e., social interaction, communication, restricted and repetitive behaviors/interests). The regression in Rett syndrome, which is a genetic disorder that occurs primarily in girls, occurs between the ages of 5 and 48 months and is characterized by decelerated head growth; loss of previously acquired purposeful hand movements, such as holding utensils or picking up objects; the development of stereotyped midline hand movements, such as hand wringing; loss of social engagement; appearance of poorly coordinated gait or trunk movements; and severely impaired language development (American Psychiatric Association, 1994).

Although approximately 20% of children with autism experience a regression in language or social behaviors (Lord, Shulman, & DiLavore, 2004; Volkmar, Chawarska, & Klin, 2005), the regressions in CDD and Rett syndrome are qualitatively distinct from the most common forms of regression in autism. First, whereas the regressions in CDD and Rett syndrome follow a period of typical development, some abnormality in children with autism is most often recognized, in hindsight, in the first year of life (Osterling & Dawson, 1994), prior to the onset of regression. Second, the regression in autism is characterized by a loss of language and/or social behaviors, without a loss of adaptive or motor skills (Volkmar & Rutter, 1995; Luyster et al., 2005), which are both typically seen in Rett syndrome and CDD. Moreover, the regression in children with autism is almost always before the age of 24 months (Lord et al., 2004; Luyster et al., 2005; Ozonoff et al., 2005; Chawarska, Paul, et al., 2007).

In addition to early regression, there are other behavioral markers that have been established as indicators of ASD in the first few years of life. Retrospective analyses of videotapes of children in their first year of life have indicated that those who later receive a diagnosis of ASD exhibit poor visual orientation and attention, limited response to name, lack of socially directed looking, excessive mouthing of objects, and aversion to social touch, relative to comparison groups of typically developing children and children with non-ASD developmental delays (Baranek, 1999; Osterling, Dawson, & Munson, 2002).

More recently, prospective studies of infant siblings of children with ASD, a population of children at high risk for developing ASD, have suggested a number of early features that are associated with a later diagnosis of ASD. Using the Autism Observation Scale for Infants (AOSI) (see below), Zwaigenbaum et al. (2005) found that at 12 months of age, children who were later diagnosed with ASD showed evidence of language delay, as well as several behavioral abnormalities, such as difficulties with eye contact, visual tracking and attention, social smiling, imitation, social interest and affect. These infants also tended to demonstrate decreased positive affect and were more likely to exhibit extreme distress reactions and to fixate on objects. Using a parent-report measure of early communication skills, the MacArthur–Bates Communicative Development Inventory–Infant Form (Fenson et al., 1993), Mitchell et al. (2006) found that infant siblings who later met criteria for ASD reportedly understood fewer phrases and demonstrated significantly fewer gestures at 12 months of age than typically developing controls or siblings who did not receive ASD diagnoses. These delays were still apparent at 18 months of age, as were reported delays in understanding and use of single words.

Studies comparing very young children with ASD to those with other types of developmental delays have made it increasingly possible for clinicians and researchers to differentiate between ASD and other non-spectrum disorders. However, obtaining agreement between diagnoses of autism, AS, and PDD-NOS has been much more difficult, particularly in young children. Several different definitions for these disorders exist, which has complicated communication between professionals in the field (Ozonoff et al., 2000; Klin, Pauls, Schultz, & Volkmar, 2005). According to DSM-IV, AS is characterized by both qualitative impairments in social interaction and the presence of RRBs that are identical to those seen in autism. However, unlike in autism, there can be no delay in language, cognitive development, or adaptive behavior (except social skills) in a diagnosis of AS (American Psychiatric Association, 1994). A diagnosis of PDD-NOS is intended for children who exhibit significant impairments in reciprocal social interaction, as well as difficulties in either communication or the presence of RRBs (or subthreshold difficulties in both areas), who do not meet criteria for another ASD.

Evidence suggests that diagnoses of PDD-NOS in early preschool are less stable than autism diagnoses (e.g., Stone et al., 1999; Lord et al., 2006). Clinicians are more reliable when making distinctions in 2-year-olds between ASD and nonspectrum diagnoses than between specific diagnoses on the spectrum, and it is not uncommon for children to have a change in diagnosis within the spectrum (e.g., from a diagnosis of PDD-NOS to autism) (Stone et al., 1999; Lord et al., 2006). What may be most important for very young children, therefore, is making a distinction between a spectrum and a nonspectrum diagnosis, because differential diagnoses within the spectrum tend to be less stable (Lord et al., 2006). Thus, the intervention that children receive should be based more on their individual profiles of strengths and weaknesses, rather than on their specific diagnostic classifications.

SCREENING FOR ASD

General Issues

Our increasing knowledge of early development in children later diagnosed with ASD has facilitated the creation of a number of screeners targeted at identifying young children with ASD. A major challenge associated with the development of these instruments is being able to discriminate children with significant developmental delays from children with less pervasive and often temporary developmental delays. In large part, the ability to do this depends on our understanding of what verbal and nonverbal skills cluster together in the first few years of typical development, and the degree to which these skills are impaired in children for whom ASD is a concern.

Clarifying these early profiles of development and using them to screen for ASD in young children has both theoretical and practical implications. First, identifying children with ASD in the first few years of life allows for the collection of data about early profiles and trajectories of development. Such information is valuable for theoretical accounts of ASD as well as for informing efforts to improve the accuracy of the screening instruments themselves. In addition, earlier detection of ASD permits prompt delivery of intervention services, and research has indicated that intervention is more effective if provided earlier (Harris & Handleman, 2000).

Different approaches have been taken in designing screeners, some using caregivers as informants and others using professionals. There are also two levels of screeners, one designed for population-based screening (i.e., level 1 screeners), and the other designed for more targeted screening of children suspected of having a developmental disorder (i.e., level 2 screeners). In general, screening is distinct from diagnostic assessment in that the former is a relatively broad-based approach intended to identify children with unrecognized or ambiguous symptoms of developmental disabilities, whereas the latter is most appropriate for children for whom there is already some clear evidence of developmental abnormality.

Level 1 screeners typically employ caregiver reports as a means of gathering information. The primary advantage of this approach is that parents and caregivers are most familiar with the skills of the child across a variety of situations, and they may be more accurate than professionals in reporting low-frequency behaviors (such as using another person's hand as a tool). However, caregivers may have less experience with children and a less refined understanding of the questions on the screener, which could potentially result in either over- or underestimating their child's skills. There is also a risk of biased reporting (if caregivers already have beliefs about the diagnostic status of their child). Finally, creating a scale that caregivers will interpret as intended can be quite difficult.

Level 2 screeners that use the reports of professionals (such as health care workers or psychologists) have a different set of advantages and disadvantages. Professionals may be more highly trained in observing and identifying certain diagnostically meaningful behaviors, and completion of the screeners can be standardized across reporters. However, they spend much less time with the child. As a result, they generally do not have the opportunity to evaluate the child across contexts and are much less likely than caregivers to note low-frequency behaviors.

In evaluating the effectiveness of level 1 and level 2 screeners, it is useful to consider the constructs of sensitivity and specificity. *Sensitivity* refers to a measure's ability to accurately "rule in" all individuals with the targeted trait, and *specificity* refers to its ability to accurately "rule out" all individuals without the targeted trait. In the context of screening for ASD, sensitivity may be more important for level 1 screeners, because high sensitivity can maximize the detection of children who are showing a behavioral profile suggestive of ASD. Regardless of whether ASD is their final diagnosis or not, these children are likely to be "at risk" for one form of disability or another and will benefit from identification and referral. Thus, even though decreasing specificity and increasing sensitivity results in more false positives, which can be expensive and potentially problematic, it is better to identify these children with developmental complications early on, rather than later or not at all. In contrast, for level 2 screeners and diagnostic measures, specificity is a higher priority, because it is at this point that the measures must be able to discriminate ASD from phenotypically similar conditions, such as language delay or intellectual disability.

Screening Instruments

Current measures for screening and diagnosis are considered here in turn, with reference to current research on their advantages and limitations for children under age 3. Population (level 1) and focused (level 2) screening are addressed (see Figure 2.1).

The CHecklist for Autism in Toddlers (CHAT; a level 1 screener) was initially introduced in the United Kingdom as a population screening measure for ASD (Baron-Cohen, Allen, & Gillberg, 1992). The CHAT emphasized joint attention and imagination and was administered to children by health nurses, who routinely visit 18-month-olds in their homes in the United Kingdom. During the visit, the parents were also asked a series of questions about their child's development. Results indicated that most children classified by the CHAT as having autism were, in fact, later diagnosed with the disorder. However, it later became clear that two-thirds of the children who eventually received an ASD diagnosis were missed by the CHAT (Baird et al., 2000). Moreover, because children with suspected developmental disabilities were eliminated even before the screening, the CHAT's effectiveness in distinguishing between ASD and other developmental disabilities was unclear.

The Modified CHecklist for Autism in Toddlers (M-CHAT), a modified version of the CHAT (Robins, Fein, Barton, & Green, 2001), was created to address some of these concerns. The M-CHAT was administered

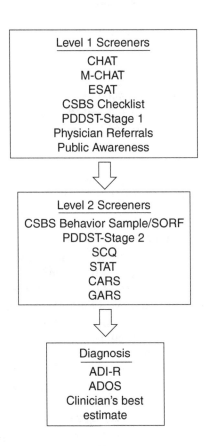

FIGURE 2.1. Levels of screening and diagnosis for children with ASD at age 3 or younger.

to parents of 24-month-old children who were recruited from pediatric practices and special education programs in the United States. In contrast to the CHAT, the M-CHAT is not administered to the child and instead relies on parent report. Like its predecessor, the M-CHAT successfully identified children with autism at age 2. The M-CHAT was tested on two groups of children, a population sample and a sample from special education programs. More than 90% of the children identified as having autism were already in special education programs (Robins et al., 2001), so the effectiveness of the M-CHAT for use in the general population is not yet clear. Initial reports of sensitivity and specificity were very high (.87 and .99, respectively), but the authors caution that absolute psychometrics for this measure cannot be determined until all follow-up evaluations are completed (Robins et al., 2001; Robins & Dumont-Mathieu, 2006). A larger study of the M-CHAT in a more representative sample is now under way, and the results of this study will be important in evaluating the effectiveness of the M-CHAT.

The Early Screening for Autistic Traits (ESAT; Swinkels et al., 2006) is a level 1 screener questionnaire with a greater emphasis on play and less on joint attention than the previous instruments. Children who earned high scores on the instrument were likely to have developmental problems. However, for children younger than 24 months of age, the ESAT did not successfully distinguish children with ASD from those with non-ASD conditions. In addition, like the CHAT and M-CHAT, it also failed to identify many children who were later diagnosed with ASD (see, e.g., Buitelaar et al., 2000). Despite the measure's problems with poor sensitivity, the use of the ESAT heightened public awareness and provided easy access to referrals. As a result of these related benefits, early identification increased.

The Communication and Symbolic Behavior Scales—Developmental Profile (CSBS-DP; Wetherby & Prizant, 2002) is a brief caregiver questionnaire intended to identify children with communication disorders (not specifically ASD) between the ages of 6 and 24 months. If a child screens positively on the questionnaire based on his or her caregiver's responses, then a direct assessment (the Behavior Sample) and an additional caregiver questionnaire are administered. Although the initial questionnaire is a level 1 screener, a level 2 screener—the Scale of Red Flags (SORF; Wetherby & Woods, 2002) for autism—was developed for use in scoring videotapes of the Behavior Sample. With the SORF, researchers were able to successfully identify most children with language delay as having or not having autism. However, because most of the children observed had screened positively on the CSBS caregiver questionnaire, there was no way to identify missed cases and determine the measure's sensitivity.

The Pervasive Developmental Disorders Screening Test (PDDST; Siegel, 1996) also offers a level 1 and a level 2 screener and is intended for children over the age of 18 months and under the age of 6 years. It is a parent report questionnaire and is designed to screen specifically for ASD. It targets areas of first concern frequently reported by parents of children with ASD, such as nonverbal communication, temperament, play, language, and social engagement. Stage 1 of the PDDST (intended for use in primary care settings) was reported to have a sensitivity of .85 and a specificity of .71 in a clinic-based sample. In a sample of children with ASD and children with other developmental disorders, sensitivity and specificity of the PDDST-Stage 2 (intended for use in developmental disorders clinics) varied according to the cutoff used, ranging from .69 to .88 and .25 to .63, respectively (Siegel, 1996; Siegel & Hayer, 1999). Research on the PDDST is ongoing to provide further details about its psychometric properties and usefulness in different populations.

The Screening Test for Autism in Two-Year-Olds (STAT; Stone, Coonrod, & Ousley, 2000) involves a direct assessment and, as a level 2 screener, is intended for children already suspected of having ASD. However, unlike the diagnostic tests described below, it is relatively brief. In addition, it is more straightforward to administer and score; consequently, it does not require extensive training on the part of the examiner. In a validation sample of 12 children with autism and 21 children with non-spectrum developmental disorders, the STAT correctly identified 10 (83%) of the children with autism and 18 (86%) of the children with other developmental disorders (Stone et al., 2000).

The Social Communication Questionnaire (SCQ; Rutter, Bailey, Lord, & Berument, 2003) is a level 2 caregiver questionnaire designed to identify participants with ASD for research purposes. Although the measure was normed on older children and adults, research has indicated that if the cutoff is modified so that fewer endorsed items are required, the SCQ works well for children as young as 3 years old (Corsello et al., 2007). However, because the children had already been referred for services, it is unclear how appropriate the SCQ is for use in the general population.

There are two other well-known scales primarily intended for level 2 screening but which may be mistaken for diagnostic instruments: the Childhood Autism Rating Scale (CARS) and the Gilliam Autism Rating Scale (GARS). The CARS (Schopler, Reichler, & Renner, 1988) is most useful with children beyond the 2-year-old level and up to 4 or 5 years in developmental skills, and it has been shown to have high sensitivity in older children and adults (Sevin, Matson, Coe, Fee, & Sevin, 1991; Eaves & Milner, 1993). Studies have yielded mixed results with regard to the utility of the CARS for use with very young children. Lord (1995) reported that the CARS overidentified autism in 2-year-olds with cognitive impairments, whereas Stone and colleagues (1999) reported good agreement with clinical diagnosis at age 2 (82% agreement). Agreement of the CARS and clinical impression is better by age 3 (Lord, 1995; Stone et al., 1999), and specificity can be improved by raising the CARS cutoff by 2 points (Lord, 1995).

The GARS (Gilliam, 1995) is a behavioral checklist that was developed to screen for autism. However, the measure was not designed for or normed on children under 3 years of age, and thus its usefulness for a young population is unknown. One study (South et al., 2002) employed the GARS in a sample of 119 preschool and school-age children with autism. Overall, the GARS underdiagnosed autism, failing to accurately classify more than half of the sample. Until revisions are made, the appropriateness of the GARS for children under 3 is limited.

EARLY DIAGNOSIS OF ASD

Once a child has been identified as being at risk for ASD, he or she should be referred to a psychologist, psychiatrist, or developmental pediatrician who specializes in early diagnosis of developmental disabilities. To aid clinicians in making accurate diagnoses, it is essential that a diagnostic assessment be multidimensional and multidisciplinary (see Figure 2.2).

This includes gathering information from different sources and assessing a child's behavior across a variety of contexts. Research has indicated that diagnoses of 2-year-olds were significantly more stable when confirmed across two or three sources (i.e., standardized parent interview, direct child observation, and clinician's best estimate diagnosis) as opposed to just one (Lord et al., 2006).

Several instruments have been designed to aid professionals in gathering information needed to make a diagnosis of ASD. (For a more comprehensive discussion of practice parameters and diagnostic instruments, see Filipek, Accardo, & Ashwal, 2000; Klinger & Renner, 2000; Lord & Corsello, 2005; and Bishop & Lord, 2006.) Standardized parent interviews and questionnaires can be useful in eliciting information from parents about their child's behavior. In contrast to the traditional open-ended interview, semistructured interviews allow for a more comprehensive assessment of communication, social, and play behaviors associated with ASD and other developmental disorders. The most widely used and well-established semistructured interview that is designed to diagnose ASD is the Autism Diagnostic Interview–Revised (ADI-R; Lord, Rutter, & Le Couteur, 1994). The ADI-R provides quantifiable scores related to severity of symptoms in the areas of communication, reciprocal social interaction, and restricted and repetitive behaviors, as well as separate algorithms for verbal and nonverbal children. In order to meet criteria for a diagnosis of autism, the child must meet cutoffs in Communication, Reciprocal Social Interaction, Restricted and Repetitive Behaviors and Interests, and Age of

---

Medical Examination

- Rule out sensory impairment (check hearing and vision).
- Conduct genetic testing if indicated based on dysmorphology or family history.
- Conduct neurological exam.

Parent Interview

- Obtain thorough developmental history (attainment and/ or loss of motor, speech, self-help milestones).
- Administer semistructured interview to gather information about social and communication development, play, restricted and repetitive behaviors, and adaptive skills.

Child Observation

- Create context in which to observe child's social-communication behaviors, play, and repetitive behaviors (with both parent and examiner).
- Consult parents and teachers about whether behaviors observed during assessment were consistent with child's behavior in other settings.

Developmental and Language Testing

- Assess verbal (expressive and receptive) and nonverbal abilities.
- Gather information about receptive and expressive language abilities.
- Evaluate gross and fine motor skills.

FIGURE 2.2. Assessing young children with suspected ASD.

Onset. In children over the age of 3, these cutoffs have been found to clearly differentiate between children with autism and those with other disorders (Lord et al., 1994).

The validity of this instrument for children under the age of 3 has not been established. Therefore, a "Toddler" version of the ADI-R is undergoing development and being used in some investigations. It includes 32 additional questions and codes specifically relevant to onset of difficulties in the early years (C. Lord, personal communication, August, 2006). Because this modified instrument is not yet available for general use, professionals may decide to use the published version of the ADI-R but should use caution when interpreting the scores for children under the age of 3. In particular, some studies have reported low sensitivity of the ADI-R for populations of young children because many children do not meet cutoffs in the Restricted, Repetitive and Stereotyped Patterns of Behavior Domain (Ventola et al., 2006; Chawarska, Klin, et al., 2007).

Although the majority of 2-year-olds with ASD exhibit RRBs (Richler et al., 2007), some of the RRB items that are currently included in the ADI-R algorithm (e.g., compulsions and rituals) may be less prevalent in very young children with ASD.

The Diagnostic Interview for Social and Communication Disorders (DISCO; Wing, Leekam, Libby, Gould, & Larcombe, 2002) is another semistructured interview designed to aid in the diagnosis of ASD. Whereas the ADI-R is a diagnostic measure of ASD, the DISCO includes questions about a wider range of difficulties and can be used to compile information necessary to diagnose other developmental and psychiatric disorders. The Development, Diagnostic and Dimensional Interview (3di; Skuse et al., 2004) is a computer-based standardized interview intended to assess autism severity, as well as symptoms of comorbid conditions, such as ADHD. Although reliability and validity estimates of the 3di were high, the original validation sample of children with ASD consisted mainly of school-age children with relatively mild symptoms. Thus, the utility of the 3di for use in young children or those with more severe symptoms of ASD is less well established.

Information obtained through parent report is an important part of any child assessment, but direct clinical observation of the child is also required in order to make an accurate diagnosis. Observations in which the clinician simply observes the child in an unstructured context do not always elicit behaviors associated with a diagnosis of ASD. Therefore, administering measures such as the Autism Diagnostic Observation Schedule—Generic (ADOS-G; Lord et al., 2000) and the Autism Observation Scale for Infants (AOSI; Bryson, Zwaigenbaum, McDermott, Rombough, & Brian, 2007) provides opportunities for the clinician to observe social, communication, and play behaviors in standardized, semistructured contexts. The ADOS-G is organized into four modules that correspond to various levels of language skills, and each module is composed of a standard series of tasks designed to elicit information in the areas of communication, reciprocal social behavior, and restricted and repetitive behaviors. Module 1 is intended for children who are nonverbal or who have single-word speech, which generally makes it most appropriate for use in very young children suspected of having ASD. Module 2 is designed for children with phrase speech, so it may also be employed in assessing highly verbal 2- and 3-year-old children with suspected ASD. Modules 3 and 4 are less relevant for the present discussion, as they are intended for children with complex sentences (i.e., sentences with two or more clauses). As with the ADI-R, a toddler version of the ADOS-G is also currently under development. In addition, new algorithms have been developed that use the existing items of the ADOS-G to improve the sensitivity and specificity of the algorithms, especially in populations that can be difficult to classify (e.g., very young children) (see Gotham, Risi,

Pickles, & Lord, 2007). Separate algorithms have been developed for children in Module 1 who use words meaningfully and spontaneously during the session and those who do not, and separate modules have been developed for children under and over age 5 years who receive Module 2. These modifications have resulted in increased specificity for autism and better sensitivity and specificity for nonautism ASD in most modules.

The AOSI is intended to elicit the same types of information as the ADOS-G, but it is specifically designed for infants under 18 months of age. Thus, in addition to play-based activities similar to those in the ADOS-G, the AOSI also includes some tasks, such as eye tracking and attention shifts, that are intended to detect very early markers of ASD. As discussed previously, initial studies using the AOSI have suggested that siblings who are later diagnosed with ASD show differences in social and communication behaviors as early as 12 months (Zwaigenbaum et al., 2005). These play-based assessment tools help the clinician to structure the assessment context such that the child is given multiple opportunities to communicate and engage in social interactions with the examiner and parent. However, both the ADOS-G and the AOSI require extensive training to ensure standardized administration procedures and coding reliability.

A number of prospective studies have suggested that children can be accurately diagnosed with ASD as young as 24 months when using standard instruments such as the ADI-R and the ADOS-G. However, although these measures produce reliable information about very young children, their diagnostic thresholds should be carefully applied to children who have nonverbal mental ages below certain cutoffs (15 months on the ADOS-G or 18 months on the ADI-R). Research has suggested that using the ADI-R and ADOS-G in this population results in a high rate of misdiagnosis for children who do not have ASD but are at very low developmental levels. Therefore, as described above, researchers are currently in the process of modifying these instruments to improve their appropriateness for use with very young children. The use of these instruments with certain special populations is also not well established, as they have not been validated for use in children with severe sensory impairments (e.g., congenital blindness, profound hearing impairment) or motor difficulties (e.g., children who are not walking).

Because the selection of appropriate diagnostic instruments depends in part on the child's developmental level and associated medical characteristics, it is essential to obtain a thorough medical and developmental history. This information is needed in order to make accurate interpretations about the child's behavior. For example, in a child who has delayed motor milestones, such as sitting upright or walking, it is necessary to assess for general developmental delay and motor problems before interpreting behaviors, such as lack of babbling or poor eye contact, that may be more indicative of ASD. An adaptive behavior measure, such as the

Vineland Adaptive Behavior Scales (VABS; Sparrow, Balla, & Cicchetti, 1984), can be helpful in providing estimates of a child's general developmental level. Some researchers even suggest that children with ASD follow a particular profile on measures of adaptive behavior, which could be used for diagnostic purposes (Carter et al., 1998; Paul et al., 2004), but this has not yet been examined in very young children with ASD. Researchers are beginning to examine whether profiles on developmental tests, such as the Mullen Scales of Early Learning (MSEL; Mullen, 1995), can be used to differentiate between young children with and without ASD (Landa & Garrett-Mayer, 2006).

Directly assessing a child's developmental level is another important component of a diagnostic evaluation for ASD. Social, communication, and play behaviors cannot be accurately assessed without first knowing what is developmentally appropriate for an individual child. A toddler with moderate to severe intellectual disability who is functioning at a 1-year-old level would not be expected to communicate or interact socially at the same level as a 2-year-old with average developmental or cognitive skills. Similarly, a toddler with a language disorder would not be expected to verbally communicate as proficiently as a toddler without language delays. Therefore, incorporating developmental and language testing into the assessment battery is required in order for a clinician to interpret a child's behavior in the context of his or her general developmental level (see Chawarska & Bearss, Chapter 3, this volume for further discussion). Because individuals on the autism spectrum often exhibit significant discrepancies between their verbal and nonverbal IQs (Joseph, Tager-Flusberg, & Lord, 2002), tests that do not rely too heavily on the use of language, such as the MSEL (Mullen, 1995), and that assess nonverbal skills separately from verbal skills, such as the Differential Ability Scales (DAS; Elliott, 1990), are ideal for testing children with suspected ASD or communication disorders. Assessing receptive and expressive language abilities separately is also important and can be accomplished through the use of measures such as the Sequenced Inventory of Communication Development (Hedrick, Prather, & Tobin, 1999), the Preschool Language Scale, fourth edition (PLS-4; Zimmerman, Steiner, & Pond, 2002) and the Reynell Developmental Language Scales (Reynell & Gruber, 1978) (see Paul, Chapter 4, this volume, for further discussion).

CONCLUSION

There is an accumulating body of evidence to suggest that by the age of 2 years, it is possible to distinguish children with ASD from typically developing infants and those with nonspectrum developmental delays. Furthermore, longitudinal studies suggest that diagnoses of ASD are relatively stable over time. However, differentiating ASD from other kinds of developmental delays requires information from multiple sources, as well as systematic observation of the child by an experienced clinician. Research has suggested that obtaining an accurate diagnosis of ASD early in life has important theoretical and practical implications. The earlier we are able to identify the symptoms of ASD, the closer we will come to understanding the etiology of the disorder on a genetic and neurobiological level. In addition, gathering information about the earliest indicators of ASD may provide insight into the core symptoms and primary deficits of the disorder. Early identification is also a crucial first step in obtaining appropriate intervention services. This is particularly important, given recent findings that earlier intervention is associated with improved outcomes.

ACKNOWLEDGMENTS

The authorship of this chapter is alphabetical. Each author contributed equally to the writing of the chapter. This work was supported by Grant Nos. R01MH066496 from the National Institute of Mental Health and HD 35482-01 from the National Institute of Child Health and Human Development to Catherine Lord. Somer L. Bishop's work was also supported in part by National Institute on Alcohol Abuse and Alcoholism Training Grant No. T32 AA 07477 to Robert Zucker, and Rhiannon Luyster's work by National Research Service Award No. F31MH73210-02 from the National Institute of Mental Health.

REFERENCES

American Psychiatric Association. (1994). *Diagnostic and statistical manual of mental disorders* (4th ed.). Washington, DC: Author.

Babad, Y. E., Alexander, I. E., Babad, E. Y., Read, P. B., Shapiro, T., Leiderman, H., et al. (1983). Returning the smile of the stranger: Developmental patterns and socialization factors. *Monographs of the Society for Research in Child Development, 48*, 1–93.

Baird, G., Charman, T., Baron-Cohen, S., Cox, A., Swettenham, J., Wheelwright, S., et al. (2000). A screening instrument for autism at 18 months of age: A 6-year follow-up study. *Journal of the American Academy of Child and Adolescent Psychiatry, 39*, 694–702.

Baldwin, D. A. (1993). Infants' ability to consult the speaker for clues to word reference. *Journal of Child Language, 20*, 395–418.

Baranek, G. T. (1999). Autism during infancy: A retrospective video analysis of sensory–motor and social behaviors at 9–12 months of age. *Journal of Autism and Developmental Disorders, 29*, 213–224.

Baron-Cohen, S., Allen, J., & Gillberg, C. (1992). Can autism be detected at 18 months?: The needle, the haystack, and the CHAT. *British Journal of Psychiatry, 161*, 839–843.

Bishop, S. L., & Lord, C. (2006). Autism spectrum disorders. In J. Luby (Ed.), *Handbook of preschool mental health: Development, disorders, and treatment* (pp. 252–279). New York: Guilford Press.

Bishop, S. L., Richler, J., & Lord, C. (2006). Association between restricted and repetitive behaviors and nonverbal IQ in children with autism spectrum disorders. *Child Neuropsychology, 12,* 247–267.

Bryson, S. E., Zwaigenbaum, L., McDermott, C., Rombough, V., & Brian, J. (2007). The Autism Observational Scale for Infants: Scale development and reliability data. *Journal of Autism and Developmental Disorders.* Retrieved from *www.springerlink.com/content/104757*

Buitelaar, J. K., Willemsen-Swinkels, S., Daalen, E., Dietz, C., Naber, F., & Van Engeland, H. (2000, October). *The screening instrument for the early detection of autism.* Paper presented at the 47th annual meeting of the American Academy of Child and Adolescent Psychiatry, New York, NY.

Carpenter, M., Nagell, K., Tomasello, M., Butterworth, G., & Moore, C. (1998). Social cognition, joint attention, and communicative competence from 9 to 15 months of age. *Monographs of the Society for Research in Child Development, 63,* 1–174.

Carter, A. S., Volkmar, F. R., Sparrow, S. S., Wang, J.-J., Lord, C., Dawson, G., et al. (1998). The Vineland Adaptive Behavior Scales: Supplementary norms for individuals with autism. *Journal of Autism and Developmental Disorders, 28,* 287–302.

Charman, T., Taylor, E., Drew, A., Cockerill, H., Brown, J. A., & Baird, G. (2005). Outcome at 7 years of children diagnosed with autism at age 2: Predictive validity of assessments conducted at 2 and 3 years of age and pattern of symptom change over time. *Journal of Child Psychology and Psychiatry, 46,* 500–513.

Chawarska, K., Klin, A., Paul, R., & Volkmar, F. (2007). Autism spectrum disorder in the second year: Stability and change in syndrome expression. *Journal of Child Psychology and Psychiatry, 48,* 128–138.

Chawarska, K., Paul, R., Klin, A., Hannigen, S., Dichtel, L. E., & Volkmar, F. (2007). Parental recognition of developmental problems in toddlers with autism spectrum disorders. *Journal of Autism and Developmental Disorders, 37,* 62–72.

Chawarska, K., & Volkmar, F. R. (2005). Autism in infancy and early childhood. In F. R. Volkmar, R. Paul, A. Klin, & D. Cohen (Eds.), *Handbook of autism and pervasive developmental disorders, Vol. 1. Diagnosis, development, neurobiology, and behavior* (3rd ed., pp. 223–246). Hoboken, NJ: Wiley.

Corsello, C., Hus, V., Pickles, A., Risi, S., Cook, E., Levanthal, B., et al. (2007). Between a ROC and a hard place: Decision making and making decisions about using the SCQ. *Journal of Child Psychology and Psychiatry, 48,* 932–940.

Courchesne, E., Carper, R., & Akshoomoff, N. A. (2003). Evidence of brain overgrowth in the first year of life in autism. *Journal of the American Medical Association, 290,* 337–344.

Cuccaro, M. L., Shao, Y., Grubber, J., Slifer, M., Wolpert, C. M., Donnelly, S. L., et al. (2003). Factor analysis of restricted and repetitive behaviors in autism using the Autism Diagnostic Interview-R. *Child Psychiatry and Human Development, 34,* 3–17.

Dawson, G., Meltzoff, A. N., Osterling, J., Rinaldi, J., & Brown, E. (1998). Children with autism fail to orient to naturally occurring social stimuli. *Journal of Autism and Developmental Disorders, 28,* 479–485.

Dawson, G., Toth, K., Abbott, R., Osterling, J., Munson, J., Estes, A., et al. (2004). Early social attention impairments in autism: Social orienting, joint attention, and attention to distress. *Developmental Psychology, 40,* 271–283.

Dixon, W., & Smith, P. H. (2000). Links between early temperament and language acquisition. *Merrill–Palmer Quarterly, 46,* 417–440.

Eaves, R. C., & Milner, B. (1993). The criterion-related validity of the Childhood Autism Rating Scale and the Autism Behavior Checklist. *Journal of Abnormal Child Psychology, 21,* 481–491.

Elliott, C. D. (1990). *Differential Ability Scales.* San Antonio, TX: Psychological Corporation.

Evans, D. W., Leckman, J. F., Carter, A., Reznick, J. S., Henshaw, D., King, R. A., et al. (1997). Ritual, habit, and perfectionism: The prevalence and development of compulsive-like behavior in normal young children. *Child Development, 68,* 58–68.

Fenson, L., Dale, P. S., Reznick, J. S., Bates, E., Thal, D., & Pethick, S. (1994). Variability in early communicative development. *Monographs of the Society for Research in Child Development, 59,* 1–185.

Fenson, L., Dale, P. S., Reznick, J. S., Thal, D., Bates, E., Hartung, J. P., et al. (1993). *The MacArthur Communicative Development Inventories: User's guide and technical manual.* San Diego: Singular Publishing Group.

Filipek, P. A., Accardo, P. J., & Ashwal, S. (2000). Practice parameter: Screening and diagnosis of autism—A report of the Quality Standards Subcommittee of the American Academy of Neurology and the Child Neurology Society. *Neurology, 55,* 468–479.

Gilliam, J. E. (1995). *Gilliam Autism Rating Scale.* Austin, TX: PRO-ED.

Gotham, K., Risi, S., Pickles, A., & Lord, C. (2007). The Autism Diagnostic Observation Schedule: Revised algorithms for improved diagnostic validity. *Journal of Autism and Developmental Disorders, 37,* 613–627.

Handleman, J. S., & Harris, S. (Eds.). (2000). *Preschool education programs for children with autism* (2nd ed). Austin, TX: PRO-ED.

Harris, S. L., & Handleman, J. S. (2000). Age and IQ at intake as predictors of placement for young children with autism: A four- to six-year follow-up. *Journal of Autism and Developmental Disorders, 30,* 137–142.

Hedrick, D., Prather, E., & Tobin, A. (1999). *Sequenced Inventory of Communication Development–Revised.* Los Angeles: Western Psychological Services.

Johnson, M. H., Griffin, R., Csibra, G., Halit, H., Farroni, T., De Haan, M., et al. (2005). The emergence of the social brain network: Evidence from typical and atypical development. *Development and Psychopathology, 17,* 509–619.

Joseph, R. M., Tager-Flusberg, H., & Lord, C. (2002). Cognitive profiles and social-communicative functioning in children with autism spectrum disorder. *Journal of Child Psychology and Psychiatry, 43,* 807–821.

Klin, A., Pauls, D., Schultz, R., & Volkmar, F. (2005). Three diagnostic approaches to Asperger syndrome: Implications for research. *Journal of Autism and Developmental Disorders, 35,* 221–234.

Klinger, L. G., & Renner, P. (2000). Performance-based measures in autism: Implications for diagnosis, early detection, and identification of cognitive profiles. *Journal of Clinical Child Psychology, 29,* 479–492.

Landa, R., & Garrett-Mayer, E. (2006). Development in infants with autism spectrum disorders: A prospective study. *Journal of Child Psychology and Psychiatry, 47,* 629–638.

Lord, C. (1995). Follow-up of two-year-olds referred for possible autism. *Journal of Child Psychology and Psychiatry, 36,* 1365–1382.

Lord, C., & Corsello, C. (2005). Diagnostic instruments in autistic spectrum disorders. In F. Volkmar, R. Paul, A. Klin, & D. Cohen (Eds.), *Handbook of autism and pervasive developmental disorders: Vol. 2. Assessment, interventions, and policy* (pp. 730–771). Hoboken, NJ: Wiley.

Lord, C., Risi, S., DiLavore, P., Shulman, C., Thurm, A., & Pickles, A. (2006). Autism from two to nine. *Archives of General Psychiatry, 63,* 694–701.

Lord, C., Risi, S., Lambrecht, L., Cook, E. H., Leventhal, B. L., DiLavore, P. C., et al. (2000). The Autism Diagnostic Observation Schedule—Generic: A standard measure of social and communication deficits associated with the spectrum of autism. *Journal of Autism and Developmental Disorders, 30,* 205–223.

Lord, C., Rutter, M., & Le Couteur, A. (1994). The Autism Diagnostic Interview—Revised: A revised version of a diagnostic interview for caregivers of individuals with possible pervasive developmental disorders. *Journal of Autism and Developmental Disorders, 24,* 659–685.

Lord, C., Shulman, C., & DiLavore, P. (2004). Regression and word loss in autistic spectrum disorders. *Journal of Child Psychology and Psychiatry, 45,* 936–955.

Luyster, R., Richler, J., Risi, S., Hsu, W. L., Dawson, G., Bernier, R., et al. (2005). Early regression in social communication in autism spectrum disorders: A CPEA study. *Developmental Neuropsychology, 27,* 311–336.

Meltzoff, A. N. (1995). Understanding the intentions of others: Re-enactment of intended acts by 18-month-old children. *Developmental Psychology, 31,* 838–850.

Meltzoff, A. N., & Moore, M. K. (1989). Imitation in newborn infants: Exploring the range of gestures imitated and the underlying mechanisms. *Developmental Psychology, 25,* 954–962.

Meltzoff, A. N., & Moore, M. K. (1994). Imitation, memory, and the representation of persons. *Infant Behavior and Development, 17,* 83–99.

Mitchell, S., Brian, J., Zwaigenbaum, L., Roberts, W., Szatmari, P., Smith, I., et al. (2006). Early language and communication development of infants later diagnosed with autism spectrum disorder. *Journal of Developmental and Behavioral Pediatrics, 27,* S69–S78.

Moore, V., & Goodson, S. (2003). How well does early diagnosis of autism stand the test of time? Follow-up study of children assessed for autism at age 2 and development of an early diagnostic service. *Autism, 7,* 47–63.

Mullen, E. (1995). *The Mullen Scales of Early Learning.* Circle Pines, MN: American Guidance Service.

Mundy, P., & Neal, A. R. (2001). Neural plasticity, joint attention, and a transactional social-orienting model of autism. In L. M. Glidden (Ed.), *International review of research in mental retardation: Autism* (Vol. 23, pp. 139–168). San Diego: Academic Press.

Osterling, J., & Dawson, G. (1994). Early recognition of children with autism: A study of first birthday home videotapes. *Journal of Autism and Developmental Disorders, 24,* 247–257.

Osterling, J., Dawson, G., & Munson, J. (2002). Early recognition of 1-year-old infants with autism spectrum disorder versus mental retardation. *Development and Psychopathology, 14,* 239–251.

Ozonoff, S., South, M., & Miller, J. N. (2000). DSM-IV-defined Asperger syndrome: Cognitive, behavioral and early history differentiation from high-functioning autism. *Autism: Special Issue: Asperger syndrome, 4,* 29–46.

Ozonoff, S., Williams, B. J., & Landa, R. (2005). Parental report of the early development of children with regressive autism: The delays-plus-regression phenotype. *Autism, 9,* 461–486.

Paul, R., Miles, S., Cicchetti, D., Sparrow, S., Klin, A., Volkmar, F., et al. (2004). Adaptive behavior in autism and pervasive developmental disorder-not otherwise specified: Microanalysis of scores on the Vineland Adaptive Behavior Scales. *Journal of Autism and Developmental Disorders, 34,* 223–228.

Reynell, J., & Gruber, C. (1978). *Reynell Developmental Language Scales–U.S. edition.* Los Angeles: Western Psychological Services.

Richler, J., Bishop, S. L., Kleinke, J., & Lord, C. (2007). Restricted and repetitive behaviors in young children with autism spectrum disorders. *Journal of Autism and Developmental Disorders, 37,* 73–85.

Robins, D. L., & Dumont-Mathieu, T. M. (2006). Early screening for autism spectrum disorders: Update on the modified CHecklist for autism in toddlers and other measures. *Journal of Developmental and Behavioral Pediatrics, 27,* S111–S119.

Robins, D. L., Fein, D., Barton, M. L., & Green, J. A. (2001). The Modified CHecklist for autism in toddlers: An initial study investigating the early detection of autism and pervasive developmental disorders. *Journal of Autism and Developmental Disorders, 31,* 131–144.

Rogers, S. J., & Ozonoff, S. (2005). Annotation: What do we know about sensory dysfunction in autism?: A critical review of the empirical evidence. *Journal of Child Psychology and Psychiatry, 46,* 1255–1268.

Rutter, M., Bailey, A., Lord, C., & Berument, S. K. (2003). *Social Communication Questionnaire.* Los Angeles: Western Psychological Services.

Schopler, E., Reichler, R. J., & Renner, B. R. (1988). *The Childhood Autism Rating Scale.* Los Angeles: Western Psychological Services.

Sevin, J. A., Matson, J. L., Coe, D. A., Fee, V. E., & Sevin, B. M. (1991). A comparison and evaluation of three commonly used autism scales. *Journal of Autism and Developmental Disorders, 21,* 551–556.

Siegel, B. (1996). *Pervasive Developmental Disorders Screening Test (PDDST).*Unpublished manuscript.

Siegel, B., & Hayer, C. (1999, April). *Detection of autism in the 2nd and 3rd year: The Pervasive Developmental Disorders Screening Test (PDDST).* Paper presented at the Society for Research in Child Development, Albuquerque, NM.

Siegel, B., Pliner, C., Eschler, J., & Elliott, G. R. (1988). How children with autism are diagnosed: Difficulties in identification of children with multiple developmental delays. *Journal of Developmental and Behavioral Pediatrics, 9,* 199–204.

Siperstein, R., & Volkmar, F. (2004). Brief report: Parental reporting of regression in children with pervasive developmental disorders. *Journal of Autism and Developmental Disorders, 34,* 731–734.

Skuse, D., Warrington, R., Bishop, D., Chowdhury, U., Lau, J., Mandy, W., et al. (2004). The developmental, dimensional and diagnostic interview (3di): A novel computerized assessment for autism spectrum disorders. *Journal of the American Academy of Child and Adolescent Psychiatry, 43,* 548–558.

Slomkowski, C., Nelson, K., Dunn, J., & Plomin, R. (1992). Temperament and language: Relations from toddlerhood to middle childhood. *Developmental Psychology, 28,* 1090–1095.

South, M., Williams, B. J., McMahon, W. M., Owley, T., Filipek, P. A., Shernoff, E., et al. (2002). Utility of the Gilliam Autism Rating Scale in research and clinical populations. *Journal of Autism and Developmental Disorders, 32,* 593–599.

Sparrow, S. S., Balla, D. A., & Cicchetti, D. V. (1984). *Vineland Adaptive Behavior Scales.* Circle Pines, MN: American Guidance Service.

Stone, W. L., Coonrod, E. E., & Ousley, O. Y. (2000). Screening Tool for Autism in Two-Year-Olds (STAT): Development and preliminary data. *Journal of Autism and Developmental Disorders, 30,* 607–612.

Stone, W. L., Lee, E. B., Ashford, L., Brissie, J., Hepburn, S. L., Coonrod, E. E., et al. (1999). Can autism be diagnosed accurately in children under 3 years? *Journal of Child Psychology and Psychiatry, 40,* 219–226.

Swinkels, S. H. N., Dietz, C., van Daalen, E., Kerkhof, I. H. G. M., van Engeland, H., & Buitelaar, J. K. (2006). Screening for autistic spectrum in children aged 14 to 15 months. I: The development of the Early Screening of Autistic Traits Questionnaire (ESAT). *Journal of Autism and Developmental Disorders, 36,* 723–732.

Thelen, E. (1979). Rhythmical stereotypies in normal human infants. *Animal Behaviour, 27,* 699–715.

Tomasello, M. (1995). Joint attention as social cognition. In C. Moore & P. J. Punham *Joint attention: Its origins and role in development* (pp. 103–130). Hillsdale, NJ: Erlbaum.

Tomasello, M., Carpenter, M., Call, J., Behne, T., & Moll, H. (2005). Understanding and sharing intentions: The origins of cultural cognition. *Behavioral and Brain Sciences, 28,* 675–735.

Tomasello, M., Farrar, M. J., & Dines, J. (1984). Children's speech revisions for a familiar and an unfamiliar adult. *Journal of Speech and Hearing Research, 27,* 359–363.

Valenza, E., Simion, F., Cassia, V. M., & Umilta, C. (1996). Face preference at birth. *Journal of Experimental Child Psychology, 22,* 315–336.

Ventola, P., Kleinman, J., Pandey, J., Barton, M., Allen, S., Green, J., et al. (2006). Agreement among four diagnostic instruments for autism spectrum disorders in toddlers. *Journal of Autism and Developmental Disorders, 36,* 839–847.

Volkmar, F., Chawarska, K., & Klin, A. (2005). Autism in infancy and early childhood. *Annual Review of Psychology, 56,* 315–336.

Volkmar, F. R., Klin, A., Siegal, B., Szatmari, P., Lord, C., Campbell, M., et al. (1994). Field trial for autistic disorder in DSM-IV. *American Journal of Psychiatry, 151,* 1361–1367.

Volkmar, F. R., & Rutter, M. (1995). Childhood disintegrative disorder: Results of the DSM-IV autism field trial. *Journal of the American Academy of Child and Adolescent Psychiatry, 34,* 1092–1095.

Vouloumanos, A., & Werker, J. F. (2004). Tuned to the signal: The privileged status of speech for young infants. *Developmental Science, 7,* 270–276.

Walden, T. A., & Ogan, T. A. (1988). The development of social referencing. *Child Development, 59,* 1230–1240.

Wetherby, A. M., & Prizant, B. M. (2002). *Communication and Symbolic Behavior Scales Developmental Profile* (first normed ed.). Baltimore: Brookes.

Wetherby, A. M., & Woods, J. (2002). *Systematic observation of red flags for autism spectrum disorders in young children.* Unpublished manual, Florida State University, Tallahassee.

Wing, L., Leekam, S. R., Libby, S. J., Gould, J., & Larcombe, M. (2002). The Diagnostic Interview for Social and Communication Disorders: Background, inter-rater reliability and clinical use. *Journal of Child Psychology and Psychiatry, 43,* 307–325.

Woodward, A. (1999). Infants' ability to distinguish between purposeful and nonpurposeful behaviors. *Infant Behavior and Development, 22,* 145–160.

World Health Organization. (1992). *International classification of diseases and related health problems* (10th ed.). Geneva, Switzerland: Author.

Zimmerman, I. L., Steiner, V. G., & Pond, R. E. (2002). *Preschool Language Scale, fourth edition (PLS-4).* San Antonio, TX: Harcourt Assessment.

Zwaigenbaum, L., Bryson, S., Rogers, T., Roberts, W., Brian, J., & Szatmari, P. (2005). Behavioral manifestations of autism in the first year of life. *International Journal of Developmental Neuroscience, 23,* 143–152.

CHAPTER 3

———•———

Assessment of Cognitive and Adaptive Skills

KATARZYNA CHAWARSKA
KAREN BEARSS

The pathogenic factors responsible for autism spectrum disorders (ASD) affect multiple areas of functioning, producing a significant overlap between clinical presentation of young children with ASD and those with other developmental problems. Approximately 25% of children seen in a primary care setting exhibit some form of developmental delay, with speech deficits as the most common concern raised by parents of children between the ages of 1 and 5 (Filipek et al., 1999). Other developmental concerns frequently reported by parents include problems with social-emotional development, adaptive behaviors (e.g., sleep or feeding problems), cognitive delays, motor skills delays, behavioral concerns (e.g., impulsivity, aggression, hyperactivity, self-stimulatory behaviors) or anxiety (Gilliam & Mayes, 2000, 2004). Moreover, owing to factors that are not fully understood, there is considerable interindividual variability of clinical presentation among young children with ASD, complicated further by notable intraindividual variation in the level of functioning in specific domains. In addition, the developmental trajectories in children with ASD vary greatly. Some children experience accelerated rates of progress over time, whereas others experience deceleration of their skill acquisition over time, resulting in significant changes in standard test scores from one assessment to another. With such a high prevalence of developmental delays both transient and enduring among young children, as well as considerable heterogeneity of the syndrome expression, discerning toddlers with ASD from those with other developmental delays can be challenging and requires careful consideration of a child's functioning in multiple areas of development (Klin, Chawarska, Rubin, & Volkmar, 2004; Lord & Risi, 2000; see also Bishop, Luyster, Richler, & Lord, Chapter 2, and Paul, Chapter 4, this volume).

This chapter reviews procedures that constitute essential components of a comprehensive developmental evaluation for young children suspected of having ASD. The assessment battery typically consists of standardized direct measures of development, standard interview procedures with parents and other caretakers, and unstructured clinical observations. This multisource, multimethod approach is necessary for obtaining the most reliable and valid appraisal of the child's levels of functioning and is essential for the diagnostic considerations and educational planning. This chapter contains descriptions of several comprehensive measures of development that can be utilized for children in their first years of life, addresses challenges associated with assessment of young children with ASD and provides a review of the existing literature on early cognitive development of children with ASD.

CORE AREAS OF DEVELOPMENT

According to the widely accepted Multidomain Developmental Assessment Model, development is an interactively unfolding, continuous process that occurs in several distinct but interrelated domains (Gesell, 1948; Mullen, 1995; Piaget, 1954; Uzgiris & Hunt, 1975). Typically identified domains are (1) nonverbal cognition (e.g., visual–spatial skills, memory, discrimination and categorization skills), (2) motor skills (fine and gross), (3) verbal cognition and communication (including receptive and expressive language skills), (4) adaptive functioning (daily living skills), and (5) personal–social skills (social competence, emotional regulation) (Gilliam & Mayes, 2000, 2004). The goal of the developmental assessment is to achieve an understanding of the child's level of functioning across a variety of domains as well as to determine how intraindividual discrepancies in skill acquisition may affect the child's overall level of functioning and well-being (Gilliam & Mayes, 2004). Toward this end, a thorough developmental assessment typically involves the administration of highly integrated and overlapping procedures, allowing the examiner to gain the information necessary for a diagnosis and for determining the child's profile of strengths and deficits in the areas of interest (Klin, Chawarska, Rubin, et al., 2004). In the assessment of a young child suspected of having an ASD, appraisal of the child's abilities in the areas of verbal and nonverbal development, as well as adaptive skills, provides a basis for clinical interpretation of specific social and communicative skills ascertained through both standard assessment and clinical observation (Klin, Chawarska, Rubin, et al., 2004; Sparrow, Carter, Racusin, & Morris, 1995; see also Bishop et al., Chapter 2, this volume).

COMPONENTS OF THE DEVELOPMENTAL ASSESSMENT

Developmental History

A clinical interview, targeting the child's medical and developmental history, onset and progression of symptoms, and family factors that may affect the child's current presentation as well as access to treatment, is central to a comprehensive developmental evaluation. Interviews are typically conducted with parents, though input of other caregivers and medical professionals involved in the child's care may provide relevant information about the child's functioning. The information gathered generally includes family structure and the child's medical history, including information regarding pregnancy, delivery, postnatal course, traumatic events, presence of neurological and genetic abnormalities, sensory impairments, allergies, and so forth. An appreciation of the relevant environmental factors having to do with family history (e.g., birth of a sibling, separation, parental illness) or exposures (e.g., to alcohol, illicit drugs, medications, or heavy metals such as lead) is critical for diagnostic purposes as well.

Furthermore, documenting the ages of attainment of the major developmental milestones, as well as the ages and circumstances of the onset of parental concerns, is crucial to an understanding of the processes that may be involved in the child's presenting symptoms (Chawarska, Paul, et al., 2007). Certain parental concerns regarding the early disruption of the developmental process, such as a slow-down, failure to progress (plateau), or loss of skills (regression), are of particular importance. Recent studies suggest that almost 90% of parents notice first concerns by the child's second birthday (Chawarska, Paul, et al., 2007; De Giacomo & Fombonne, 1998). Children who are later diagnosed with Pervasive Developmental Disorder-Not Otherwise Specified (PDD-NOS) rarely trigger parental concerns in the first year of life; in contrast, approximately 30% of parents whose children were later diagnosed with autism report the first concerns prior to or around the first birthday (Chawarska, Paul, et al., 2007). Approximately 25–30% of parents of children with ASD report the loss of some skills between 18 and 24 months; this phenomenon is much more frequently reported in toddlers with autism than in those with PDD-NOS (Chawarska, Paul, et al., 2007). It should be noted that reports of loss of language skills or social interests during a certain developmental period do not preclude the presence of developmental delays manifesting earlier in the child's development (Luyster et al., 2005; Siperstein &

Volkmar, 2004). Thus, the "pre-regression" period of development needs to be carefully documented as well. Parents of toddlers with autism or PDD-NOS tend to be initially concerned about their children's limited responsivity to language, delays in speech, and limited social interests. The frequency of other concerns appears to differ, depending on the child's specific spectrum diagnosis. In children diagnosed later with autism, concerns regarding delays in attainment of motor milestones or the presence of unusual sensory interests are more prevalent than in those later diagnosed with PDD-NOS. Conversely, parents of toddlers diagnosed with PDD-NOS report more concerns related to regulatory functions involved in feeding, sleeping, and the overall activity level, as compared with parents of toddlers with autism (Chawarska, Paul, et al., 2007). It is not clear whether the latter finding is due to an actual higher prevalence of these problems in children diagnosed with PDD-NOS, or whether these perhaps milder difficulties are overshadowed by more severe problems experienced in toddlers with autism.

A skillfully conducted interview also provides information regarding parents' perception of the child's strengths and difficulties, as well as the parents' fears associated with the process of the assessment and ideas about what the child's symptoms may signify (Gilliam & Mayes, 2004). It is crucial for the clinicians involved in the case to fully appreciate parental ideations regarding the etiology of the observed symptoms. These can range from genetic (e.g., related to having another child with ASD), neurological (e.g., linked to a complicated perinatal course or brain structure abnormalities), environmental exposures (e.g., to specific agents such as gluten or mercury), to specific life events such as the birth of another sibling, child care arrangements, or other factors associated with family functioning. These ideas can be enduring and have an impact on the parents' ability to cope with the diagnosis, as well as on the selection of and subsequent adherence to treatment (Levy, Mandell, Merhar, Ittenbach, & Pinto-Martin, 2003; see also Smith & Wick, Chapter 9, this volume). Information regarding the extent of the social support network within the family and broader community that is available to the parents is also essential for assisting in treatment planning for the child.

Developmental Assessment

Parent-report developmental measures are often employed by professionals as screening devices aimed at clarifying whether children with suspected developmental delays require further testing, or as an aid in validating and contextualizing the results of direct standardized testing (Filipek et al., 1999). Among the scales with the strongest psychometric properties are the Ages and Stages Questionnaires, second edition (ASQ; Bricker & Squires, 1999), the Brigance Screens (Brigance, 1986; Glascoe,

1996), and the Child Development Inventories (CDIs; Ireton, 1992; Ireton & Glascoe, 1995; see Gilliam & Mayes, 2004, for review).

For diagnostic reasons and treatment planning purposes, the developmental assessment of young children presenting for a differential diagnosis of an ASD requires a direct assessment approach. The reason for such an approach is not only the possible limitations of a parental report with regard to early development, but also the need for a detailed and systematic observation of the child's behavior in response to standard probes. Furthermore, although a parental report typically reflects behaviors that are likely to occur in less structured environments, such as the home, the structured form of the assessment procedures resembles a format more typically encountered in the context of a therapy session. The aim of the developmental assessment is not only to determine whether the child is meeting the expected developmental milestones in the targeted domains, but also to observe the child's problem-solving strategies in action so as to elucidate a host of attentional, motivational, and cognitive factors that are likely to affect his or her performance and influence the child's amenability to treatment. Interactive testing also allows for documenting low-frequency and less severe symptoms that are likely to be missed by parents and can be elicited through selected behavioral probes.

Two of the most widely used developmental scales with very young children are the Bayley Scales of Infant and Toddler Development, Third Edition (Bayley-III; Bayley, 2006) and the Mullen Scales of Early Learning (Mullen Scales; Mullen, 1995). The Bayley-III and Mullen Scales are performance-based scales that assess a child's development in several domains as they occur in the context of direct interaction and goal-oriented activities. Both measures have been designed to meet federal and state guidelines for early childhood assessment (e.g., Individuals with Disabilities Education Improvement Act of 2004) in order to determine whether a child is developing normally or may have a qualified developmental delay.

The Bayley-III has been designed to assess the developmental functioning of infants between 1 and 42 months of age. It consists of five scales: the Cognitive, Language, Motor, Social-Emotional, and Adaptive Behaviors scales. Bayley-III normative data were collected in 2004 and based on a U.S. sample of 1,700 children stratified on key demographic variables (see Bayley, 2006, for more details regarding the validity and reliability of the revised test). Of the five scales, only three are administered directly to the child: the Cognitive, Language, and Motor scales. The primary goal of the Bayley-III Cognitive Scale is to assess information-processing skills, including habituation, memory, speed of processing, novelty preference, problem solving, and number concepts. The Language Scale consists of the Receptive and Expressive Communication subtests. The Receptive Communication subtest assesses responsiveness to sounds as well as the ability to comprehend and respond appropriately to words and requests. The Expressive Communication subtest captures the ability to vocalize (e.g., cooing, babbling, consonant and vowel production) as well as to imitate sounds and words. For older children, the focus turns to assessing the use of one-word approximations and naming pictures of objects and actions, as well as the ability to communicate needs, respond to questions, and produce multiple-word sentences. The Motor Scale consists of the Fine and Gross Motor subtests, which focus on the child's movement, sensory integration, perceptual–motor integration, and basic milestones of prehension and locomotion.

The two remaining scales, the Social-Emotional and Adaptive Behavior scales are in parent questionnaire format and inquire about day-to-day observations of the child's behavior. The Social-Emotional Scale is based on the Social-Emotional Growth Chart (Greenspan, 2004), which identifies various stages of social-emotional development for children from birth to 42 months of age, including self-regulation, affective expression, and so forth. The Adaptive Behavior Scale, based on the Adaptive Behavior Assessment System, Second Edition (ABAS-II; Harrison & Oakland, 2003), is designed to evaluate the attainment of practical, everyday skills required for children to function and meet environmental demands. Examples of these demands include the ability to effectively and independently take care of oneself (e.g., eating, dressing, safety skills) and the ability to interact with others (e.g., peer interactions).

The second most widely used standardized and direct measure of early development is the Mullen Scales of Early Learning (Mullen, 1995). The Mullen Scales is an individually administered multidomain measure of cognitive functioning for children from birth through 68 months. Like the newly revised Bayley-III Scales, the Mullen Scales were developed on the basis of the theory that child intelligence is most accurately conceptualized as a network of interrelated but functionally distinct developmental skills (Mullen, 1995). The scale structure differs somewhat from that advanced in the Bayley-III. Cognitive functioning is assessed on the Mullen Scales using four core scales (Visual Reception, Receptive Language, Expressive Language, and Fine Motor). Further, a Gross Motor scale covering skills between birth and 33 months was also included because of the central role that motor control and mobility play in the development of skills relevant to the four cognitive domains of the Mullen Scales. Normative data were based on a sample of 1,849 children from the U.S. population (see Mullen, 1995, for details on reliability and validity).

The primary targets of the Visual Reception scale are nonverbal visual discrimination, categorization, and visual memory skills. The scale minimizes the role of language in terms of instructions and response modality, with most responses involving simple manipulation(s) of objects (e.g., searching, sorting, or matching) or pointing to or touching pictures to indicate choice. The Fine Motor scale provides a measure of visual–motor planning and control. The primary ability areas covered are unilateral and bilateral manipulation of objects and writing readiness, with a considerable emphasis on the ability to imitate actions modeled by the examiner. Whereas the Visual Reception and Fine Motor scales place little emphasis on the understanding of language or the ability to vocalize or verbalize in order to complete the tasks, the two language scales of the Mullen Scales focus on these abilities. The Receptive Language scale emphasizes the child's auditory comprehension and memory. As in the Bayley-III, tasks probe for responsiveness to sounds and the ability to follow simple adult-driven instructions with, and without, gestural prompting. For younger children, probes target overall responsivity to speech and nonspeech sounds, response to name, understanding of communicative gestures, and so forth. For older children, tasks require following two- and three-step directions and understanding verbal concepts (e.g., position, size, length, color, and shape). Minimal verbal output is required of the child; pointing or touching is sufficient for most items, except for general knowledge questions, which require one- to three-word responses. The Expressive Language scale evaluates the child's spontaneous use of language. In young children, the focus is primarily on the ability to spontaneously produce vocalizations and words. For older children, demands for language production increase, with tasks involving naming pictures, repeating numbers and phrases, and answering vocabulary and practical reasoning questions.

Adaptive Skills

The term *adaptive skills* refers to a set of conceptual, social, and practical skills that are acquired and enable people to function in everyday situations (American Association on Mental Retardation [AAMR], 2002). Adaptive skills are typically age related, defined by expectations or standards of other people, modifiable, and defined by typical performance (Sattler & Hoge, 2006). The importance of an assessment of adaptive skills is emphasized by the AAMR (2002). Legal and professional standards have been outlined regarding the development of adaptive functioning, and these standards are taken into account by a number of special education and disability classification systems (e.g., the Individuals with Disabilities Education Improvement Act of 2004 [IDEA] and DSM-IV). During infancy and early childhood, expected adaptive behavior skills include the appropriate use of expressive and receptive language, the ability to interact with others, the emergence of social reasoning and social comprehension, basic self-care such as dressing and bathing, and participation in basic household chores. The inclusion of the assessment of adaptive functioning in the battery for young children is crucial, considering that one of the characteristic features of ASD is the observed discrepancy, both in children and in adults, between the levels of cognitive functioning and the ability to translate these skills into real-world functioning (Klin et al., 2007; Saulnier & Klin, 2007).

One of the most widely used and comprehensive measures of adaptive behaviors is the recently revised Vineland Adaptive Behavior Scales, second edition (Vineland-II; Sparrow, Ciccetti, & Balla, 2005). The Vineland-II is appropriate for ages birth through age 90. The Vineland-II has four forms: Survey Interview Form, Parent/Caregiver Rating Form, Expanded Interview Form, and Teacher Rating Form. The Survey and Expanded Interview Forms are clinician-administered semistructured interviews, and the Parent/Caregiver and Teacher Rating Forms are questionnaires designed to capture the adaptive behavior of the child in the home or school setting, respectively.

The Survey and Caregiver Rating Forms contain eleven subdomains, grouped into four adaptive behavior domains: Communication, Daily Living Skills, Socialization, and Motor Skills. These versions also include a Maladaptive Behavior Domain that measures undesirable behaviors that may interfere with a child's adaptive behavior. Normative scores as well as age-equivalent scores are provided for each of the subdomains and domains, allowing a detailed analysis of a child's individual profile of strengths and weaknesses. The recent revision resulted in an increased item density in the birth–3 years age range, thus enhancing the scales' validity and reliability in this population. Finally, the revised version includes supplementary norms for children with autism ages 3–16 (Sparrow et al., 2005). A nationally representative sample of 3,695 individuals from birth through 90 years of age provided normative data (see Sparrow et al., 2005, for details on validity and reliability).

CHALLENGES IN TESTING YOUNG CHILDREN WITH ASD

Due to specific deficits in social attention and motivation, nonverbal communication, and imitation, as well as the presence of self-stimulatory behaviors, the administration of standardized tests to young children with ASD can be challenging, though the types of difficulties vary widely from child to child (Akshoomoff, 2006; Koegel, Koegel, & Smith, 1997; National Research Council, 2001). For some toddlers with ASD, the highly structured and well-defined context of a developmental test plays to their strengths, which may include good response to novelty and an interest in visual discrimination and perceptual matching skills. Thus, these toddlers may have little difficulty in completing a developmental test. In other cases, the extent of difficulties a child experiences during an assessment may raise a question as to whether the testing is capturing the child's test-taking difficulties rather than his or her cognitive disability (see, e.g., Neisworth & Bagnato, 2004). Thus, the testing of young children with ASD requires not only extensive knowledge of typical and atypical development in general, but also familiarity with strategies that can be employed to enhance the children's attention and motivation without compromising the standardized test administration procedures.

As an inherent part of their disability, young children with autism exhibit decreased orienting to social stimuli, such as faces (Dawson, Meltzoff, Osterling, Rinaldi, & Brown, 1998; Klin, Jones, Schultz, Volkmar, & Cohen, 2002; Volkmar & Mayes, 1990), as well as to human speech and gestures (Adamson, McArthur, Markov, Dunbar, & Bakeman, 2001; McArthur & Adamson, 1996; Mundy & Burnette, 2005; Paul, Chawarska, Fowler, Cicchetti, & Volkmar, 2007; Wetherby et al., 2004). This limited ability to respond to social cues, limited motivation to master and "show off" new skills, and difficulty in regulating attention often leads to a significant amount of the assessment time spent "on break," out of the chair (Chawarska, Klin, Paul, & Volkmar, 2007) or whining (Akshoomoff, 2006). Infants and toddlers with ASD do not typically monitor the attention of others (e.g., have difficulties looking at pictures or objects that others look at, touch, or point to) (Charman et al., 2001; Chawarska, Klin, et al., 2007; Cox et al., 1999; Wetherby et al., 2004), which reflects their inherent difficulty in responding to bids for joint attention (Tomasello, 1995). Consequently, these children have difficulty in completing probes whereby the examiner attempts to redirect a child's attention to an object or a picture, in order to, for example, examine his or her language skills. Furthermore, the completion of a number of tasks on developmental tests requires some level of motor imitation (e.g., building block structures, drawing following a model) and the use of gestures (e.g., pointing, giving, showing). These skills typically are impaired in young children with ASD (Rogers, Hepburn, Stackhouse, & Wehner, 2003).

Even when taking into account these obstacles related to both age and type of disability, standardized assessments of young children with ASD are necessary, and there are no "untestable" children. Problems with testing usually stem from the selection of an inappropriate assessment instrument, insufficient time allotted to the assessment, or the limited experience of a clinician (Ozonoff, Goodlin-Jones, & Solomon, 2005). Moreover, the difficulties experienced by a child during standardized assessment are not simply barriers, but constitute a vital source of clinical information relevant to diagnosis and treatment planning.

Considering that for each individual toddler, different factors may influence his or her ability to participate in testing, it is necessary to obtain information about such factors through direct observation and parent interview prior to the testing session (Koegel et al., 1997). Unstructured behavioral observations (e.g., during an interaction with the parent or solitary play) provide an opportunity to gather information about the child's interests, predominant mode of object exploration, ability to attend to and monitor behaviors of others, ability to initiate social and communicative exchanges, and ability to regulate emotions. An opportunity to determine the presence and intensity of self-stimulatory behaviors and motor mannerisms is also likely to aid in the assessment process by providing clues regarding environmental modifications that may facilitate the child's participation in the testing procedures. Furthermore, a brief interview with a parent may provide additional information regarding specific aspects of the testing situation that are likely to interfere with test administration (e.g., presence of mirrors, background noises such as air-conditioning, or specific objects of strong attachment such as balls or spoons, that are likely to consume the child's entire attention).

Parents can also identify a list of possible reinforcers that are likely to enhance the child's attention to and compliance with the task demands. Owing to a child's lack of intrinsic social orientation and motivation to engage in interactions, standard methods of encouraging performance (i.e., verbal praise and affective cues such as smiling) may not be effective for maintaining attention and on-task behaviors. Thus, other forms of reinforcement may be more useful. The choice of reinforcer is often idio-syncratic. An opportunity to momentarily hold a preferred toy upon completion of a task (e.g., an object of a strong attachment), repeat a preferred activity (e.g., dropping blocks into a container or lining up cars), gain access to a preferred physical routine (e.g., "row, row, row your boat" or tickle game), or have a small snack (e.g., a sip of juice) may provide additional motivational support and facilitate completion of the test. For some children, encouragement strategies such as applause, cheering, and touching may seem overwhelming or aversive and actually contribute to their difficulty in completing the test. For other children, high affect and physical contact (e.g., tickling) may prove very effective in maintaining their optimal level of arousal and attention. Furthermore, the use of specific phrases (e.g., "first . . . then") or visual supports (e.g., picture schedules) may provide the child with a certain degree of predictability and create expectation of a reward, which in turn may help to maintain an alert and engaged state. It should be noted that these strategies usually work with toddlers who have had experience with structured intervention programs and have acquired the cognitive skills necessary for grasping and benefiting from such contingencies. Adopting a fast pace, with one task or trial swiftly following another in a play-like manner, and avoiding superfluous breaks in between tasks helps young children with ASD to remain engaged and may prevent them from drifting into off-task behaviors. Physical prompting such as gentle touching, tapping, and redirecting can also be used as needed to promote on-task behavior. Furthermore, a vast majority of children with ASD in this age range have very limited attention to speech and difficulty in understanding language (Chawarska, Klin, et al., 2007; Wetherby et al., 2004). Thus, instructions often have to be simplified and, whenever possible, accompanied by multiple non-verbal (e.g., gestural), physical (e.g., tapping on table to attract attention or moving testing materials into the child's visual field), and affective cues.

Despite these efforts, the examiner may still encounter instances when the child refuses to attempt completion of a task. Although fatigue or noncompliance can play a role and needs to be ruled out before the test results are deemed valid, studies of neuropsychological task performance among preschoolers suggest that test refusals typically reflect poor skills in a given area or an attempt to avoid failure. Higher rates of refusal on cognitive tasks are often predictive of lower scores on cognitive tests later in development (Mantynen, Poikkeus, Ahonen, Aro, & Korkman, 2001).

THE ROLE OF PARENTS IN STRUCTURED ASSESSMENT

Parents play an important role in the developmental and diagnostic assessment process. Parental presence may help the child adjust to the new situation and reassure the child throughout the testing. Incidental parent–child interactions provide essential information to the clinician regarding the child's spontaneous functional social and communication skills. Parents can also provide information necessary for judging the typicality of behaviors observed during the standardized testing. Finally, their involvement can be crucial in revealing contextualized skills, which may become apparent only with a specific interactive partner or with use of specific prompts. Although these aspects of the child's performance rarely find their way into the standard scoring procedures, they provide rich clinical information regarding the child's learning and affective style and the ability to generalize skills across contexts.

Although parental involvement in the assessment is important for the child's success and the clinician's overall impressions, participation in an assessment of a child suspected of having a developmental disorder can be very stressful for parents. Parental stress may stem from the fact that many delays and abnormalities often become painfully apparent in the process (see Bailey, Chapter 11, this volume; Gilliam & Mayes, 2004). Briefing parents on the nature of the tests can help alleviate some stress. Explaining that in order to fully appreciate the child's developmental skills, tasks that seem easy as well as difficult will be administered, and thus, because of the nature of the test, several failures are expected. Toddlers in general can be quite self-directed; their moods change quickly and so do their levels of cooperation. This is particularly true of toddlers with developmental disabilities. One of the chief concerns of parents entering a diagnostic process with their toddler is whether the examiners will be able to obtain a representative sample of their child's behavior and, consequently, whether their conclusions will be valid. It is absolutely essential to reassure parents that special care will be taken to obtain the child's optimal performance and that their input regarding whether the behaviors observed during testing are representative of those seen on a daily basis will play an important role in the diagnostic process. The formation of an alliance with the parents at the beginning of the assessment process can facilitate discussion regarding specific test results, their implications for the diagnosis, and the strategies that will need to be adopted to remedy the documented problems. Parents who are convinced as to the validity of the assessment are more likely to follow up on the recommendations, become active members of the therapeutic team, and advocate more effectively on behalf of their children (see Bishop et al., Chapter 2; Wetherby & Woods, Chapter 7; and Bailey, Chapter 11, this volume).

INTERPRETATION AND REPORTING OF THE DEVELOPMENTAL FINDINGS

Reporting the developmental findings in infants and toddlers with ASD usually involves synthesizing the medical and developmental history, reviewing behavioral observations throughout the course of testing, describing the results of individual tests in terms of the child's capacities in different functional areas (e.g., motor, cognitive, language, and social skills), and integrating these findings with the parental report regarding the child's typical behaviors and repertoire of adaptive skills (Gilliam & Mayes, 2004; Filipek et al., 1999; Klin, Chawarska, Rubin, et al., 2004; National Research Council, 2001). The primary purpose of documenting the child's clinical presentation is to communicate to parents and professionals, in the most accessible and precise manner possible, the information necessary for designing a treatment plan and for monitoring the child's rate of progress over time as a function of treatment and maturation. It is extremely important that the summary place emphasis not only on the child's delays and abnormalities, but also on his or her unique strengths, relative to peers and to the child's other areas of functioning (e.g., relative strength in visual discrimination skills, marked curiosity and ability to learn means–ends contingencies, or the ability to handle novel situations and transitions), as they are highly consequential for designing effective individualized treatment plans. In the interpretation of the child's profile of verbal, nonverbal, motor, and adaptive skills, it is often necessary to consider the limitations inherent to each of the assessment instruments. For instance, although a young child may score in the average range on the formal testing of receptive and expressive language, these scores may not be reflective of the child's functional communication skills—that is, the ability to use language to share ideas and make requests. In fact, dissociation between the ability to produce speech and to use it functionally is one of the core features of communication disorder in ASD. Therefore, supplementing the standardized developmental assessment with an appraisal of the levels of functional verbal and nonverbal communication usually constitutes an integral part of a developmental assessment (see Paul, Chapter 4, this volume).

DEVELOPMENTAL SKILLS
OF YOUNG CHILDREN WITH ASD

Early observations (Kanner, 1943/1968) and more recent experimental studies (Charman et al., 1997; Cox et al., 1999; Dawson & Adams, 1984; Dawson, Meltzoff, Osterling, & Rinaldi, 1998; Dawson et al., 2002; Mundy, Sigman, & Kasari, 1990; Mundy, Sigman, Ungerer, & Sherman, 1986; Sigman & Ungerer, 1981, 1984) suggest that in the first years of life, the development of children with autism is characterized by significant intraindividual scatter. In older children, the scatter may be reflected, for instance, in a split between verbal and nonverbal skills, greater delays in adaptive than cognitive functioning, and selective impairments in executive functioning, nonverbal communication, pragmatics of language, and social interactions (Ehlers et al., 1997; Freeman, Del'Homme, Guthrie, & Zhang, 1999; Joseph, Tager-Flusberg, & Lord, 2002; Klin, Volkmar, & Sparrow, 1992; Klin, Volkmar, Sparrow, Cicchetti, & Rourke, 1995; Saulnier & Klin, 2007; Volkmar et al., 1994).

Several recent studies provide direct insights into the developmental functioning of children with ASD in the first 3 years of life. The evidence suggests that a considerable proportion of infants and toddlers with ASD experience significant delays in one or more areas. For instance, Akshoomoff (2006) examined developmental skills in a small group of young (mean age 30 months) children with ASD and noted that almost 75% of toddlers experienced very significant delays in at least one of the areas tapped by the Mullen Scales. The delays in the area of verbal functioning are often much more severe than those in the nonverbal domain (Akshoomoff, 2006; Carter et al., 2007; Charman, Baron-Cohen, et al., 2003; Charman et al., 1997; Eaves & Ho, 2004; Landa & Garrett-Mayer, 2006; Wetherby et al., 2004). However, this type of verbal–nonverbal discrepancy has also been noted in children with other developmental disabilities, and thus, in and of itself, does not appear to be syndrome-specific (Eaves & Ho, 2004; Landa & Garrett-Mayer, 2006). The extent of cognitive delays appears to be associated with the degree of autistic psychopathology even in very young children. Chawarska (2007) reported that although less than 20% of infants diagnosed with autism prior to the second birthday had significant delays (2 *SD* below the mean) in nonverbal functioning on the Mullen Scales, almost 70% had significant delays in expressive and receptive language skills. In comparison, those later diagnosed with PDD-NOS tended to have relatively spared nonverbal skills; still, more than 40% received verbal scores in the very low range (Chawarska, 2007).

Furthermore, studies on older children with ASD document the presence of a significant discrepancy between receptive and expressive language on standardized tests (Charman, Drew, Baird, & Baird, 2003; Joseph et al., 2002; Lord & Paul, 1997). Recent studies suggest that a similar pattern can be observed in toddlers with ASD (Paul, Chawarska, Klin, & Volkmar, 2006; see also Paul, Chapter 4, this volume). These findings are not surprising, as early receptive language skills encompass general responsivity to speech, orientation to name and other high-frequency words imbued with affective content (e.g., "no," "mama"), as well as response to social smile and conventional gestures. These particular skills have been found to be deficient in infants and toddlers with autism (Baranek, 1999; Baron-Cohen, Cox, Baird, Swettenham, & Nighingale, 1996; Lord, 1995; Mundy, Sigman, & Kasari, 1994; Osterling, Dawson, & Munson, 2002; Stone, Ousley, Yoder, Hogan, & Hepburn, 1997). At the same time, these children often are capable of producing a range of consonant sounds as well as single words (Charman, Drew, et al., 2003; Paul et al., 2006; see also Paul, Chapter 4, this volume), which is reflected in the expressive language scores, even though these vocalizations may be only rarely used communicatively.

Stability and Change in the Levels of Functioning in the First Years

Several longitudinal studies provide insight into the developmental trajectories of young children with ASD. As compared with typical peers and children with other developmental difficulties, children with ASD may show a relatively slow rate of development that becomes particularly noticeable early in the second year of life (Landa & Garrett-Mayer, 2006). Landa and Garret-Mayer (2006) followed a large group of infants at 6, 14, and 24 months of age. A majority of the infants belonged to a high-risk group, as defined by having an older sibling with an ASD, and the remaining group was considered low-risk because of a family history negative for ASD. At 24 months of age, some of the infants were diagnosed with ASD or language delay, and a majority of infants were deemed unaffected.

Although there were no significant differences between the ASD and control groups in performance on the Mullen Scales at 6 months, differences began to emerge at 14 months. Infants with ASD had lower raw scores in the verbal and motor domains but not in the nonverbal cognitive domain as compared with unaffected infants. A comparison with infants with language delays revealed that infants with ASD had significantly greater delays in the receptive language and fine motor domains, but not in the expressive language or nonverbal domains. As time progressed, the gap between the ASD and language-delayed groups, as well as the unaffected groups, widened further owing to the slow rate of progress in the ASD group.

There also appear to be differences in the rate of development among infants with various subtypes of ASD. Differences in cognitive functioning between autism and PDD-NOS groups are usually apparent in older children; however, in toddlers these differences are somewhat less pronounced (Chawarska, Klin, et al., 2007; Lord et al., 2006). In one study (Chawarska, Klin, et al, 2007) a group of infants diagnosed with an ASD prior to their second birthday was followed until the age of 3–4 years, at which point some of them received a diagnosis of autism, and others PDD-NOS. Although prior to the second birthday, toddlers in the two diagnostic groups performed comparably on a developmental test, by the follow-up assessment the differences in developmental levels between the two diagnostic groups became apparent. By the age of 3 years, toddlers diagnosed with PDD-NOS had higher verbal and nonverbal scores on the Mullen Scales than their peers with autism. The trend leading to divergent outcomes in terms of IQ and adaptive skills continues as children grow older, so that when evaluated at the age of 9 years, children with PDD-NOS show consistently higher levels of verbal, nonverbal, and adaptive functioning as compared with their peers with autism, even though their initial levels of functioning at the age of 2 were rather similar (Lord et al., 2006).

Exclusive focus on changes at the level of group means can mask the presence of significant individual variability in the early developmental trajectories of children with ASD (Charman et al., 2005; Chawarska, 2007; Eaves & Ho, 2004; Klin, Chawarska, Paul, et al., 2004). The period between the ages of 2 and 4 years appears to be particularly notorious for limited stability of cognitive skills. Although some suggest that the limited predictive value of developmental tests administered prior to the age of 3 may be due to the nature of a specific measure, similar results have been reported using instruments such as the Griffiths Scales (Charman et al., 2005), the Mullen Scales (Chawarska, 2007), and the Bayley Scales (Eaves & Ho, 2004; Yang, Huang, Schaller, Wang, & Tsai, 2003). Charman and colleagues (2005) documented that a correlation between verbal and nonverbal cognitive scores at 2 and 3 years was only moderate and that the correlation between 2 and 7 years scores was close to zero. The scores began to stabilize after the age of 3 years and were moderately predictive of the scores at the age of 7 years.

Several other studies documented specific change patterns in the levels of cognitive functioning within the first 3–4 years of life. For instance, Eaves and Ho (2004) reported that in a group of toddlers with ASD evaluated at the age of 2 and followed up approximately 2 years later, 20% of the children declined dramatically in standard verbal and nonverbal scores, and approximately 30% showed significant gains in verbal scores. The remaining 50% of the children showed less dramatic changes in either direction. Another study of a relatively large cohort of children diagnosed with ASD in the second year and followed into the third to fourth year suggested that the individual change patterns depend on both the area of functioning and the extent of autistic pathology (Chawarska, 2007). When assessed prior to the second birthday, only 30% of toddlers with autism had verbal scores in the average to below average range as measured by the Mullen Scales. When their verbal skills were evaluated 1–2 years later, 20% of the children maintained their average to below average scores and an additional 30% improved their verbal skills, reaching the average to below average range. However, the remaining 50% of the toddlers with autism tested very poorly at the age of 3–4: Forty percent maintained their very low scores and almost 10% showed a very slow rate of skill acquisition, leading to a decline in standard scores. As far as nonverbal skills were concerned, even though a majority of infants (75%) with autism tested within the average to below average range at their first assessment, at follow-up this rate dropped to approximately 50%. In contrast, toddlers with PDD-NOS showed much more encouraging individual skill acquisition patterns. Although at the first visit verbal skills were significantly delayed in approximately 45% of children, at follow-up all toddlers with PDD-NOS had verbal scores in the average to below average range, with 55% maintaining their relatively good scores and 45% making significant improvements. A similar pattern was noted in the nonverbal domain for this diagnostic group.

These observations suggest that the rates of progress between the second and third years of life are highly variable. The short-term outcomes in terms of verbal and nonverbal skills in toddlers with autism is relatively good in about 50% of cases, with the remaining toddlers evidencing either maintenance of very low scores or a decline in standard scores by the early preschool age. Toddlers with PDD-NOS typically show a relatively good rate of progress, reflected either in the maintenance of average to below average scores or in gains in standard scores in both verbal and nonverbal domains. Extending such prospective studies into adolescence can allow the examination of long-term outcomes in infants diagnosed early with ASD and can provide crucial information regarding predictors of outcome as well as moderating and mediating factors.

ADAPTIVE LEVELS OF FUNCTIONING
OF YOUNG CHILDREN WITH ASD

For most children, adaptive behavior skills that are learned in one setting are readily generalized to other situations or environments. The application of such skills across contexts, or skill generalization, presents a significant challenge for children with ASD. A number of studies (Bolte & Poustka, 2002; Gillham, Carter, Volkmar, & Sparrow, 2003; Freeman, Ritvo, Yokota, Childs, & Pollard, 1988; Klin et al., 2007; Saulnier & Klin, 2007; Stone, Ousley, Hepburn, Hogan, & Brown, 1999; Volkmar, Carter, Sparrow, & Cicchetti, 1993) have documented a characteristic pattern of adaptive skills in children with autism. Many children with autism exhibit adaptive behavior scores that are almost 1 *SD* lower than what would be expected for their intellectual level (Carter et al., 1998; Klin et al., 2007; Saulnier & Klin, 2007; Williams et al., 2006). This discrepancy exists even for children with below average cognitive functioning and within the restricted skill range of young children, so that some children are failing to achieve even elemental skills that are otherwise normally acquired in the first months of life (Klin et al., 1992). The reasons for this cognitive–adaptive functioning gap may differ, depending on the specific domain. Difficulties in socialization and communication constitute core deficits in autism, so it is not surprising that they typically fall below the child's cognitive levels. For children with autism, daily living skills such as practicing self-care (e.g., getting dressed) and following household routines may be directly affected by noncompliance (Kraijer, 2000). Determining a child's current adaptive functioning is vital for subsequent programming development, as it should focus on minimizing the disparity between what the child should be able to do (based on cognitive functioning) and what he or she actually does on a daily basis (as illustrated by the child's adaptive skill set).

Currently, there are only a few peer-reviewed reports focused on Vineland profiles for preschool-age children with autism. Most studies include preschool-age children as part of a larger sample, thus limiting the ability to comment on the characteristics of Vineland profiles specifically within preschoolers. For example, Carter and colleagues (1998) developed supplementary normative data on the Vineland for individuals with autism, but categorized their normative data based on the children under 10 years of age versus children 10 years or older. Carpentieri and Morgan (1996) compared the adaptive and intellectual functioning of autistic and nonautistic children with a sample that included preschool age children, but the mean age of the entire sample was 8. Nonetheless, although still limited, the evidence suggests that children with autism under the age of 3 years begin to demonstrate a characteristic profile of deficits in adaptive skills seen in older children (Stone et al., 1999). Stone and colleagues compared adaptive skills in 30 toddlers with autism with 30 children with global delays or language impairments. Toddlers with autism had significantly lower scores in the Socialization and Communication domains of the Vineland and greater adaptive skills versus mental age discrepancies than their nonautistic peers. Although there is evidence from both longitudinal (Freeman et al., 1999) and cross-sectional studies (Klin, et al., 2007) suggesting that children with ASD acquire adaptive skills over time, information on the rate of skill acquisition is relatively limited. When standard rather than age-equivalent scores are considered, significant declines over time are typically reported. For instance, Szatmari, Bryson, Boyle, Streiner, and Duku (2003) documented a decline in Vineland Socialization standard scores and relatively stable scores in the Communication domain in a sample seen initially at 4–6 years and followed at 12–14 years. The decline in standard scores in the Vineland Socialization and Communication domains, but not in the Daily Living Skills domain, has been reported recently in two independent cross-sectional samples of 7- to 18-year-old high-functioning children with ASD (Klin et al., 2007). Thus, although children with ASD continue to acquire new adaptive skills, their rate of progress tends to be slow, leading to a widening of the gap in adaptive functioning as compared with typical peers. Both early language and nonverbal skills have been found to predict outcomes as captured by the Vineland Communication and Socialization domains (Szatmari et al., 2003; Saulnier & Klin, 2007). Considering the importance of acquiring adaptive skills for the overall quality of life for children with ASD, future studies should evaluate not only the developmental trajectories of children with ASD in regard to these skills, but also factors that affect rates of progress besides initial IQ and extent of the autistic disability (McGovern & Sigman, 2005).

THE ROLE OF DEVELOPMENTAL ASSESSMENT IN DIAGNOSTIC CONSIDERATIONS

The assessment of cognitive and adaptive skills constitutes an integral element of diagnostic assessment (American Psychiatric Association, 2000; see also Bishop et al., Chapter 2, this volume). Interpreting results of the diagnostic measures within the child's specific developmental context represent a cornerstone of best practices in the early diagnosis of developmental disorders. At present, the responsibility for integrating information from multiple sources and weighing their relative significance with regard to diagnosis falls to experienced clinicians. It is hoped that the growing numbers of prospective studies of children identified as having ASD in the second and third years of life will result in identification of performance profiles involving multiple areas of functioning that are specific to various subtypes within ASD and will allow for differentiating them from toddlers with other developmental disabilities. This knowledge, in turn, can inform and enrich the diagnostic process. Preliminary results of a prospective study on early diagnosis of ASD highlight the utility of such an approach (Chawarska, Klin, & Volkmar, 2003). Simultaneous consideration of the child's level of verbal and nonverbal skills along with the levels of dysfunction in the areas of socialization, communication, play, and stereotyped behaviors, greatly enhanced the diagnostic classification procedure allowing for more accurate differentiation of toddlers with autism, PDD-NOS, global developmental delay, and specific language disorders. Identifying dimensions relevant for differential diagnosis of ASD in early development, as well as unique performance profiles characteristic of various subtypes of ASD, would greatly advance the field of early diagnosis, and further work on this important topic is necessary.

CONCLUSIONS

Developmental assessment of infants and toddlers with developmental disabilities is a complex and multileveled process. It results typically in establishing a child's levels of verbal, nonverbal, exploration, adaptive, and motor skills, as well as ascertaining the role of arousal, attention, affect regulation, and motivational factors that might have an impact on the child's learning style and the level of adaptive functioning. Furthermore, documenting the possible impact of biological and environmental factors, including family circumstances and access to services, provides complementary information necessary for the interpretation of test findings and designing an intervention plan.

Although data on early developmental trajectories of young children with ASD are still limited, a coherent picture is beginning to emerge. A vast majority of infants and toddlers with ASD experience significant delays in at least one key area of development. It is likely that their developmental trajectories in verbal and nonverbal domains do not begin to diverge markedly from those with other developmental difficulties until the second year of life. The magnitude of the delay is often much greater in the verbal than in the nonverbal domain. Furthermore, very young children with autism appear to have more profound delays in the ability to respond to and understand language than in the ability to produce vocalizations and speech sounds. The rate of progress in the first 3–4 years of life among children with ASD is highly variable, with a considerable proportion of toddlers either making very significant gains or experiencing a slowdown in the rate of skill acquisition within a 1- to 2-year period. Thus, the early scores on developmental tests in toddlers with ASD are not very good predictors of the cognitive levels observed in the early school years. The individual trajectories begin to stabilize after the age of 4, at which time cognitive scores become more predictive of later developmental functioning.

The differences in the levels of verbal and nonverbal functioning between toddlers with autism and those with PDD-NOS are relatively minor early in development; nonetheless, toddlers with PDD-NOS show, in general, a better rate of progress and are more likely to achieve scores in the normative range than their peers with autism by early preschool age. Changes in cognitive functioning are, in most cases, accompanied by the acquisition of adaptive skills necessary for functioning in day-to-day situations. However, the acquisition rates of adaptive skills lag behind those observed in the verbal and nonverbal cognitive domains, emphasizing the necessity of including adaptive skills training into the early intervention program.

The upcoming several years will bring to light a fascinating body of evidence regarding early developmental trajectories of children with ASD, as the currently ongoing prospective studies of younger siblings of children with ASD reach their conclusions. Particularly important will be further clarification regarding the areas of cognitive development that are the most relevant for diagnostic, prognostic, and treatment purposes, possibly with greater differentiation into specific skills related to attention, learning, memory, concept development, imitation, and exploration. The identification of specific performance profiles linked to specific developmental disorders as they are expressed at various early stages of development can lead to early and more accurate diagnosis and earlier implementation of the most appropriate intervention strategies for a given disorder.

ACKNOWLEDGMENTS

Preparation of this chapter was supported by STAART Center Grant No. U54 MH66494 funded by the National Institute on Deafness and Communication Disorders, the National Institute of Environmental Health Sciences, the National Institute of Child Health and Human Development, and the National Institute of Neurological Disorders and Stroke, and by research grants funded by the National Alliance for Autism Research and the Korczak Foundation.

REFERENCES

Adamson, L., McArthur, D., Markov, Y., Dunbar, B., & Bakeman, R. (2001). Autism and joint attention: Young children's responses to maternal bids. *Applied Developmental Psychology, 22,* 439–453.

Akshoomoff, N. (2006). Use of the Mullen Scales of Early Learning for the assessment of young children with autism spectrum disorders. *Child Neuropsychology, 12,* 269–277.

American Association on Mental Retardation. (2002). *Mental retardation: Definition, classification, and systems of support* (10th ed.). Washington, DC: Author.

American Psychiatric Association. (2000). *Diagnostic and statistical manual of mental disorders* (4th ed., text rev.). Washington, DC: Author.

Baranek, G. T. (1999). Autism during infancy: A retrospective video analysis of sensory-motor and social behaviors at 9–12 months of age. *Journal of Autism and Developmental Disorders, 29*(3), 213–224.

Baron-Cohen, S., Cox, A., Baird, G., Sweettenham, J., & Nighingale, N. (1996). Psychological markers in the detection of autism in infancy in a large population. *British Journal of Psychiatry, 168*(2), 158–163.

Bayley, N. (2006). *Bayley Scales of Infant and Toddler Development, Third Edition.* San Antonio, TX: Harcourt Assessment.

Bolte, S., & Poustka, F. (2002). The relation between general cognitive level and adaptive behavior domains in individuals with autism with and without comorbid mental retardation. *Child Psychiatry and Human Development, 33*(2), 165–172.

Bricker, D., & Squires, J. (1999). *The Ages and Stages Questionnaires (ASQ): A direct completed child monitoring system* (2nd ed.). Baltimore: Brookes.

Brigance, A. (1986). *The BRIGANCE® Screens.* North Billerica, MA: Curriculum Associates.

Carpentieri, S., & Morgan, S. B. (1996). Adaptive and intellectual functioning in autistic and nonautistic retarded children. *Journal of Autism and Developmental Disorders, 26,* 611–620.

Carter, A. S., Black, D., Tewani, S., Connolly, C., Kadlec, M., & Tager-Flusberg, H. (2007). Sex differences in toddlers with autism spectrum disorders. *Journal of Autism and Developmental Disorders, 37*(1), 87–98.

Carter, A. S., Volkmar, F. R., Sparrow, S. S., Wang, J. J., Lord, C., Dawson, G., et al. (1998). The Vineland Adaptive Behavior Scales: Supplementary norms for individuals with autism. *Journal of Autism and Developmental Disorders, 28,* 287–302.

Charman, T., Baron-Cohen, S., Swettenham, J., Baird, G., Cox, A., & Drew, A. (2001). Testing joint attention, imitation, and play as infancy precursors to language and theory of mind. *Cognitive Development, 15*(4), 481–498.

Charman, T., Baron-Cohen, S., Swettenham, J., Baird, G., Drew, A., & Cox, A. (2003). Predicting language outcome in infants with autism and pervasive developmental disorder. *International Journal of Language and Communication Disorders, 38*(3), 265–285.

Charman, T., Drew, A., Baird, C., & Baird, G. (2003). Measuring early language development in preschool children with autism spectrum disorder using the MacArthur Communicative Development Inventory (Infant Form). *Journal of Child Language, 30*(1), 213–236.

Charman, T., Swettenham, J., Baron-Cohen, S., Cox, A., Baird, G., & Drew, A. (1997). Infants with autism: An investigation of empathy, pretend play, joint attention, and imitation. *Developmental Psychology, 33*(5), 781–789.

Charman, T., Taylor, E., Drew, A., Cockerill, H., Brown, J.-A., & Baird, G. (2005).

Outcome at 7 years of children diagnosed with autism at age 2: Predictive validity of assessments conducted at 2 and 3 years of age and pattern of symptom change over time. *Journal of Child Psychology and Psychiatry, 46*(5), 500–513.

Chawarska, K. (2007). *Longitudinal study of syndrome expression: ASD from the second to the fourth year.* Paper presented at the Society for Child Development Conference, Boston, MA.

Chawarska, K., Klin, A., Paul, R., & Volkmar, F. R. (2007). Autism spectrum disorder in the second year: Stability and change in syndrome expression. *Journal of Child Psychology and Psychiatry, 48*(2), 128.

Chawarska, K., Klin, A., & Volkmar, F. (2003, November). *Developmental profiles of 2-year-old children with autism.* Poster presented at the 7th Congress Autism–Europe, Lisbon, Portugal.

Chawarska, K., Paul, R., Klin, A., Hannigen, S., Dichtel, L., & Volkmar, F. (2007). Parental recognition of developmental problems in toddlers with autism spectrum disorders. *Journal of Autism and Developmental Disorders, 37*(1), 62–73.

Cox, A., Klein, K., Charman, T., Baird, G., Baron-Cohen, S., Swettenham, J., et al. (1999). Autism spectrum disorders at 20 and 42 months of age: Stability of clinical and ADI-R diagnosis. *Journal of Child Psychology and Psychiatry and Allied Disciplines, 40*(5), 719–732.

Dawson, G., & Adams, A. (1984). Imitation and social responsiveness in autistic children. *Journal of Abnormal Child Psychology, 12*(2), 209–225.

Dawson, G., Meltzoff, A. N., Osterling, J., & Rinaldi, J. (1998). Neuropsychological correlates of early symptoms of autism. *Child Development, 69*(5), 1276–1285.

Dawson, G., Meltzoff, A., Osterling, J., Rinaldi, J., & Brown, E. (1998). Children with autism fail to orient to naturally occurring social stimuli. *Journal of Autism and Developmental Disorders, 28,* 479–485.

Dawson, G., Munson, J., Estes, A., Osterling, J., McPartland, J., Toth, K., et al. (2002). Neurocognitive function and joint attention ability in young children with autism spectrum disorder versus developmental delay. *Child Development, 73*(2), 345–358.

De Giacomo, A., & Fombonne, E. (1998). Parental recognition of developmental abnormalities in autism. *European Child and Adolescent Psychiatry, 7*(3), 131–136.

Eaves, L. C., & Ho, H. H. (2004). The very early identification of autism: Outcome to age 4½–5. *Journal of Autism and Developmental Disorders, 34*(4), 367–378.

Ehlers, S., Nyden, A., Gillberg, C., Sandberg, A. D., Dahlgren, S. O., Hjelmquist, E., et al. (1997). Asperger syndrome, autism and attention disorders: A comparative study of the cognitive profiles of 120 children. *Journal of Child Psychology and Psychiatry and Allied Disciplines, 38*(2), 207–217.

Filipek, P. A., Accardo, P. J., Baranek, G. T., Cook, E. H., Dawson, G., Gordon, B., et al. (1999). The screening and diagnosis of autistic spectrum disorders. *Journal of Autism and Developmental Disorders, 29*(6), 439–484.

Freeman, B., Del'Homme, M., Guthrie, D., & Zhang, F. (1999). Vineland Adaptive Behavior Scale scores as a function of age and initial IQ in 210 autistic children. *Journal of Autism and Developmental Disorders, 29*(5), 379–384.

Freeman, B., Ritvo, E. R., Yokota, A., Childs, J., & Pollard, J. (1988). WISC–R and Vineland Adaptive Behavior Scale scores in autistic children. *Journal of the American Academy of Child and Adolescent Psychiatry, 27*(4), 428–429.

Gesell, A. (1948). *Studies in child development.* Oxford, UK: Harper.

Gillham, J. E., Carter, A. S., Volkmar, F. R., & Sparrow, S. S. (2003). Toward a developmental operational definition of autism. In M. E. Hertzig & E. A. Farber (Eds.), *Annual progress in child psychiatry and child development: 2000–2001* (pp. 363–381). New York: Brunner-Routledge.

Gilliam, W. S., & Mayes, L. C. (2000). Developmental assessment of infants and toddlers. In C. H. Zeanah, Jr. (Ed.), *Handbook of infant mental health* (2nd ed., pp. 236–248). New York: Guilford Press.

Gilliam, W. S., & Mayes, L. C. (2004). Integrating clinical and psychometric approaches: Developmental assessment and the infant mental health evaluation. In R. DelCarmen-Wiggins & A. Carter (Eds.), *Handbook of infant, toddler, and preschool mental health assessment* (pp. 185–203). New York: Oxford University Press.

Glascoe, F. P. (1996). *A validation study and the psychometric properties of the BRIGANCE® Screens.* North Billerica, MA: Curriculum Associates.

Greenspan, S. (2004). *The Greenspan Social Emotional Growth Chart: A screening questionnaire for infants and young children.* San Antonio, TX: Harcourt Assessment.

Harrison, P. L., & Oakland, T. (2003). *Adaptive Behavior Assessment System–II.* San Antonio, TX: Psychological Corporation.

Individuals with Disabilities Education Improvement Act of 2004, Public Law No. 108-446, §632, 118 Stat. 2744.

Ireton, H. (1992). *Child Development Inventories.* Minneapolis: Behavior Science Systems.

Ireton, H., & Glascoe, F. P. (1995). Assessing children's development using parents' reports: The Child Development Inventory. *Clinical Pediatrics, 34,* 248–255.

Joseph, R. M., Tager-Flusberg, H., & Lord, C. (2002). Cognitive profiles and social-communicative functioning in children with autism spectrum disorder. *Journal of Child Psychology and Psychiatry and Allied Disciplines, 43*(6), 807–821.

Kanner, L. (1943/1968). Autistic disturbances of affective contact. *Acta Paedopsychiatrica: International Journal of Child and Adolescent Psychiatry, 35*(4–8), 98–136.

Klin, A., Chawarska, K., Paul, R., Rubin, E., Morgan, T., Wiesner, L., et al. (2004). Clinical case conference: Autism at the age of 15 months. *Archives of General Psychiatry, 161,* 1–8.

Klin, A., Chawarska, K., Rubin, E., & Volkmar, F. (2004). Clinical assessment of young children at risk for autism. In R. DelCarmen-Wiggins & A. Carter (Eds.), *Handbook of infant, toddler, and preschool mental health assessment* (pp. 311–336). New York: Oxford University Press.

Klin, A., Jones, W., Schultz, R., Volkmar, F., & Cohen, D. (2002). Visual fixation patterns during viewing of naturalistic social situations as predictors of social competence in individuals with autism. *Archives of General Psychiatry, 59*(9), 809–816.

Klin, A., Saulnier, S., Sparrow, S., Cicchetti, D., Volkmar, F., & Lord, C. (2007).

Social and communication abilities and disabilities in higher functioning individuals with autism spectrum disorders: The Vineland and the ADOS. *Journal of Autism and Developmental Disorders, 37*(4), 748–759.

Klin, A., Volkmar, F. R., & Sparrow, S. S. (1992). Autistic social dysfunction: Some limitations of the theory of mind hypothesis. *Journal of Child Psychology and Psychiatry and Allied Disciplines, 33*(5), 861–876.

Klin, A., Volkmar, F., Sparrow, S., Cicchetti, D., & Rourke, B. P. (1995). Validity and neuropsychological characterization of Asperger syndrome: Convergence with nonverbal learning disabilities syndrome. *Journal of Child Psychology and Psychiatry and Allied Disciplines, 36*(7), 1127–1140.

Koegel, L. K., Koegel, R. L., & Smith, A. (1997). Variables related to differences in standardized test outcomes for children with autism. *Journal of Autism and Developmental Disorders, 27*(3), 233–243.

Kraijer, D. (2000). Review of adaptive behavior studies in mentally retarded persons with autism/pervasive developmental disorder. *Journal of Autism and Developmental Disorders, 30*, 39–47.

Landa, R., & Garrett-Mayer, E. (2006). Development in infants with autism spectrum disorders: A prospective study. *Journal of Child Psychology and Psychiatry, 47*(6), 629–638.

Levy, S. E., Mandell, D. S., Merhar, S., Ittenbach, R. F., & Pinto-Martin, J. A. (2003). Use of complementary and alternative medicine among children recently diagnosed with autistic spectrum disorder. *Journal of Developmental and Behavioral Pediatrics, 24*(6), 418–423.

Lord, C. (1995). Follow-up of two-year-olds referred for possible autism. *Journal of Child Psychology and Psychiatry and Allied Disciplines, 36*(8), 1365–1382.

Lord, C., & Paul, R. (1997). Language and communication in autism. In F. R. V. D. J. Cohen (Ed.), *Handbook of autism and developmental disorders* (pp. 195–225). New York: Wiley.

Lord, C., & Risi, S. (2000). Diagnosis of autism spectrum disorders in young children. In A. M. Wetherby & B. M. Prizant (Eds.), *Autism spectrum disorders: A transactional developmental perspective* (pp. 11–30). Baltimore: Brookes.

Lord, C., Risi, S., DiLavore, P. S., Shulman, C., Thurm, A., & Pickles, A. (2006). Autism from 2 to 9 years of age. *Archives of General Psychiatry, 63*(6), 694–701.

Luyster, R., Richler, J., Risi, S., Hsu, W.-L., Dawson, G., Bernier, R., et al. (2005). Early regression in social communication in autism spectrum disorders: A CPEA study. *Developmental Neuropsychology, 27*(3), 311–336.

Mantynen, H., Poikkeus, A.-M., Ahonen, T., Aro, T., & Korkman, M. (2001). Clinical significance of test refusal among young children. *Child Neuropsychology, 7*(4), 241–250.

McArthur, D., & Adamson, L. B. (1996). Joint attention in preverbal children: Autism and developmental language disorder. *Journal of Autism and Developmental Disorders, 26*(5), 481–496.

McGovern, C. W., & Sigman, M. (2005). Continuity and change from early childhood to adolescence in autism. *Journal of Child Psychology and Psychiatry, 46*(4), 401–408.

Mullen, E. (1995). *Mullen Scales of Early Learning–AGS Edition.* Circle Pines, MN: American Guidance Service.

Mundy, P., & Burnette, C. (2005). Joint attention and neurodevelopmental models of autism. In F. Volkmar, R. Paul, A. Klin, & D. Cohen (Eds.), *Handbook of autism and pervasive developmental disorders: Diagnosis, development, neurobiology, and behavior* (Vol. 1, 3rd ed., pp. 650–681). New York: Wiley.

Mundy, P., Sigman, M., & Kasari, C. (1990). A longitudinal study of joint attention and language development in autistic children. *Journal of Autism and Developmental Disorders, 20*(1), 115–128.

Mundy, P., Sigman, M., & Kasari, C. (1994). Joint attention, developmental level, and symptom presentation in autism. *Development and Psychopathology, 6*(3), 389–401.

Mundy, P., Sigman, M., Ungerer, J., & Sherman, T. (1986). Defining the social deficits of autism: The contribution of non-verbal communication measures. *Journal of Child Psychology and Psychiatry and Allied Disciplines, 27*(5), 657–669.

National Research Council. (Ed.). (2001). *Educating children with autism.* Washington, DC: National Academy Press.

Neisworth, J., & Bagnato, S. (2004). The mismeasure of young children: The authentic assessment alternative. *Infants and Young Children, 17*(3), 198–212.

Osterling, J., A., Dawson, G., & Munson, J. A. (2002). Early recognition of 1-year-old infants with autism spectrum disorder versus mental retardation. *Development and Psychopathology, 14*(2), 239–251.

Ozonoff, S., Goodlin-Jones, B., & Solomon, M. (2005). Evidence-based assessment of autism spectrum disorders in children and adolescents. *Journal of Clinical Child and Adolescent Psychology, 34*(3), 523–540.

Paul, R., Chawarska, K., Fowler, C., Cichetti, D., & Volkmar, F. (2007). "Listen, my children, and you shall hear": Auditory preferences in toddlers with autism spectrum disorders. *Journal of Speech, Language, and Hearing Research, 50*, 1–15.

Paul, R., Chawarska, K., Klin, A., & Volkmar, F. (2006). Dissociations in the development of early communication in autism spectrum disorders. In R. Paul (Ed.), *Language disorders from a developmental perspective* (pp. 163–194). Mahwah, NJ: Erlbaum

Piaget, J. (1954). *The construction of reality in the child.* New York: Basic Books.

Rogers, S. J., Hepburn, S. L., Stackhouse, T., & Wehner, B. (2003). Imitation performance in toddlers with autism and those with other developmental disorders. *Journal of Child Psychology and Psychiatry, 44*(5), 763–781.

Sattler, J. M., & Hoge, R. D. (2006). *Assessment of children: Behavioral, social, and clinical foundations* (5th ed.). San Diego: Sattler.

Saulnier, S., & Klin, A. (2007). Brief report: Social and communication abilities and disabilities in higher functioning individuals with autism and Asperger syndrome. *Journal of Autism and Developmental Disorders, 37*(4), 788–793

Sigman, M., & Ungerer, J. (1981). Sensorimotor skills and language comprehension in autistic children. *Journal of Abnormal Child Psychology, 9*(2), 149–165.

Sigman, M., & Ungerer, J. A. (1984). Cognitive and language skills in autistic, mentally retarded, and normal children. *Developmental Psychology, 20*(2), 293–302.

Siperstein, R., & Volkmar, F. (2004). Brief report: Parental reporting of regression in children with pervasive developmental disorders. *Journal of Autism and Developmental Disorders, 34*(6), 731–734.

Sparrow, S. S., Carter, A. S., Racusin, G., & Morris, R. (1995). Comprehensive psychological assessment through the life span: A developmental approach. In

D. Cicchetti & D. J. Cohen (Eds.), *Developmental psychopathology: Vol. 1. Theory and methods* (pp. 81–105). Oxford, UK: Wiley.

Sparrow, S. S., Cicchetti, D. V., & Balla, D. A. (2005). *Vineland Adaptive Behavior Scales–Second Edition (Vineland II), Survey Interview Form/Caregiver Rating Form.* Livonia, MN: Pearson Assessments.

Squires, J., Bricker, D., & Potter, L. (1997). Revision of a parent-completed developmental screening tool: Ages and Stages Questionnaires. *Journal of Pediatric Psychology, 22,* 313–328.

Stone, W. L., Ousley, O. Y., Hepburn, S. L., Hogan, K. L., & Brown, C. S. (1999). Patterns of adaptive behavior in very young children with autism. *American Journal on Mental Retardation, 104*(2), 187–199.

Stone, W. L., Ousley, O. Y., Yoder, P. J., Hogan, K. L., & Hepburn, S. L. (1997). Nonverbal communication in two- and three-year-old children with autism. *Journal of Autism and Developmental Disorders, 27*(6), 677–696.

Szatmari, P., Bryson, S. E., Boyle, M. H., Streiner, D. L., & Duku, E. (2003). Predictors of outcome among high functioning children with autism and Asperger syndrome. *Journal of Child Psychology and Psychiatry, 44*(4), 520–528.

Tomasello, M. (1995). Joint attention as social cognition. In C. Moore & P. J. Dunham (Eds.), *Joint attention: Its origins and role in development* (pp. 103–130). Hillsdale, NJ: Erlbaum.

Uzgiris, I., & Hunt, J. (1975). *Assessment in infancy. Ordinal scales of psychological development.* Urbana: University of Illinois Press.

Volkmar, F. R., Carter, A., Sparrow, S. S., & Cicchetti, D. V. (1993). Quantifying social development in autism. *Journal of the American Academy of Child and Adolescent Psychiatry, 32*(3), 627–632.

Volkmar, F. R., Klin, A., Siegel, B., Szatmari, P., Lord, C., Campbell, M, et al. (1994). Field trial for autistic disorder in DSM-IV. *American Journal of Psychiatry, 151*(9), 1361–1367.

Volkmar, F. R., & Mayes, L. C. (1990). Gaze behavior in autism. *Development and Psychopathology, 2*(1), 61–69.

Wetherby, A. M., Woods, J., Allen, L., Cleary, J., Dickinson, H., & Lord, C. (2004). Early indicators of autism spectrum disorders in the second year of life. *Journal of Autism and Developmental Disorders, 34*(5), 473–493.

Williams, S. K., Scahill, L., Vitiello, B., Aman, M. G., Arnold, L. E., McDougle, C. J., et al. (2006). Risperidone and adaptive behavior in children with autism. *Journal of the American Academy of Child and Adolescent Psychiatry, 45,* 431–439.

Yang, N. K., Huang, T.-A., Schaller, J. L., Wang, M. H., & Tsai, S.-F. (2003). Enhancing appropriate social behaviors for children with autism in general education classrooms: An analysis of six cases. *Education and Training in Developmental Disabilities, 38*(4), 405–416.

CHAPTER 4

———•———

Communication Development and Assessment

RHEA PAUL

Communication deficits are one of the core symptoms of autism spectrum disorders (ASD). Therefore, tracing the development of communication in this syndrome is central to understanding its early course and trajectory of impairment. Although the terms *language* and *communication* are sometimes used synonymously, it is important in this context to be aware that deficits in the ability to communicate are evident prior to the acquisition of language in very young children with ASD. Although children with ASD are frequently delayed in their acquisition of first words and in their use of words and sentences to express needs and interact with others, this delay is foreshadowed by early-appearing deficits in the use of gaze, gestures, and vocalizations to accomplish the same goals, as well as in the tendency to orient and listen to speech. In this chapter, the early communication of infants and toddlers with typical development is outlined and contrasted with what is known about this sequence in ASD. In addition, communication development is discussed in three areas: preverbal development, understanding of spoken language, and first use of words and word combinations.

PREVERBAL COMMUNICATIVE DEVELOPMENT

From the moment of birth, communication is an active process between the child and the social environment. Far from being a passive recipient

76

of adult speech, even the newborn infant engages in behaviors that rivet the adult's attention and elicit social interaction.

Early Perceptual Propensities

Although, of course, young infants do not understand the literal meaning of language addressed to them, it does appear that newborns begin life with attentional preferences for human, linguistic interaction and with a set of social behaviors that can elicit this stimulation. These abilities appear, because of their emergence so soon after birth, to be innately programmed and, as such, provide a great deal of economy in the task of mastering language. Certain propensities present from the first days of life include a preference for sounds in the frequency range of the human voice (Hutt, Hutt, Lenard, Bernuth, & Jewerff, 1968), for speech over other rhythmic or musical sounds (Butterfield & Siperstein, 1974), and for child-directed over adult-directed speech (Fernald, 1983; Cooper & Aslin, 1994; Moon, Pennton-Cooper, & Fifer, 1993; Pegg, Werker, & McLeod, 1992). Newborns look for the source of a voice they hear, register pleasure with facial expression when they identify the source, and remain quiet, inhibiting their movements, until the voice ceases (Owens, 2000). They do not show this kind of recognition when a nonhuman auditory stimulus is heard. Three-day-old infants are able to recognize their own mothers' voices, as opposed to the voices of other women (Hepper, Scott, & Shahidulla, 1993), probably as a result of prenatal experience with the mother's voice heard through the amniotic sac (Jusczyk, 1999b). Newborns are also attracted to and prefer to look at faces (Kagan & Lewis, 1965). Parents, conveniently, interpret this preference as a sign of willingness to interact. The newborn appears, then, to be biologically organized to attract language input and tune in to the linguistic environment.

There is evidence that speech perception begins at a very early age and may, in fact, be biologically determined in human infants (Eimas, 1975). For example, infants only weeks old are able to discriminate among a variety of speech sounds, including /pa/ versus /ba/, /ta/ versus /da/, /ba/ versus /ga/, to name a few (Aslin & Smith, 1988; Eimas, Siqueland, Jusczyk, & Vigorito, 1971; Graham, Bashir, & Stark, 1999), and make these distinctions along the same categorical boundaries as adults do. These distinctions are likely to be part of the human auditory system, as Werker and Tees (1984) found that infants in English-speaking environments were able to distinguish sounds that are not used in English, but are in Hindi. By 1 year of age, though, this ability to discriminate sounds not heard in the native language has all but disappeared. These findings suggest that the infant does have some "built-in" capacity to make discriminations among sounds that are important in speech, but that this ability is modified with experience. Rather than learning to make these distinctions from the language that he or she hears, though, it seems that the infant comes to the task of language with some discriminations "preset." Depending on what particular distinctions are used by the ambient language, some of these innately programmed distinctions are maintained by the child's experience, whereas others are extinguished. The acceleration of this process toward the end of the first year may also signal a shift in focus for the language learner, from sound discrimination to the mapping of sound to meaning (Werker & Tees, 1999).

Children also acquire a range of differentiated responses to the sounds of language throughout their first year. By 4 months of age, they respond to different tones of voice; by 6 months, they show evidence of selective listening (choosing to respond to some sounds and ignore others). In the latter half of the first year, babies inhibit their behavior if told "no" in a loud, sharp voice, but they do the same if they hear "yes" spoken in the same tone (Spitz, 1957). Their response at this stage, then, is not to a specific lexical item, but to an emotional tone in the speech.

Young babies also appear to be able to coordinate acoustic information about speech with visual information about oral posture. Kuhl and Meltzoff (1988) showed that infants looked for a significantly longer time at the picture of the face whose oral gesture corresponded to the vowel the 6-month-old babies were hearing at the time (retracted lips for /i/; open lips for /a/). This surprising finding suggests a very early ability to integrate visual and auditory cues in perceiving speech and would seem to provide children with an excellent foundation for learning the articulatory movements associated with the speech sounds they will eventually learn to produce.

Although children do not understand words per se until near the end of the first year, they appear to begin to develop the bases for the grammatical and semantic categories, with which these words will be associated, much earlier. Infants are able to use acoustic and phonological cues to distinguish words based on grammatical class. Shi, Werker, and Morgan (1999) showed that infants presented with lists of lexical (content; e.g., *dog, shoe*) and grammatical (function; e.g., *the*) words could detect a switch to a word from a different category, although they were not sensitive to changes within the same grammatical category.

Colombo and associates (Colombo, O'Brien, Mitchell, Roberts, & Horowitz, 1987) showed babies 6–7 months of age slides of various kinds of birds until the children habituated to these stimuli and reduced their visual fixation time. These researchers then showed two new slides simultaneously, one of a parakeet and one of a horse, for example. Babies reliably looked longer at the horse, suggesting that it was more novel to them than the parakeet, which they had also not seen before. Thus, it appears that the children included the parakeet in the category they had formed for the objects viewed previously (i.e., birds). These findings suggest that even at this early age, babies are able to organize their perceptions into conceptual categories that eventually can be mapped onto words.

Infants also appear to have specialized abilities that facilitate the task of segmenting words from the ongoing stream of speech. Saffran, Aslin, and Newport (1996) showed that by 8 months of age, infants are able to recognize word-like sound units from an ongoing acoustic field, based on expectations they have developed for the likelihood that certain sounds will appear together. Moreover, they accomplish this task, using nonsense syllables presented by examiners, after only 2 minutes of exposure.

Jusczyk, Houston, and Newsome (1999) also reported that infants at 7–10 months of age can use stress patterns in a similar way to recognize word-like elements within an acoustic stream. When presented, for example, with a series of syllables that have a strong–weak syllable pattern (*hamster*), they show preferences for listening to new combinations that have the same pattern and are more likely to react to strong–weak patterns as if they were words, than to weak–strong patterns (*giraffe*). As they develop, children acquire increasingly sophisticated means of locating word boundaries in fluent speech. By 11 months of age, children's sensitivity to word boundaries depends on multiple sources of information, including the order of sounds in the word, the stress pattern in the word, and the way in which individual sounds are pronounced (Jusczyk, 1999a; Myers et al., 1996). This ability to use a variety of acoustic cues to segment words from a speech stream by relying on probabilities of sound structure abstracted from a relatively small amount of listening experience helps to explain how children learn to pick out words from the many sounds they hear in their environments.

Infants also appear to be sensitive to auditory information that is associated with syntactic boundaries. Hirsh-Pasek and associates (Hirsh-Pasek et al., 1987) showed that babies of this age preferred to look toward a speaker that played sentences containing pauses at clause or phrase boundaries (*Cinderella lived in a great big house/but it was sort of dark/ because she had a mean . . .*), as opposed to sentences with pauses in the middle of a clause (*Cinderella lived in a great big house but it was/ sort of dark because she had/a mean . . .*). These results suggest that babies as young as 7 months can detect syntactic boundaries, an ability that would greatly economize the amount of information they ultimately need to acquire in order to understand sentences. Recent studies (Kuhl, Coffey-Corina, Padden, & Dawson, 2005; Tsao, Liu, & Kuhl, 2004; Werner, Dawson, Osterling, & Dino, 2000) have shown that these early-developing speech perception capacities, and particularly the ability to "tune in" to sounds that are relevant for learning the ambient language, are related to outcomes in vocabulary size and sentence complexity at age 2.

Perceptual Capacity in Infants with ASD

What about children with ASD? Do they demonstrate the early perceptual capacities that help them "tune in" to the relevant stimuli in the ambient language and use this experience to break into the language code? It seems reasonable to hypothesize that one source of the pervasive difficulty in language learning evidenced by children with ASD may be a reduced amount of relevant language experience caused by diminished attention to and preference for native language sound patterns during infancy. Many parents of children with ASD report that these babies sometimes seemed deaf and did not respond to voices or their names, and retrospective studies of videotapes of infants who turn out to have ASD support the observations that these children show poorer responses to their own names than do peers (Osterling & Dawson, 1994; Werner et al., 2000). Although few studies have investigated early auditory perception in infants who turn out to have autism, one case study (Dawson, Osterling, Meltzoff, & Kuhl, 2000) found some difficulty in the ability to discriminate consonants, though not vowels, at the end of the first year of life in a child found later to have ASD. Data on toddlers with ASD also suggest that there is a reduced preference for child-directed speech, and that this reduction is related to measures of understanding language (Paul, Chawarska, Klin, & Volkmar, 2007), as well as to measures of understanding language a year later (Paul, Chawarska, Fowler, Cicchetti, & Volkmar, 2007). Older children with autism also have been shown to have a reduced preference for child-directed speech (Klin, 1992). Just as studies of visual preferences show a reduced preference for social stimuli in young children with autism (Klin, 2003), these early studies suggest something analogous may be going on in the auditory realm, and these failures to orient to important visual and auditory information in the first year of life could have cascading consequences for later development.

Infant Sound Production

Crying is the newborn's principal form of vocal behavior. Beginning in the first month after birth, the infant masters the ability to produce cries that differentiate among affective states. Pain versus hunger cries are differentiated within the first week of life (Graham et al., 1983). Other noncry vocalizations also emerge early in life. Contentment vocalizations can be distinguished from distress sounds in typically developing children within the first month (Ricks & Wing, 1975).

The quality of infant vocalizations changes drastically throughout the first year of life. Stark (1979) has presented a framework for describing infant vocal behavior, which appears in Table 4.1. According to this framework, the infant from birth to 2 months of age produces primarily reflex-

TABLE 4.1. A Summary of Stark's (1979) Stages of Infant Vocalization

Stage	Age range	Vocalization types
I	0–2 months	Reflexive cries and vegetative sounds
II	2–5 months	Cooing and laughing
III	4–8 months	Vocal play and beginning babbling
IV	6–9 months	Reduplicated babbling
V	9–18 months	Jargon babbling

ive cries and other vegetative sounds. Although the newborn's cries have a profound effect on the adults who hear them, the infant is not using the crying in any intentional way to attract the adults' notice. Rather, the cry is an instinctual response to an internal state such as hunger, cold, or boredom. Vegetative sounds such as burps, coughs, and sneezes are also reflexive, but adults respond to these noises as if they were communicative, as well. This willingness on the part of an adult to attribute intentionality to the infant's early reflexive sound production may be one of the ways in which infants are "taught" to use sound to communicate.

As the baby grows, the head and neck anatomy changes, resulting in a greater diversity of sounds that can be produced and a more speech-like resonance associated with vocalization. Between 2 and 5 months of age, babies begin two behaviors that are important for the development of speech and communication. One is the pleasant, somewhat speech-like sound that babies produce primarily in response to social interactions, known as *cooing*, or "comfort" sounds. The name arises from the "oo"-like quality of most of the vowels heard during this type of vocalizing and from the fact that most of the consonants produced sound like /k/ and /g/. Again, the reasons for the "coo" quality of these vocalizations are anatomic. As the baby lies in a prone or semiprone position, gravity operates most strongly on the relatively large posterior portion of the tongue, pulling it back toward the roof of the mouth. This oral posture produces the consonants we recognize as /g/ and /k/, as well as the vowel we recognize as "oo."

A second new vocal behavior in this stage is the infant's laugh, which emerges at about the same time as cooing. Usually accompanied by a social smile, infant laughing is produced in response to an interaction the infant perceives as pleasurable, very often because it is a known routine whose components are predictable. Thus, a baby may laugh when the mother plays "peek-a-boo" for him or her or when she assumes a posture as if ready to tickle the baby. Crying becomes less frequent during this period of increasingly diverse and speech-like vocalization.

The next stage of vocal development begins at about 4 months of age and extends to about 8 months. Stark (1979) refers to this period as "vocal play." In this phase the infant begins to pronounce what sound like single syllables with vowel-like and consonant-like components. Although not approximations of words and not meant to convey any referential meaning, these early forms of babbling continue the infant's progress toward increasingly speech-like sounds. The consonants produced tend to be made more toward the front of the mouth than were those used for cooing, including sounds such as /b/, /p/, and /m/.

At the next stage, infants use vocal play as a means of responding to or initiating contact with adults, so that proto-"conversations" can take place in which parent and infant babble back and forth to each other. Babies also engage in vocal play when alone, and this play may function as a means for the infant to "practice" the new sounds.

There is also evidence that vocal learning begins to be shaped in the middle of the first year by imitation of sound patterns in the ambient language. Kuhl and Meltzoff (1996) presented audio and video recordings of three vowel sounds to infants at 12 and 20 weeks and analyzed their vocalizations. By 20 weeks, infants were able to imitate specific vowels with appropriate relative format frequencies. Moreover, Kuhl and Meltzoff (1996) showed that providing infants with enhanced opportunities to imitate sounds increased their production of speech-like vocalizations. In general, vocal imitation appears to be an important means by which typically developing children move toward speech. Infants begin attempting to imitate others' productions in back-and-forth babbling games during the vocal play period and continue to use imitation, first of sounds and intonation contours, and later of words, throughout the second year of life.

Stark (1979) reported that a new form of vocal behavior, which she referred to as "reduplicated babbling," appears in the second half of the first year of life. This type of vocalization includes consonant–vowel combinations, such as /bababa/ or /nanana/, in which the same syllable is repeated over and over. Consonants most likely to appear include /b/, /p/, /t/, /d/, /m/, /n/, and the glide y. Like vocal play, reduplicated babbling occurs both when the baby is alone and as a form of interaction. Oller and associates (Oller, Eilers, Neal, & Cobo-Lewis, 1998) report that this form of vocalization, which they refer to as "canonical babble," is an important milestone of communication development. Their research suggests that children who do not develop canonical babbling by 10 months of age are at risk for later language disorders.

Toward the end of the first year of life, many babies begin to use "vocables," or phonetically consistent forms. These are productions that are unique to the child in that they do not closely resemble any adult word, but are used reliably in certain situations. For example, Carter

(1979) reported that one child consistently used an /m/ sound along with reaching to indicate that he wanted something. These early consistent forms are sometimes referred to as "protowords."

Preverbal Production in Infants with ASD

Again, there is a paucity of direct data on the development of vocal productions of infants who go on to have ASD. Most of the literature on vocalization in ASD describes vocal production in children who remain at prelinguistic levels of communication into the preschool years, rather than in children during the first year of life. Ricks and Wing (1975), for example, showed that adults had trouble distinguishing the meaning of the cries of their preverbal preschoolers with ASD, although they could correctly interpret typical children's cries. Wetherby, Yonclas, and Bryan (1989), in a study of three prelinguistic preschoolers with ASD, found few well-formed syllables and many atypical vocalizations, such as growling and tongue clicking. Sheinkopf, Mundy, Oller, and Steffens (2000) reported on a group of preschool age-children with language levels at 15 months and found a similar rate of production of atypical sounds, although they did find that well-formed syllables were also produced. Wetherby et al. (2004) reported that atypical intonation in prelinguistic vocalizations was a significant discriminator of toddlers with ASD from those with either typical development or other developmental disabilities.

Heilmann, Ullstadius, Dahlgren, and Gillberg (1992) showed that preschoolers with ASD were less likely than peers matched for mental age to imitate adult vocal productions. Similarly, Rogers, Hepburn, Stackhouse, and Wehner (2003) found that 2-year-olds with autism were significantly more impaired in overall imitation abilities, as well as in oral–facial imitation, as compared with age mates with other developmental disabilities. Thus, although echolalia is a behavior commonly attributed to speakers with ASD, at the very early stages of communication, when echoing is a typical and useful strategy for learning speech, children with ASD are less likely than other toddlers to copy the speech they hear. Despite the suggestions of the findings cited here, the trajectory of early vocal development from the first weeks to the end of the first year of life has not yet been studied in infants who go on to show ASD.

Prelinguistic Interaction and Communication

Infants' early vocalizations appear to constitute proto-conversations with parents (Bateson, 1975). Other early forms of interaction include making eye contact with the parents (at about 1 month of age), smiling and laughing in response to speech (at 2 months), and vocalizing in response to sounds (at 4 months). These very early patterns of back-and-forth activity lay the basis for many later developing forms of reciprocity, including participation in interactive games, such as "pat-a-cake," and eventually in turn taking in conversation. Babies may also begin to imitate some of the parent's intonation patterns (Trevarthen, 1979), and by 3 months of age show more vocal responsiveness to their mothers than to other adults. As a baby gains better motor coordination, more formal interactions occur, such as pat-a-cake or peek-a-boo games, waving bye-bye, or "following" conversations by looking first at one person and then another.

Babies use gaze extensively to regulate interactions. They look at the parent when they are interested in interacting and avert their gaze when they become tired or overstimulated (Stern, 1977). Likewise, babies are sensitive to changes in parental gaze during interactions. Infants as young as 14 weeks smile significantly more when an adult's gaze is directed toward them than during periods of averted gaze (Hains & Muir, 1996). It seems likely that, from very early on, typically developing babies are sensitive to gaze as a signal of initiation and termination of social interaction. Babies can also follow their parents' gaze to attend to an object they look and/or point at, and appear to do so reliably by 1 year of age (Moore & Corkum, 1998; Morissette, Ricard, & Decarie, 1995). They also begin to direct the parents' attention by looking at objects themselves. Parents then follow the infant's line of regard and look at what the baby looks at. Frequently, parents comment on this object of the baby's gaze. These interactions, in which the parent and child share focus on an object, have been called "joint attention routines" (Bruner, 1977) and are thought to be very important in laying the foundation for the basic topic–comment structure of language in which one speaker directs the other's attention to a focus of interest, on which the conversation then elaborates. Several studies (e.g., Baldwin, 1995; Brookes & Meltzoff, 2005) have shown that infants' ability to engage in joint attention is related to their later language development.

At about 8 months of age, babies begin to develop the representational and intentional skills that allow them to hold goals in mind long enough to pursue them through action. Cognitive development at this time also supports the ability to understand actions as a means to an end, and babies begin to use communication as a means to the outcomes—in gaining parental attention or the acquisition of objects—that they desire. Such communicative acts generally become manifest at the same time other forms of intentional behavior emerge—about 8–10 months of age.

Communication at this stage is expressed primarily with gestures, such as holding an object up for the mother to view, or pointing. Acredolo and Goodwyn (1988) reported that the communicative use of symbolic gestures, often invented by the child, is quite common during the last half of the first year of life. They found that some children as young as 11 months of age used relatively stable gestures that resembled manual signs to stand for objects or actions for the purpose of communication, without having been taught any gestural system. For example, a child may bounce up and down to indicate "rabbit" or press on the eyes to indicate "sun." Often these gestures are accompanied by a look at the parent to see that he or she is attending. Capone and McGregor (2004) report that early use of gestures is a significant predictor of language acquisition in both typical and atypical development.

Bates (1976) categorized early intentional behaviors into two broad types based on their communicative function: *protoimperatives* and *protodeclaratives*. Protoimperative speech acts are those in which the child attempts to get the listener to do something for him or her, or to stop doing something, and appear to evolve into linguistic imperatives or commands. Protoimperative speech acts include requests for objects, which the child can indicate by pointing or reaching. Requests for actions, which the child can convey by miming some part of a familiar ritual, also fall into this category. For example, a child may climb on the mother's lap and touch his nose to indicate that he wants his mother to play the "body-part-naming game" that is frequently a part of interactive routines at this stage. Protests or rejections also occur, in which the child communicates, by pushing away or turning away, the desire to turn down some object or activity the mother is attempting to offer. Protodeclarative speech acts direct the mother's attention to an object of the child's interest; the child points to it, holds it up, shows, or gives it to accomplish this act. These acts are thought to lay the basis for the later use of referential language. Protodeclarative speech acts are thought to evolve out of the earlier-established joint attentional routines that appear to be very important for later language development.

As babies begin to evidence intentional communication, parents "up the ante" (Bruner & Garton, 1978), requiring a more sophisticated form of response in order for it to "count" as the child's turn. Whereas we saw earlier that parents accepted any child behavior, such as a burp or a cough, as a communicative act, when true intentionality does develop, they begin to require the child to do something more intentional in order to fulfill a turn. The child is now expected to imitate the parent, produce a conventional gesture, and eventually to vocalize. In this way, the baby's communication is "shaped" into language.

Prelinguistic Communication in Infants with ASD

Studies of early communication in children with ASD reveal that their rates of communicative expression are lower and that they are less likely to engage people visually or direct their acts to the communication partners with gaze (Stone, Ounsley, Yoder, Hogan, & Hepburn, 1997; Wetherby, Cain, Yonclas, & Walker, 1988). A failure to develop the ability to follow others' gaze and to use gaze to direct others and share attention to objects is one of the most frequent findings in studies of young children with ASD (Stone et al., 1997; Wetherby et al., 2004; see Mundy & Burnette, 2005, for review), and these joint attention behaviors have been found to have a strong predictive relationship to language development in children with ASD (Charman, Drew, Baird, & Baird, 2003; Rogers et al., 2003; Sigman & Ruskin, 1999; Wetherby et al., 2004), as they do in children with typical development.

Studies of early gestural expression in young children with ASD show this to be another area of significant difference. Toddlers with ASD have been shown to fail either to respond to communicative gestures of others, or to use conventional gestures, especially pointing, as a means of communication. These children often employ gestures that appear to use another as a tool, such as grabbing an adult's hand and moving it toward a desired object, and fail to pair these gestures with gaze directed to the adult. However, 2-year-olds with ASD were not shown to differ from peers with intellectual disability in their production of reaching, giving, or touching objects (Stone et al., 1997).

When they do communicate, children with ASD have been shown in several studies (Curcio, 1978; Dawson, Meltzoff, Osterling, Rinaldi, & Brown, 1998; Mundy, Sigman, & Kasari, 1994; Sigman, Mundy, Sherman, & Ungerer, 1986; Wetherby et al., 2004) to be able to express wants and needs with a variety of means, including their atypical gestures, with a frequency similar to that seen in typical peers. However, their communicative acts are disproportionately proto-imperative. Children with ASD frequently request objects and actions, as well as reject and protest proffered objects and activities. They differ from children with typical development, however, in producing a greatly reduced frequency of the proto-declarative acts that emerge from early joint attentional interactions. Thus, delays in the development of language that are so common in young children with ASD are forecast by significant deficits in the development of prelinguistic communication skills that allow typical children to make the transition to conventional language.

UNDERSTANDING LANGUAGE

Although parents often act as if they believe their child understands language almost from the first day of life, true lexical comprehension does not emerge until somewhat later. By 6 months, typically developing children respond to their names and to "no" (Spitz, 1957). By 8 months, a few words associated with games such as "pat-a-cake" or "so big" are recognized. Infants gradually become more active responders to these routines (Bruner, 1977). This early comprehension is contextually bound, however.

If the baby is used to playing pat-a-cake on the changing table but is told to clap hands in the bathtub, the child will probably not comply.

By 12 months, merely saying the words ("Let's play pat-a-cake!" or "Show me your nose") often elicits a spontaneous action from the child such as clapping or touching the nose (Chapman, 2000). At this age, children also show clear evidence of understanding some words or even simple phrases, responding appropriately to specific words outside the context of routine games (Huttenlocher, 1974; Tomasello & Kruger, 1992). Parents often believe that their toddlers understand everything they hear; however, studies of early language comprehension in highly structured settings have suggested that young children do not understand many more words than they are able to say (Bloom, 1993; Chapman, 2000). When parents are asked to report the kinds of words and instructions that their young children are able to understand, they typically give much higher estimates than is observed during formal testing. Using a standard questionnaire (Fenson et al., 1993), parents estimated that their 8-month-olds understood an average of 6 phrases and about 20 words, increasing to an average of 23 phrases and 169 words by 16 months.

Comprehension in ordinary situations may be achieved by a variety of nonlinguistic strategies that allow children to respond to what their parents say, when in fact they are responding to what their parents do or what they know about the way things usually happen. Chapman (1978) pointed out that this contextually bound comprehension often leads parents to believe that babies at 8–12 months understand much more of language than they actually do. Chapman described a set of strategies for comprehension that are frequently used by infants of this age to comply with parental requests and that give the parent the impression the child is actually understanding language. These are summarized in Table 4.2. Few parents truly test their children's language comprehension by asking them to do things completely out of context (e.g., asking a child to go get Mommy's keys from the bedroom during a family meal), and this "conspiracy" between the parent, who asks the child to do things he or she was likely to do anyway, and the child, who marshals information from several sources in order to interact cooperatively with the parent, results in children's having many opportunities to hear words that match the actions they are performing—and thus to learn more language—as well as to engage in social interactions that are rewarding for both parties.

Children in the second year of life do acquire knowledge of a large number of word meanings, with the average receptive vocabulary size at 50 words by 15 months, and in the hundreds by the second birthday (Fenson et al., 1993). Ability to understand word combinations is limited to one or two words per utterance, but the strategies outlined above allow the child to engage successfully with adults who choose their instructions judiciously to match the child's predilections.

TABLE 4.2. Summary of Comprehension Abilities in Children Younger Than 2 Years

Age	Comprehension ability	Comprehension strategy	Example
8–12 months	Understands a few single words in routine contexts	• Looks at objects mother looks at • Acts on objects noticed • Imitates ongoing action	• Baby looks at ball Mom is looking at when she says, "Get the ball! Throw it to Mommy!" • Baby moves toward ball Mom is looking at. • Baby imitates Mom's gesture for throwing ball.
12–18 months	Understands single words outside of routine but still requires some contextual support	• Locates objects mentioned • Gives evidence of notice • Does what you usually do	• Baby finds ball among toys on floor when she says, "Get the ball! Throw it to Mommy!" • Baby picks up ball. • Baby throws ball.
18–24 months	Understands words for absent objects, some two-term combinations	• Puts objects in containers, on surfaces • Acts on objects in the way mentioned (child as agent)	• Baby puts ball in cup when Mom says, "Put the ball in the cup!" • Baby pushes ball when Mom says, "Make the dolly push the ball!"

Note. Data from Chapman (1978).

Language Comprehension in ASD

One of the most frequently reported early signs of ASD in the first year of life is a reduced tendency to respond to others' speech, particularly to the child's own name, and this observation is consistent in the second and third years as well (Lord, 1995; Osterling & Dawson, 1994). Gosse, Paul, and Chawarska (2006) reported that 2-year-olds with ASD differed from peers with typical or delayed development in the number of words and phrases parents reported they understood; however, they differed significantly from mental-age (MA)-matched children with other developmental disorders only in the ability to respond to common phrases, such as "come here." These findings suggest that toddlers with ASD may be as able as mental-age mates to form associations between objects and their verbal labels, but are less able than children without ASD to make the contextually appropriate responses that children with typical development use as strategies to "fool" parents into believing they have high levels of understanding. In fact, formal testing of children with ASD at this age finds scores on language comprehension that were as low as those seen in expressive language (DiLavore, Lord, & Rutter, 1995; Paul, Chawarska, Klin, et al., 2007), both of which are significantly delayed relative to both chronological and mental age. Moreover, an aberrant pattern of higher expressive than receptive test performance was seen in some toddlers with ASD, a pattern very rarely observed in children with typical development or in those with other developmental disabilities (Paul, Chawarska, Klin, et al., 2007). Part of the reason for this finding may be that these children showed a reduced tendency, relative to same-age peers, to attend to child-directed speech when tested in a laboratory situation (Nadig, Ozonoff, Singh, Young, & Rogers, 2006; Paul, Chawarska, Fowler, et al., 2007). Thus, toddlers with ASD may be less inherently interested in speech than are typical peers, spend less time actively listening to it, and thus have less experience with making sense of speech in the context of ongoing events. This reduction in experience may be one of the reasons for the slow growth of receptive vocabulary seen in these children, which in turn may help to account for the protracted course of language development typical of this population, even in children with relatively strong nonverbal cognition.

FIRST WORDS

The conventional use of language begins at about 12 months in typical development, when toddlers usually say their first recognizable words. This development is closely related to the acquisition of the consonant sounds used in a language (Stoel-Gammon, 2003). Research in the area of sound development has shown that between 12 and 24 months of age, typical children produce most of the consonant sounds of their language and are beginning to produce a range of syllable structures to support the production of words (Stoel-Gammon, 2002). Typical children say their first words at 12–15 months of age. During the 12- to 18-month period, there is a gradual increase in both receptive and expressive vocabulary. The words children learn in this period name objects and people, usually those on which the child acts (e.g., *daddy, mommy, cookie, ball*) and describe relationships between objects (e.g., *all gone, more*) (Fenson et al., 1993). Children also learn social words to be used in rituals such as greetings. Much like early gestures, first words are often used to express ideas such as appearance ("Uh-oh"), disappearance ("All gone") and recurrence ("More"), related to the child's developing notions of object permanence (Bloom & Lahey, 1978; Gopnik & Meltzoff, 1987).

By the age of 18 months, expressive vocabulary size typically reaches an average of about 50–100 words (Fenson et al., 1994; Nelson, 1973) and the "word explosion" begins. This period may be punctuated by many requests from children for adults to label things in the world around them, and words are now learned very quickly, often after only a single exposure without any explicit instruction. This stage marks an important turning point, as children are no longer learning via association; instead, they understand the referential nature of words (Nazzi & Bertoncini, 2003) and are able now to use words to get new information about the world (Halliday, 1975). By 16–19 months infants are able to use nonverbal cues, such as an adult's eye gaze, to make quite fine distinctions between an object that an adult is naming and another object that happens to be present (Baldwin, 1991; Fernald, Marchman, Hurtado, & Zangl, 2006), suggesting that they can now understand the intentions of others within language contexts. Similar findings for learning words to describe actions have been reported for 2-year-olds (Tomasello & Kruger, 1992).

Between 18 and 24 months, typical children begin combining words to form two-word "telegraphic" utterances (Brown, 1973) encoding a small set of meanings. Children talk about objects by naming them and by discussing their locations or attributes, who owns them, and who is doing things to them. They also talk about other people, their actions, their locations, their own actions on objects, and so forth. Objects, people, actions, and their interrelationships preoccupy the typically developing young child. Thus, early language development, from gestures to single words to beginning sentences, is in many ways a remarkably organized process that reflects both how young children think about the world (e.g., recognition of the coming and going of things and people) and what is important to them (e.g., things that they can act on, interesting events such as going outside or wiping up a spill). Individual differences exist among typically developing children, but language development follows a generally consistent pattern, with forms being acquired and put to use in order to interact more elaborately with others.

Early Language in Children with ASD

Children with ASD, as we have seen, produce fewer vocalizations and do less vocal imitation than peers with typical development. They also produce a narrower range of consonant sounds than their age mates (Schoen, Paul, Chawarska, Klin, & Volkmar, 2004). Given the close relationship between sound and word production in early language development, it should not be surprising that children with ASD, who have fewer sounds available to them, produce fewer words than typically developing peers.

Parents' most pressing concerns in the second year of life for children with ASD are typically in the area of speech. Acquisition of first words is usually delayed. Paul, Chawarska, Klin, et al. (2007), for example, reported that 36% of children with ASD over the age of 2 still had no expressive language. Parents may also become concerned at this time because the child has learned a few words but has never gone farther, or has lost the early words acquired. About 20% of children who are later included on the autism spectrum are reported to experience a regression in skills, usually a loss of the ability to say words, during their second year (Chawarska et al., 2007; Hoshino et al., 1987; Kobayashi, 1993; Kurita, 1985; Lord, Shulman, & DiLavore, 2004; Rogers & DiLalla, 1990; Tuchman & Rapin, 1997). Even when children begin acquiring words, expressive vocabulary size tends to lag about 6 months behind nonverbal mental age for toddlers on the ASD spectrum with both average and delayed nonverbal cognitive development (Paul, Chawarska, Klin, et al., 2007).

Children with ASD are also delayed in making the transition from single words to multiword speech. Paul, Chawarska, Klin, et al. (2007) reported that even children who had begun using single words and who had, on average, more than 100 words in their expressive vocabularies, were not routinely combining words by 28 months of age, even though typically developing children with this expressive vocabulary size do use multiword utterances (Fenson et al., 1993). Children in this sample who were not speaking at age 2 but had acquired some speech by age 4 were just beginning to combine words in their utterances at the latter age. Moreover, throughout the second and third years of life, children with ASD continued to show the deficits in use of gaze, imitation, joint attention, conventional gestures, attention to speech and faces, and interest in sharing interests and feelings that characterized their earlier development (see Chawarska & Volkmar, 2005, and Mundy & Burnette, 2005, for reviews). Although some children do make significant progress in language during this period, acquiring a large number of words and scoring within their mental-age-appropriate range on expressive and receptive language testing (Paul, Chawarska, Klin, et al., 2007), their communication remains problematic. They use echolalia excessively, their speech is often self-directed, repetitive, and without communicative function, oddities of prosody may begin to appear, and the content of their language is impoverished and insufficient to sustain age-appropriate conversation or play (Tager-Flusberg, Paul, & Lord, 2005). Although the achievement of functional language use continues to be associated with better outcomes for children with ASD (Howlin, Goode, Hutton, & Rutter, 2004), and a larger proportion of children than previously reported are currently acquiring some language during the preschool period (Paul, Chawarska, Klin, et al., 2007; Rogers, 2006), perhaps as a response to earlier identification and intervention, the acquisition of spoken language does not erase the more fundamental deficits in communication that characterize the autism spectrum.

ASSESSING EARLY COMMUNICATION IN ASD

As we have seen, communicative behaviors are significantly impaired in very young children with ASD. At the prelinguistic level of communication, impairments are prominent in the following areas:

- Depressed rate of preverbal communicative acts (Wetherby, Prizant, & Hutchinson, 1998; Wetherby et al., 2004).
- Delayed development of pointing gestures, in terms of both use and responsiveness (Dawson et al., 1998).
- Use of nonconventional means of communicating, such as pulling a person by the hand instead of pointing or looking (Stone et al., 1997).
- Reduced responsiveness to speech and to (children's) hearing their names called (Mundy & Stella, 2000; Nadig et al., 2006; Osterling & Dawson, 1994; Paul, Chawarska, Fowler, et al., 2007).
- Restricted range of communicative behaviors, limited primarily to regulatory functions (getting people to do or not do things), with very limited use of communication for social interaction or to comment or establish joint attention (Mundy & Stella, 2000; Wetherby et al., 2004).
- Atypical preverbal vocalizations (Sheinkopf et al., 2000).
- Deficits in pretend and imaginative play (Rogers, 2005).
- Limited ability to imitate (Heilmann et al., 1992; Rogers et al., 2003).

In order to identify patterns of communication consistent with a diagnosis of ASD in children under 3, assessment at this stage focuses on these areas. Standard early communication assessments can be used to, first, substantiate the presence of a significant delay in communication development. Both direct observation and parent report measures are valuable at this stage, inasmuch as very young children may not be able to demonstrate their full repertoires of behaviors in a brief, unfamiliar setting. As a result, parent report measures provide an important check on the observations made during the clinical evaluation. Instruments like those listed in Table 4.3 can be used for this phase of assessment.

Following the establishment of a significant delay by means of standard measures like those shown in Table 4.3, the communication evaluation of infants and toddlers suspected of ASD can focus more sharply on the areas known to be particularly impaired in these syndromes. These areas, as we have discussed, include rate of communication (verbal or nonverbal), use of communicative gaze and gestures, quality of vocalization, responsiveness to speech and gestures, range of communicative

TABLE 4.3. Communication Assessment Instruments for Infants and Toddlers

Assessment instrument	Age range	Area(s) assessed	Assessment method
Clinical Linguistic and Auditory Milestone Scale (Capute et al., 1986)	0–36 months	Expressive/receptive language	Observational scale
Communicative Development Inventory–III (Fenson et al., 2006)	8–36 months	Expressive/receptive vocabulary, gestures, play, early sentences	Parent report
Early Language Milestone Scale (Coplan, 1993)	0–36 months	Expressive/receptive language	Pass/fail screening
Initial Communication Processes Scale (Schery & Wilcoxen, 1982)	0–36 months	Preverbal and verbal communication	Observational scale
Language Development Survey (Rescorla, 1989)	12–36 months	Expressive vocabulary	Parent report
Mullen Scales of Early Learning	0–5 years	Expressive/receptive language	Standardized test
Preschool Language Scale–4 (Zimmerman et al., 2002)	0–7 years	Expressive/receptive language	Standardized test
Receptive-Expressive Emergent Language Scale (Bzoch, League, & Brown, 2003)	0–36 months	Expressive/receptive language	Parent report
Reynell Developmental Language Scale (Reynell & Gruber, 1990)	0–7 years	Expressive/receptive language	Standardized test
Rosetti Infant Toddler Language Scale–2nd Ed. (Rosetti, 2001)	0–36 months	Preverbal and verbal communication	Criterion-referenced measure
Vineland Adaptive Behavior Scale–II (Sparrow, Cicchetti, & Balla, 2005)	0–18 years	Expressive/receptive/written language	Caregiver report/ structured interview

functions expressed (whether restricted to regulatory functions or including social interaction and joint attentional functions), and use of play schemes. Although standard assessments can be used to demonstrate a significant delay in communicative functioning, they do not provide the information necessary to differentiate children with ASD from children with other kinds of developmental difficulties. To make this distinction, it is necessary to employ naturalistic interactions that maximize the child's opportunity for demonstrating his or her most typical interaction style, and that tap the aspects of social interaction that are most likely to be impaired in ASD. Several instruments have been developed to structure play-like interactions that allow the sampling and assessment of these preverbal communicative behaviors. These instruments include:

- Communication and Symbolic Behavior Scales (CSBS; Wetherby & Prizant, 2003).
- Early Scale of Communication and Socialization (Mundy et al., 2003).
- Communication Intention Inventory (Paul, 2007).
- Prelinguistic Communication Assessment (Stone, 1997).
- Autism Diagnostic Observation Schedule–Generic, Module 1 (Lord et al., 2000).

These scales use a variety of techniques, such as communicative "temptations," to elicit the target behaviors, then compare the rate of production of these behaviors in children with suspected autism to the rates seen in similar elicitation conditions with typically developing children. By observing a child in these structured play settings and noting the child's responses to the proffered activities, an evaluator can discern the communicative patterns that are typical of children with autism. This information, combined with scores on the standard communication measures, can be used to document deficits in the key areas of social communicative functioning that characterize the autism spectrum in the period before age 3. These assessments can then be used to document:

- That even when "tempted" to communicate, the child initiates communication infrequently (less than one act/minute [Chapman, 2000]).
- That the child does not spontaneously point or use other conventional gestures, and/or shows a low level of response to the conventional gestures of others.
- That the child uses unconventional gestures, such as pulling a person by the hand.
- That the child shows inconsistent orientation to speech and name.

- An imbalance between frequency of protoimperative and proto-declarative communicative productions.
- That even when tempted to show and share, with the availability of interesting objects, the child does not seek to engage others in his or her interests or enjoyment.
- That the child shows deficits in functional and pretend play, even when these schemes are modeled directly.
- The use of atypical vocalizations, such as a high prevalence of squeaks, squeals, and growls.
- Unusual features such as atypical vocal and intonational behavior, echoing, and stereotyped phrases, when speech is present.

Not all the instruments listed earlier provide specific contexts for observing all of these behaviors. Thus, clinicians may need to supplement the standard elicitation contexts provided by these measures with additional informal probes in order to have an opportunity to observe the full spectrum of behaviors associated with early communication in ASD. The results of these observations, in combination with more formal assessments of language and communication on standard instruments, can serve both to document the presence of deficits in social communication and to provide information on areas of communicative strengths and needs that can serve as a basis for developing a therapeutic program to address these deficits.

SUMMARY AND IMPLICATIONS

Although there are few direct empirical data on the development of autism in the earliest months of life, the information that is available suggests that children with this condition show very early-occurring deficits, relative to typical peers, in several areas that are likely to impact the development of both language and communication. These include reduced preferences for faces and voices and subsequent reduced responses to speech and people; failure to use gaze to regulate interaction through mutual gaze and engagement in joint attention routines; poor imitation of both gestures and sounds, with concomitant reductions in the use of conventional gestures (especially pointing) and the development of the sound-making skills necessary for expressive language acquisition; a range of early communicative acts restricted primarily to requesting and protesting; and reduced interest in back-and-forth activities that lay the basis for conversation. Communicative deficits do not disappear with development, and they impact the acquisition of conventional language. Significant delays are present at each of the important transitions in early language development: the emergence of first preverbal communicative acts, the production of single words, the development of knowledge or word meaning, the vocabulary "spurt," and the acquisition of multiword utterances. But even when these milestones are achieved, the language of children with ASD continues to function in the context of restricted social motivation and interpersonal connection.

For clinicians who address the needs of very young children with ASD, the necessity of assessing and managing not only conventional language, but its foundations in communication, is paramount. Nonspeaking children suspected of autism should be evaluated for the frequency, range, and functions of their preverbal communicative acts, and their means of communication documented. Children with limited communicative intentions need to experience intensive, rewarding opportunities for engaging in joint attention, using and responding to gestures, and imitating vocal productions as a foundation for language acquisition. Once speech emerges, its use must be carefully guided and organized, so that its communicative value is constantly stressed and reinforced. Teaching speech outside the context of communication is unlikely to result in optimal social functioning.

For researchers, the task of finding earlier identifiers that differentiate children with ASD from those with other developmental disorders remains. It is unlikely that one marker, such as gaze preference, speech perception, or imitative ability, will be sufficient, but perhaps a combination of these markers may be shown to be discriminative. Ongoing research with children at risk for autism because of its presence in an older sibling will undoubtedly contribute to this effort. However, identifying ASD earlier in life will not be helpful unless effective intervention strategies that are practicable at the earliest phases of development can be found. Here an in-depth understanding of the ways in which typical children integrate the multiple strands of development that enable successful social communication will be crucial. Thus, a major challenge to clinical researchers in the next decade will be the development and empirical validation of methods to "teach" children with ASD to do what comes entirely naturally to other children: to listen to speech, to look at people, to imitate what others do. Such methods will most likely involve placing artificial contingencies, such as reinforcement, on the engagement in these behaviors that typical children find rewarding for their own sake. But evidence from early intervention research in disorders more easily recognized in the first year of life (Guralnick, 1998) suggests that intensifying developmentally appropriate experiences and engaging families in early intervention can have significant and long-lasting effects in ameliorating the level of impairment for children with developmental disorders. Similar outcomes for young children with ASD may be on the horizon.

ACKNOWLEDGMENTS

Preparation of this chapter was supported by Research Grant No. P01-03008 funded by the National Institute of Mental Health; by STAART Center Grant No. U54 MH66494 funded by the National Institute on Deafness and Communication Disorders (NIDCD), the National Institute of Environmental Health Sciences, the National Institute of Child Health and Human Development, and the National Institute of Neurological Disorders and Stroke; by Research Grant No. R01 DC07129 from the NIDCD; by MidCareer Development Grant No. K24 HD045576 funded by the NIDCD; as well as by the National Alliance for Autism Research.

REFERENCES

Acredolo, L. P., & Goodwyn, S. (1988). Symbolic gesturing in normal infants. *Child Development, 59*(2), 450–466.

Aslin, R. N., & Smith, L. B. (1988). Perceptual development. *Annual Review of Psychology, 39*, 435–473.

Baldwin, D. A. (1991). Infants' contribution to the achievement of joint reference. *Child Development, 62*, 875–890.

Baldwin, D. A. (1995). Understanding the link between joint attention and language. In C. Moore & P. J. Dunham (Eds.), *Joint attention: Its origins and role in development* (pp. 131–158). Hillsdale, NJ: Erlbaum.

Bates, E. (1976). *Language in context.* New York: Academic Press.

Bateson, M. C. (1975). Mother–infant exchanges: The epigenesis of conversational interaction. *Annals of the New York Academy of Sciences, 263*, 101–113.

Bloom, L. (1993). *The transition from infancy to language.* New York: Cambridge University Press.

Bloom, L., & Lahey, M. (1978). *Language development and language disorders.* New York: Wiley.

Brookes, R., & Meltzoff, A. (2005). The development of gaze following and its relation to language. *Developmental Science, 8*(6), 535.

Brown, R. (1973). *A first language, the early stages.* Cambridge, MA: Harvard University Press.

Bruner, J. (1977). Early social interaction and language acquisition. In R. Schaffer (Ed.), *Studies in mother–infant interaction* (pp. 247–263). New York: Academic Press.

Bruner, J. S., & Garton, A. (1978). *Human growth and development: Wolfson College Lectures 1976* (p. viii). Oxford, UK: Oxford University Press.

Butterfield, E., & Siperstein, G. (1974). *Influence of contingent auditory stimulation upon non-nutritional suckle.* Paper presented at the Proceedings of the Third Symposium on Oral Sensation and Perception: The Mouth of the Infant, Springfield, IL.

Bzoch, K., League, R., & Brown, V. (2003). *The Receptive Expressive Emergent Language Test–third edition.* Austin, TX: PRO-ED.

Capone, N. C., & McGregor, K. K. (2004). Gesture development: A review for clinical and research practices. *Journal of Speech, Language, and Hearing Research,* *47*(1), 173–186.

Capute, A., Palmer, F., Shapiro, B., Wachtel, R., Schmidt, S., & Ross, A. (1986). Clinical Linguistic and Auditory Milestone Scale: Prediction of cognition in infancy. *Developmental Medicine and Child Neurology,* *28,* 762–771.

Carter, A. (1979). Prespeech meaning relations: An outline of one infant's sensorimotor development. In P. Fletcher & M. Garman (Eds.), *Language acquisition* (pp. 320–361). Cambridge, MA: Cambridge University Press.

Chapman, R. (1978). Comprehension strategies in children. In J. F. Cavanagh & W. Strange (Eds.), *Speech and language in laboratory, school, and clinic* (pp. 308–327). Cambridge, MA: MIT Press.

Chapman, R. (2000). Children's language learning: An interactionist perspective. *Journal of Child Psychology and Psychiatry,* *41,* 33–54.

Charman, T., Drew, A., Baird, C., & Baird, G. (2003). Measuring early language development in preschool children with autism spectrum disorder using the MacArthur Communicative Development Inventory (infant form). *Journal of Child Language,* *30*(1), 213–236.

Chawarska, K., Paul, R., Klin, A., Hannigen, S., Dichtel, L., & Volkmar, R. (2007). Parental recognition of developmental problems in toddlers with autism spectrum disorder. *Journal of Autism and Developmental Disorders,* *37,* 62–72.

Chawarska, K., & Volkmar, F. (2005). Autism in infancy and early childhood. In F. Volkmar, R. Paul, A. Klin, & D. Cohen (Eds.), *Handbook of autism and pervasive developmental disorders* (Vol. 1, pp. 223–246). New York: Wiley.

Colombo, J., O'Brien, M., Mitchell, D., Roberts, K., & Horowitz, F. (1987). A lower boundary for category formation in preverbal infants. *Journal of Child Language,* *14*(2), 383–385.

Cooper, R., & Aslin, R. (1994). Developmental differences in infant attention to the spectral properties of infant-directed speech. *Child Development,* *65,* 1663–1678.

Coplan, J., (1993). *Early Language Milestone Scale (ELM Scale-2).* Austin, TX: PRO-ED.

Curcio, R. (1978). Sensorimotor functioning and communication in mute autistic children. *Journal of Autism and Childhood Schizophrenia,* *8,* 281–292.

Dawson, G., Meltzoff, A., Osterling, J., Rinaldi, J., & Brown, E. (1998). Neuropsychological correlates of early symptoms of autism. *Child Development,* *69*(5), 1276–1285.

Dawson, G., Osterling, J., Meltzoff, A. N., & Kuhl, P. (2000). Case study of the development of an infant with autism from birth to two years of age. *Journal of Applied Developmental Psychology,* *21*(3), 299–313.

DiLavore, P., Lord, C., & Rutter, M. (1995). Prelinguistic Autism Diagnostic Observation Schedule. *Journal of Applied Developmental Psychology,* *25*(4), 355–379.

Eimas, P. D. (1975). Auditory and phonetic coding of the cues for speech: Discrimination of the (r–l) distinction by young infants. *Perception and Psychophysics,* *18*(5), 341–347.

Eimas, P. D., Siqueland, E. R., Jusczyk, P., & Vigorito, J. (1971). Speech perception in infants. *Science,* *171*(3968), 303–306.

Fenson, L., Dale, P. S., Reznick, J., Bates, E., Thal, D., & Pethick, S. (1994). Variability in early communicative development. *Monographs of the Society for Research in Child Development, 59*(5), v-173.

Fenson, L., Dale, P., Reznick, J., Thal, D., Bates, E., Hartung, J. P., et al. (1993). *The MacArthur Communicative Development Inventories: User's guide and technical manual.* San Diego: Singular.

Fernald, A. (1983). The perceptual and affective salience of mothers' speech to infants. In L. Feagans (Ed.), *The origins and growth of communication.* (pp. 5-29). New Brusnwick, NJ: Ablex.

Fernald, A., Marchman, V., Hurtado, N., & Zangl, R. (2006, November). *Online speech processing efficiency is related both to early vocabulary growth and to later language accomplishments.* Paper presented at the Boston University Conference on Child Language Development, Boston.

Gopnik, A., & Meltzoff, A. (1987). The development of categorization in the second year and its relation to other cognitive and linguistic developments. *Child Development, 58*(6), 1523-1531.

Gosse, C., Paul, R., & Chawarska, K. (2006, November). *Come here and come hear: Understanding of phrases in toddlers with ASD.* Paper presented at the National Convention of the American Speech, Language, and Hearing Association, Miami, FL.

Graham, J. M., Bashir, A. S., & Stark, R. E. (1999). Communicative disorders. In M. D. Levine, W. B. Carey, A. C. Crocker, et al. (Eds.), *Developmental-behavioral pediatrics* (3rd ed., pp. 847-864). Philadelphia: Saunders.

Guralnick, M. J. (1998). Effectiveness of early intervention for vulnerable children: A developmental perspective. *American Journal on Mental Retardation, 102*(4), 319-345.

Hains, M. J., & Muir, D. W. (1996). Infant sensitivity to adult eye direction. *Journal of Child Language, 67*, 1940-1951.

Halliday, M. (1975). *Learning how to mean: Explorations in the development of language.* New York: Arnold.

Heilmann, M., Ullstadius, E., Dahlgren, S., & Gillberg, C. (1992). Imitation in autism: A preliminary research note. *Behavioural Neurology, 5*, 219-227.

Hepper, P. G., Scott, D., & Shahidullah, S. (1993). Newborn and fetal response to maternal voice. *Journal of Reproductive and Infant Psychology, 11*, 147-153.

Hirsh-Pasek, K., Kemler Nelson, D. G., Jusczyk, P. W., Cassidy, K. W., Druss, B., & Kennedy, L. (1987). Clauses are perceptual units for young infants. *Cognition, 26*(3), 269-286.

Hoshino, Y., Kaneko, M., Yashima, Y., Kumashiro, H., Volkmar, F. R., & Cohen, D. J. (1987). Clinical features of autistic children with setback course in their infancy. *Japanese Journal of Psychiatry and Neurology, 41*, 237-245.

Howlin, P., Goode, S., Hutton, J., & Rutter, M. (2004). Adult outcome for children with autism. *Journal of Child Psychology and Psychiatry and Allied Disciplines, 45*(2), 212-213.

Hutt, S., Hutt, C., Lenard, H., Bernuth, H., & Jewerff, W. (1968). Auditory responsivity in the human newborn. *Nature, 218*, 888-890.

Huttenlocher, J. (1974). The origins of language comprehension. In J. Huttenlocher & R. L. Solso (Eds.), *Theories in cognitive psychology: The Loyola Symposium.* Hillsdale, NJ: Erlbaum.

Jusczyk, P. W. (1999a). How infants begin to extract words from speech. *Trends in Cognitive Science, 3*, 323–328.

Jusczyk, P. W. (1999b). Narrowing the distance to language: One step at a time. *Journal of Communication Disorders, 32*(4), 207–222.

Jusczyk, P., Houston, D., & Newsome, M. (1999). The beginning of word segmentation in English-learning infants. *Cognitive Psychology, 39*, 159–207.

Kagan, J., & Lewis, M. (1965). Studies of attention in the human infant. *Merrill–Palmer Quarterly, 11*(2), 95–127.

Klin, A. (1992). Listening preference in regard to speech: A possible characterization of the symptom of social withdrawal. *Journal of Autism and Developmental Disorders, 21*, 29–42.

Klin, A. (2003). *Visual attention in toddlers with autism.* Paper presented at the Yale Child Study Center Associates Meeting, New Haven, CT.

Kobayashi, R. (1993). Setback phenomena and the long-term prognoses for autistic children. *Japanese Journal of Child and Adolescent Psychiatry, 34*(3), 239–248.

Kuhl, P. K., Coffey-Corina, S., Padden, D., & Dawson, G. (2005). Links between social and linguistic processing of speech in preschool children with autism: Behavioral and electrophysiological measures. *Developmental Science, 8*(1), F1–F12.

Kuhl, P. K., & Meltzoff, A. N. (1988). Speech as an intermodal object of perception. In A. Yonas (Ed.), *Perceptual development in infancy* (pp. 235–266). Hillsdale, NJ: Erlbaum.

Kuhl, P. K., & Meltzoff, A. N. (1996). Infant vocalizations in response to speech: Vocal imitation and developmental change. *Journal of the Acoustical Society of America, 100*, 2425–2438.

Kurita, H. (1985). Infantile autism with speech loss before the age of thirty months. *Journal of the American Academy of Child Psychiatry, 24*(2), 191–196.

Lord, C. (1995). Follow-up of two-year-olds referred for possible autism. *Journal of Child Psychology and Psychiatry and Allied Disciplines, 36*, 1365–1382.

Lord, C., Risi, S., Lambrecht, L., Cook, E., Leventhal, B., DiLavore, P., et al. (2000). The Autism Diagnostic Observation Schedule—Generic: A standard measure of social and communication deficits associated with the spectrum of autism. *Journal of Autism and Developmental Disorders, 30*, 205–223.

Lord, C., Shulman, C., & Dilavore, P. (2004). Regression and word loss in autistic spectrum disorders. *Journal of Child Psychology and Psychiatry, 45*, 936–955

Moon, C., Pennton-Cooper, R., & Fifer, W. (1993). Two day olds prefer their native language. *Infant Behavior and Development, 16*, 495–500.

Moore, C., & Corkum, V. (1998). Infant gaze following based on eye direction. *British Journal of Developmental Psychology, 16*(4), 495–503.

Morissette, P., Ricard, M., & Decarie, T. G. (1995). Joint visual attention and pointing in infancy: A longitudinal study of comprehension. *British Journal of Developmental Psychology, 13*(2), 163–175.

Mundy, P., & Burnette, C. (2005). Joint attention and neurodevelopmental models of autism. In F. Volkmar, R. Paul, A. Klin, & D. Cohen (Eds.), *Handbook of autism and pervasive developmental disorders* (Vol. 1, pp. 65–681). New York: Wiley.

Mundy, P., Delgado, C., Block, J., Venezia, M., Hogan, A., & Seibert, J. (2003).

Early social communication scale. Retrieved June 4, 2006, from *www.psy. miami.edu/faculty/pmundy*.

Mundy, P., Sigman, M., & Kasari, C. (1994). Joint attention, developmental level, and symptom presentation in autism. *Development and Psychopathology, 6*(3), 389–401.

Mundy, P., & Stella, J. (2000). Joint attention, social orienting, and nonverbal communication in autism. In A. M. Wetherby & B. M. Prizant (Eds.), *Autism spectrum disorders: A transactional developmental perspective* (pp. 55–77). Baltimore: Brookes.

Myers, J., Jusczyk, P. W., Kemler Nelson, D. G., Charles-Luce, J., Woodward, A. L., & Hirsch-Pasek, K. (1996). Infants' sensitivity to word boundaries in fluent speech. *Journal of Child Language, 23*(1), 1–30.

Nadig, A., Ozonoff, S., Singh, L., Young, G., & Rogers, S. (2006, November). *Do 6-month-old infants at risk for autism display an infant-directed speech preference?* Paper presented at the Boston University Conference on Child Language Development, Boston.

Nazzi, T., & Bertoncini, J. (2003). Before and after the vocabulary spurt: Two modes of word acquisition? *Developmental Science, 6*(2), 136–142.

Nelson, K. (1973). Structure and strategy in learning to talk. *Monographs of the Society for Research in Child Development, 38*, 1–2.

Oller, D., Eilers, R. E., Neal, A., & Cobo-Lewis, A. B. (1998). Late onset canonical babbling: A possible early marker for abnormal development. *American Journal on Mental Retardation, 103*(3), 249–263.

Osterling, J., & Dawson, G. (1994). Early recognition of children with autism: A study of first birthday home videotapes. *Journal of Autism and Developmental Disorders, 24*(3), 247–257.

Owens, R. (2000). *Language development* (5th ed.). Boston: Allyn & Bacon.

Paul, R. (2007). *Language disorders from infancy through adolescence: Assessment and intervention* (3rd ed.). St. Louis: Mosby.

Paul, R., Chawarska, K., Fowler, C., Cicchetti, D., & Volkmar, F. (2007). "Listen my children and you shall hear": Auditory preferences in toddlers with ASD. *Journal of Speech, Language and Hearing Research, 50*, 1350–1364.

Paul, R., Chawarska, K., Klin, A., & Volkmar, F. (2007). Dissociations in the development of early communication in ASD. In R. Paul (Ed.), *Language disorders from a developmental perspective: Essays in honor of Robin Chapman* (pp. 163–194). Hillsdale, NJ: Erlbaum.

Pegg, J., Werker, J., & McLeod, P. (1992). Preference for infant-directed over adult-directed speech: Evidence from 7-week-old infants. *Infant Behavior and Development, 15*, 325–345.

Rescorla, L. (1989). The Language Development Survey: A screening tool for delayed language in toddlers. *Journal of Speech and Hearing Disorders, 54*, 587–599.

Reynell, J., & Gruber, C. (1990). *Reynell Developmental Language Scales (American Edition)*. Los Angeles: Western Psychological Services.

Ricks, D., & Wing, L. (1975). Language, communication and use of symbols. In L. Wind (Ed.), *Early childhood autism* (pp. 93–134). Oxford, UK: Pergamon Press.

Rogers, S. (2005). Play interventions for young children with autism spectrum disorders. In L. A. Reddy, T. M. Files-Hall, C. E. Schaefer (Eds.), *Empirically based play interventions for children* (pp. 215–239). Washington, DC: American Psychological Association.

Rogers, S. (2006). Evidence-based intervention for language development in young children with autism. In T. Charman & W. Stone (Eds.), *Social and communication development in autism spectrum disorders: Early identification, diagnosis, and intervention* (pp. 143–179). New York: Guilford Press.

Rogers, S. J., & DiLalla, D. L. (1990). Age of symptom onset in young children with pervasive developmental disorders. *Journal of the American Academy of Child and Adolescent Psychiatry, 29*(6), 863–872.

Rogers, S., Hepburn, S., Stackhouse, T., & Wehner, E. (2003). Imitation performance in toddlers with autism and those with other developmental disorders. *Journal of Child Psychology and Psychiatry, 44*(5), 763–781.

Rossetti, L. (2001). *Communication intervention: Birth to three* (2nd ed.). San Diego: Singular.

Saffran, J. R., Aslin, R. N., & Newport, E. L. (1996). Statistical learning by 8-month-old infants. *Science, 274*(5294), 1926–1928.

Schery, T., & Wilcoxen, A. (1982). *The Initial Communication Processes Scale.* Monterey, CA: CTB/McGraw-Hill.

Schoen, L., Paul, R., Chawarska, K., Klin, A., & Volkmar, F. (2004). *Speech and nonspeech patterns in toddlers with autism spectrum disorders.* Paper presented at the National Convention of the American Speech, Language, and Hearing Association, Philadelphia.

Sheinkopf, J., Mundy, P., Oller, D. K., & Steffens, M. (2000). Vocal atypicalities of preverbal autistic children. *Journal of Autism and Developmental Disorders, 30,* 345–354.

Shi, R., Werker, J. F., & Morgan, J. L. (1999). Newborn infants' sensitivity to perceptual cues to lexical and grammatical words. *Cognition, 72*(2), B11–B21.

Sigman, M., Mundy, P., Sherman, T., & Ungerer, J. (1986). Social interactions of autistic, mentally retarded and normal children and their caregivers. *Journal of Child Psychology and Psychiatry and Allied Disciplines, 27,* 647–656.

Sigman, M., & Ruskin, E. (1999). Continuity and change in the social competence of children with autism, Down syndrome, and developmental delays. *Monographs of the Society for Research in Child Development, 64*(1), 114.

Sparrow, S., Cicchetti, D., and Balla, D. (2005). *Vineland Adaptive Behavior Scales-II.* Circle Pines, MN: American Guidance Service.

Spitz, R. A. (1957). *No and yes: On the genesis of human communication.* Oxford, UK: International Universities Press.

Stark, R. (1979). Prespeech segmental feature development. In P. Fletcher & M. Garman (Eds.), *Language acquisition* (pp. 149–173). New York: Cambridge University Press.

Stern, D. (1977). *The first relationship.* Cambridge, MA: Harvard University Press.

Stoel-Gammon, C. (2002). Intervocalic consonants in the speech of typically developing children: Emergence and early use. *Clinical Linguistics and Phonetics, 16*(3), 155–168.

Stoel-Gammon, C. (2003). The emergence of the speech capacity. *Journal of Child Language, 30*(3), 731–734.

Stone, W. (1997). Autism in infancy and early childhood. In D. J. Cohen & F. R. Volkmar (Eds.), *Handbook of autism and pervasive developmental disorders* (2nd ed., pp. 266–282). New York: Wiley.

Stone, W., Ounsley, O., Yoder, P., Hogan, K., & Hepburn, S. (1997). Nonverbal communication in two- and three-year old children with autism. *Journal of Autism and Developmental Disorders, 27*(6), 677–696.

Tager-Flusberg, H., Paul, R., & Lord, C. (2005). Language and communication in autism. In F. Volkmar, R. Paul, A. Klin, & D. Cohen (Eds.), *Handbook of autism and pervasive developmental disorders* (Vol. 1, pp. 335–364). New York: Wiley.

Tomasello, M., & Cale Kruger, A. (1992). Joint attention on actions: Acquiring verbs in ostensive and non-ostensive contexts. *Journal of Child Language, 19*(2), 311–333.

Trevarthen, C. (1979). Prespeech in communication of infants with adults. *Journal of Child Language, 1*, 335–337.

Tsao, F.-M., Liu, H.-M., & Kuhl, P. K. (2004). Speech perception in infancy predicts language development in the second year of life: A longitudinal study. *Child Development, 75*(4), 1067–1084.

Tuchman, R. F., & Rapin, I. (1997). Regression in pervasive developmental disorders: Seizures and epileptiform electroencephalogram correlates. *Pediatrics, 99*, 560–566.

Werker, J. F., & Tees, R. C. (1984). Phonemic and phonetic factors in adult cross-language speech perception. *Journal of the Acoustical Society of America, 75*, 1866–1878.

Werker, J. F., & Tees, R. C. (1999). Influences on infant speech processing: Toward a new synthesis. *Annual Review of Psychology, 50*, 509–535.

Werner, E., Dawson, G., Osterling, J, & Dino, N. (2000). Brief report: Recognition of autism spectrum disorders before one year of age—A retrospective study based on home videotapes. *Journal of Autism and Developmental Disorders, 30*(2), 157–162.

Wetherby, A., Cain, D., Yonclas, D., & Walker, V. (1988). Analysis of intentional communication of normal children from the prelingusitic to the multiword stage. *Journal of Speech and Hearing Research, 31*, 240–252.

Wetherby, A., & Prizant, B. (2003). *Communication and Symbolic Behavior Scales—Developmental profile.* Baltimore: Brookes.

Wetherby, A., Prizant, B., & Hutchinson, T. (1998). Communicative, social\affective, and symbolic profiles of young children with autism and pervasive developmental disorders. *American Journal of Speech-Language Pathology, 7*(2), 79–91.

Wetherby, A., Woods, J., Allen, L, Cleary, J., Dickinson, H., & Lord, C. (2004). Early indicators of autism spectrum disorders in the second year of life. *Journal of Autism and Developmental Disorders, 34*, 473–493.

Wetherby, A., Yonclas, D., & Bryan, A. (1989). Communication profiles of preschool children with handicaps: Implications for early identification. *Journal of Speech and Hearing Disorders, 54*, 148–158.

Zimmerman, I., Steiner, V., & Pond, R. (2002). *Preschool Language Scale–4.* San Antonio, TX: Psychological Corporation.

CHAPTER 5

Understanding, Assessing, and Treating Sensory–Motor Issues

GRACE T. BARANEK
LINN WAKEFORD
FABIAN J. DAVID

In addition to the defining social and communicative features of autism, many young children with this disorder demonstrate differences in sensory processing and motor performance that may impact upon social participation and daily routines. Questions about the sensory–motor features of autism continue to intrigue scientists, practitioners, and families of children with autism inasmuch as they have implications for delineating specific autism phenotypes, making intervention choices, and directing research endeavors. This chapter addresses the relevance of sensory–motor processes to understanding the development of children with autism during the first 3 years of life, and implications of sensory–motor dysfunctions for development, social participation, and engagement in daily activities. A review of current research findings and theoretical information, as well as a summary of assessments and interventions targeting sensory–motor issues, are presented. Case vignettes and excerpts from interviews are provided to illustrate specific concepts or serve as examples.

LITERATURE REVIEW

Development of Sensory–Motor Systems

Very little is known about sensory–motor functions in children with autism during infancy, because early development is often characterized in hindsight after a clinical diagnosis of autism is made during the pre-school years for the majority of these children. A knowledge of typical developmental processes is key to understanding where difficulties may arise. Many sensory–motor functions are established at birth but continue to rapidly develop and reorganize throughout the early childhood years—a process that is dependent on continued and meaningful experiences in naturally complex physical and social environments. Full-term healthy babies are born with the capacity to react to sensory stimuli such as voices and touch, can visually focus on high contrasts in close proximity, and manifest a variety of motor reflexes such as sucking, grasping, and startle. At birth, some sensory systems (e.g., touch, movement, sensation) are more developed than others (e.g., smell, hearing, vision). Sensory differ-entiation and integration processes occur across all sensory systems throughout infant development, but are dependent on continued sensory input and experiences (Lewkowicz, 2002).

Early developmental theories viewed sensory–motor development as a linear process that proceeded invariantly across children (Gesell & Thomp-son, 1943). This conceptualization led to practices of assessing the integrity of the sensory–motor systems solely through attainment of developmental motor milestones or hardwired neurological reflexes. Although a subgroup of children with autism are reported to have delays in acquisition of early motor milestones (e.g., sitting, first steps) (Johnson, Siddons, Frith, & Mor-ton, 1992) and motor delays may progressively increase with age (Ohta, Nagai, Hara, & Sasaki, 1987), the majority of these children reach motor milestones within normal ranges. Although such milestones provide impor-tant developmental records, sensory–motor development is much more complex than a series of hardwired behaviors to check off a list.

Sensory–motor systems provide a necessary foundation for percep-tion and action, as well as many important cognitive and social processes throughout life (Thelen & Smith, 1994). Adequate sensory modulation is needed to maintain appropriate physiological arousal for self-maintenance (e.g., eating, sleeping), to foster development of self-regulatory behaviors (e.g., sucking to pacify, self-talk during challenging tasks), and to support motivational systems to engage in meaningful activities (e.g., play prefer-ences) (Dunn, 1997; Parham & Ecker, 2002). Multisensory integration processes are critical to retrieving perceptions of objects and events as well as to ideation and execution of most human actions, also known as praxis (Ayres, 1985; Fogassi & Gallese, 2004). For example, the process of a young child learning to button his shirt depends on adequate neural integration of separate sensory modalities, including visual, tactile, and proprioceptive information. Multisensory stimuli that are temporally and/or spatially congruent (i.e., separate stimuli occur in close proximity, simultaneously in time, and/or are similar in context) enhance neural activity and reaction times during cognitive or motor tasks. Successful completion of a complex task, such as buttoning, for example, also requires motor control and planning. Specifically, feedforward motor systems plan movement based on prior experience, thus dictating the most efficient grasp and bimanual patterns for the child beginning to button his shirt, whereas feedback motor systems adjust for subtle errors in coordination based on incoming sensory information, such as the child feeling that he missed the buttonhole and needs to try again.

Furthermore, multisensory integration processes continually shape a child's view of his or her world by allowing perception of objects, people, and events as integrated wholes and not just as separate sensory modalities (Lewkowicz, 2002; Wallace, 2004). For instance, the perception of an object such as an apple cannot be reduced solely to its separate visual (red color), tactile (smooth skin), gustatory (sweet taste) and auditory (crunchy sound) features, although all of these attributes play an important role in the gestalt perceptual experience and inform potential actions (e.g., pick the apple; eat the apple). Research with children with autism has identified difficulties with being able to formulate gestalt perceptions, sometimes referred to as weak central coherence (Happe, 1994). Some children with autism are quite adept at parsing objects or events into component features (e.g., reproducing block designs by shape or color), but less able to arrive at the overall contextual meaning (e.g., deciphering the pattern in the design), a process that is at least partially dependent on adequate multisensory integration.

Sensory–perceptual functions and executive functions for control of action appear to be separate but interrelated functions, made possible by numerous reciprocal connections in the parietal and frontal regions of the brain, as well as through interconnections with lower-order structures in the brainstem, nerves, and muscles (Fogassi & Gallese, 2004). Neurological processes enabling the retrieval of representations of objects, individuals, or actions greatly benefit from information arriving through different and multiple sensory modalities and parallel streams of processing information. For example, a preschool-age child can speculate that another person is dribbling a basketball just by hearing the sound of the ball bouncing against the pavement, without actually seeing the person bouncing the ball. Research confirming the existence of "mirror neurons" reinforces this point, as specific regions of the brain (e.g., Broca's area [Brodmann's 44 and 45] and inferior parietal cortex) may activate not only during our own manual actions with objects, but in just watching other people perform intentional manual actions with objects (Rizzolatti & Craighero, 2004). Thus, multisensory integration is a process that helps to support a child's ability to understand human action and intention, or "theory of mind"—a function that may be more difficult for young children with autism (Happe & Frith, 1995; Baron-Cohen, 2000).

Theoretically, disruptions in the integrity of the sensory–motor systems at any point in development may result in distorted perceptions of events or contribute to a narrower action repertoire. Sensory–motor learning processes are especially critical early in development when the nervous system is most malleable and much neuronal pruning takes place to make cognitive processing more efficient. In infancy, excessive neural connections between various sensory-specific regions are gradually pruned over the course of development and replaced by experience-dependent connections from repeated and meaningful sensory–motor experiences. Interestingly, head circumference (and presumably brain volume) of many children later diagnosed with autism is of normal size at birth, but increases dramatically during the first 3 years of life (Hazlett et al., 2005; Lainhart et al., 1997; Redcay & Courchesne, 2005). These findings implicate deficits in the neural pruning process and resultant functional connectivity very early in the development of children with autism. The cause of this abnormality and the extent to which specific sensory-motor or cognitive experiences can alter neurological functions and early developmental trajectories is unknown.

Although dividing *sensory* and *motor* processes into mutually exclusive entities is naive from a neurological perspective, much of the autism literature separates studies of "sensory features" (or sensory processing disruptions) from those of "motor features" (or movement disorders) (cf. Baranek, Parham, & Bodfish, 2005). Thus, for the sake of clarity, our review of these studies is similarly divided into the two sections that follow.

Sensory Features

Although unusual sensory features are not thought to be universal in autism (Dawson & Watling, 2000), they appear to be highly prevalent, early emerging, and contributory to differential diagnosis and intervention planning (Dawson & Watling, 2000; Baranek et al., 2005). Research conducted with preschoolers with autism confirms higher rates of some sensory features in autism, as compared with both typically developing children (Kientz & Dunn, 1997; Watling, Deitz, & White, 2001) and children with other developmental disabilities (Baranek, David, Poe, Stone, & Watson, 2006; Rogers, Hepburn, & Wehner, 2003). Traditionally, these studies used parent-report instruments, which have some inherent subjective bias, but good ecological validity. Rogers, Hepburn, and Wehner

(2003) used the Short Sensory Profile and demonstrated that tactile sensitivity, taste/smell sensitivity, and underreactivity were most often endorsed by parents of children ages 26–41 months with autism. Baranek et al. (2005) utilized the Sensory Experiences Questionnaire (SEQ) and concluded that approximately 69% of a preschool-age sample of children with autism showed significantly increased levels of sensory features. Two patterns (not mutually exclusive) were identified, with 56% of the sample showing hyperresponsiveness and 63% showing hyporesponsiveness to sensory experiences. Approximately 38% of this autism sample evidenced high levels of both patterns, which was much less likely (~2%) in children with other developmental disabilities.

A few studies have presented clinical chart reviews with similar findings. For example, Greenspan and Wieder (1997) reviewed medical records of 200 clinical cases of preschoolers with autism and reported similar patterns of hyperresponsiveness, hyporesponsiveness, and mixed patterns. Psychophysiological findings from older children with autism and related developmental disorders support these behavioral findings (e.g., McAlonan et al., 2002; Hirstein, Iversen, & Ramachandran, 2001). However, some studies measuring sensory gating have failed to show autism-specific deficits (Tecchio et al., 2003; Frankland et al., 2004; Kemner, Oranje, Verbaten, & Van Engeland, 2002). In contrast, there is very little information available from observational studies of very young children with autism.

Although not universal, unusual sensory features are recounted by many parents of children with autism early in development. In some cases, sensory symptoms as recollected by parents, accompanied or preceded the emergence of social-communicative features of autism.

> "When he was around 7 months of age I started taking my child to a play group and noticed that he didn't like to be put down in the grass. He would get upset at the grass touching his body . . . he would visibly tense up. If I lowered him into a sandbox he would lift his feet and legs up as long as he could to keep the sand from touching him, take a break, then do it again."—Interview with a parent of a young child with autism, Sensory Experiences Project (SEP), University of North Carolina–Chapel Hill

Such idiosyncratic observations have been endorsed by many parents in systematic parent-report studies (e.g., Ohta et al., 1987; Hoshino et al., 1982; Ornitz & Ritvo, 1968), as well as through observation of behaviors in retrospective video analyses of home movies of 8- to 12-month-old infants later diagnosed with autism (e.g., Baranek, 1999a; Adrien et al., 1993; Werner, Dawson, Osterling, & Dinno, 2000). Symptoms have included lack of orienting to auditory and visual stimuli, excessive mouthing of objects, and gaze and social touch aversions, to name a few. Recent research on high-risk samples of infant siblings of children with autism also confirm the presence of unusual sensory features such as difficulties with visual tracking and disengagement of visual attention, and sensory-oriented object manipulations by 12–18 months of age (Wetherby et al., 2004; Zwaigenbaum et al., 2005). Prospective longitudinal studies on sensory features are nonexistent. Cross-sectional studies demonstrate mixed findings with respect to whether sensory symptoms increase (Talay-Ongan & Wood, 2000), decrease (Baranek, Foster, & Berkson, 1997; Baranek et al., 2006), or do not change (Rogers, Hepburn, & Wehner, 2003) with developmental maturation. Utilizing the Sensory Processing Assessment for Young Children (SPA; Baranek, 1999c) researchers found that younger or cognitively delayed children, regardless of their diagnoses, evidenced greater avoidance and adverse reaction to sensory experiences than older and more developmentally mature children (Baranek, Boyd, Poe, David, & Watson, 2007). Thus, some sensory features may not be specific to autism, but may still have significant implications for intervention, especially when the level of experienced distress impacts upon family members' ability to care for their child or participate in community activities.

A variety of conceptual frameworks discuss the likelihood that altered sensory thresholds may decrease/increase sensitivity to specific sensory experiences and constrict optimal engagement in play, environmental exploration, and social interaction that form the basis for further learning opportunities (Dunn, 1997; Baranek, Reinhartsen, & Wannamaker, 2001; Miller, Reisman, McIntosh, & Simon, 2001). Anecdotally, many young children with autism are reported to have difficulties in tolerating specific sensory experiences such as noisy environments, messy materials, or physical affection (Grandin, 1996; Smith, Roux, Naidoo, & Venter, 2005; Watling et al., 2001).

> "She hates for me to clean her ears, and that can be just with a Q-tip or washing her ears. I mean she really pulls at the washcloth. She throws the Q-tips away or hides the Q-tips. I've even tried giving her the washcloth and letting her clean her own ears. She just really hates for anything to be around her ears. Even if I wait until she's been asleep for hours and try to go wash her ears, she'll still wake up. And she gets *really* upset, I mean to the point where she can be in tears. . . . I ask her if it's painful and she says 'no.' She says it doesn't hurt, 'It feels funny' is the way she would answer, 'It feels funny.' "—Interview with a parent of a young child with autism, SEP, University of North Carolina–Chapel Hill

Although less obvious, many children with autism have difficulties in sufficiently responding to salient sensory stimuli, as evidenced by hyposensitivity to pain, delay in orienting to name, or lack of attention to novel visual events (Baranek et al., 2006). In rarer cases, sensory input may be atypically combined across modalities, as in the case of synesthesia, or altered to form an idiosyncratic perception of an event (Cytowic, 2002; Jones, Quigney, & Huws, 2003). It is possible that neurological maturation as well as learned self-regulatory strategies and environmental adaptations may play a role in helping to modulate such hyper- and hyporesponsive reactions over time. The ability of parents or other caregivers to adapt to a child's sensory features can impact the number, type, or quality of shared social experiences, both good and bad. For example, "good" sensory experiences for the child also lead to feelings of contentment for the parents:

> "A good experience is usually when he is playing outside on the swing set. He is more relaxed, happy. The motion of it relaxes him. Oh, it is great—I love it when he is outside . . . he has so much fun!"—Interview with a parent of young child with autism, SEP, University of North Carolina–Chapel Hill

whereas "bad" sensory experiences cause distress and lead to avoidance and constraints on family routines. In some cases these experiences may be interpreted as behavioral inflexibility, inasmuch as the young child with autism strives to make his or her sensory experience more predictable.

> "Vacuum, loud noises . . . she covers her ears. . . . It's like she wants to get away from it. I don't run the vacuum cleaner when she's around, that's for sure! I use the broom. She likes to play with it when it is not on. . . . Her dad has loud music on when we come home, but I make him turn it down before we come in the door because I know it would set her off."—Interview with a parent of young child with autism; SEP, University of North Carolina–Chapel Hill

Motor Features

Now we turn our attention to the nature of motor features, including voluntary and involuntary movement disorders, in young children with autism. Although some children with autism have motor skills that appear relatively stronger than their social and communication skills (Stone, Ousley, Hepburn, Hogan, & Brown, 1999), subtle motor difficulties are frequently noted in children with autism as compared with typical reference norms (Ghaziuddin & Butler, 1998; Manjiviona & Prior, 1995). Specifically, Manjiviona and Prior reported that 50–67% of high-functioning children with autism in their sample had significant gross and fine motor impairments on a standardized test. On the contrary, Rogers, Hepburn, and Wehner (2003) did not find significant differences in standardized measures of general fine and gross motor skills of toddlers with autism relative to mental-age-matched controls.

Motor abnormalities may interfere with adaptive tasks such as buttoning and writing, as well as social-communicative functions, such as speech articulation, gesturing, and eye gaze coordination (Gilotty, Kenworthy, Sirian, Black, & Wagner, 2002; Leary & Hill, 1996; Takarae, Minshew, Luna, Krisky, & Sweeney, 2004). Motor issues may be intertwined with the core features of autism and have implications for early development of intersubjectivity and communicative intent (Rogers & Pennington, 1991; Hobson & Lee, 1999). For example, interpersonal synchrony of bodies, facial expressions, eye movements, voices, and movements is important to emotional expression and social exchanges.

Case Vignette

Charlie is a verbal, high-functioning boy with autism. Charlie's gait pattern is unusual—he walks on his toes with a little extra "bounce" in his step. Articulation errors make his speech somewhat harder to understand out of context. Charlie drools a bit, particularly during mealtimes, and has difficulty chewing textured foods and sucking through a straw. During music class, Charlie's hand motions seem a little out of sync with the accompanying song lyrics. Art activities are avoided as he struggles with the use of tools for drawing and cutting.

A variety of subtle motor abnormalities may be present in children with autism (Leary & Hill, 1996; Sweeney, Takarae, Macmillan, Luna, & Minshew, 2004; Rinehart, Bradshaw, Brereton, & Tonge, 2001; Schmitz, Martineau, Barthelemy, & Assaiante, 2003; Mari, Castiello, Marks, Marraffa, & Prior, 2003), with prevalence estimates ranging as high as 85–90% (Miyahara et al., 1997; Wing, 1981), at least in older samples of children. Clinical observations often report specific difficulties in praxis and smooth coordination of movements (DeMyer, Barton, & Norton, 1972; Trecker, 2001), but empirical studies with very young children are lacking. Praxis requires ideation, planning, and execution of skills in novel ways (Ayres, 1985) and may impact a child's ability to use tools, imitate human actions, and play sports, for example. Motor planning and coordination between various components of a motor task are essential for efficient movement. Greenspan and Wieder (1997) reported that in 100% of the cases reviewed in their study, the children manifested some difficulties with motor planning/sequencing, with 48% demonstrating severe difficulties in this area. DeMyer and colleagues (1972) found that children with autism had strengths in repetitive gross motor skills such as stair climbing, but had difficulties in complex skills requiring imitation of arm movements or complex ball play. Parham, Mailloux, and Roley (2000) noted that oral praxis, which is critical for speech articulation, was particularly problematic for children with autism relative to matched controls.

It is unclear as to which aspects of praxis may or may not be specifically affected in autism—for example, difficulties in establishing motor patterns, changing movement patterns in response to sensory cues, timing/sequencing movements, inhibiting actions, or using sensory feedback to guide movement. Two studies (Rinehart et al., 2001; Mari et al., 2003) showed that deficits may be more noticeable in movement preparation then in the execution phase once the movement begins for high-functioning persons with autism. David et al. (2007) demonstrated evidence for temporal dyscoordination during a precision grip task that most typically developing 7-year-olds accomplish fluidly, and found that older children with autism tended to utilize compensatory strategies, such as gripping harder to lift the object, to aid successful completion of the task. Such deficits have also been found in persons with cerebellar dysfunctions (Fellows, Ernst, Schwarz, Topper, & Noth, 2001). Questions arise about whether or not certain motor features or deficits in movement control are specific to autism, inasmuch as children with other disorders manifest similar motor problems.

Imitation of actions and body postures is an aspect of praxis that is important for social-communicative development in children with autism (Smith & Bryson, 1994). Researchers have suggested that imitation difficulties in children with autism may not be the result of problems in abstracting the meaning of the actions (Rogers, Bennetto, McEvoy, & Pennington, 1996; Stone, Ousley, & Littleford, 1997; Hughes & Russell, 1993), but rather may reflect difficulties in generating or using internal somatosensory representations, because children with autism have greater difficulties in imitating body postures and oral movements than in imitating object manipulations (Stone et al., 1997; DeMyer et al., 1972; Page & Boucher, 1998; Parham et al., 2000; Adams, 1998; Rogers, Hepburn, Stackhouse, & Wehner, 2003). Such "proprioceptive" deficits affecting praxis require further research but may have implications for treatment such that reproduction of actions may be facilitated in the context of ongoing visual cues. Because there appears to be a correlation between aspects of imitative praxis, particularly sequencing of oral and/or fine motor movements, and expressive speech development (Rogers & Bennetto, 2000), later language abilities (Stone et al., 1997; Sigman & Ungerer, 1984), as well as sign vocabulary (Seal & Bonvillian, 1997) in children with autism, these issues have ramifications for early intervention and general prognosis.

How early are motor features evident in children with autism? Descriptive reports, including case studies (e.g., Dawson, Osterling, Meltzoff, & Kuhl, 2000) and parent surveys (e.g., Ornitz, Guthrie, &

Farley, 1977) often endorse unusual motor aspects of children with autism such as hypotonia and repetitive movements that are first evident during infancy. Impaired motor imitation has been reported in numerous studies of toddlers with autism (Stone et al., 1997; Charman et al., 1997) and these skills seem to improve over the course of development or perhaps with treatment. Stereotyped movements may become more apparent during the preschool years for children with autism (Cox et al., 1999; Lord, 1995) and may be associated with less environmental exploration in novel situations (Pierce & Courchesne, 2001).

"I really don't understand it. I think there's some thing that he gets in his body, because now that he can communicate a little bit more, I can ask him. Sometimes he jumps when I don't want him to jump, and I'll say, 'Freddy, can you stop your body? Can you stop jumping?' And the other day for the first time he actually went like this and hugged himself tightly. I think sometimes he jumps when he's excited. From what I've read, proprioceptive input . . . I think there's something in the way his brain gets messages from his body that jumping satisfies for him. I've read a number of things by adults with autism about their sensory experience, and I've really tried to be more understanding and more respectful of the fact that his body is different than mine. His brain works differently than mine, and the things that I may not understand may actually be very important to him, and very pleasurable to him. So, just trying to, you know, come to terms with that as we live our lives together."—Interview with a parent of a young child with autism, SEP, University of North Carolina–Chapel Hill

"Abnormal" stereotypies are more difficult to separate out in infancy, because most typically developing children also manifest a variety of rhythmic motor movements (e.g., leg kicking, arm flapping) and repetitive object explorations (banging, mouthing, waving) in their first year of life (Baranek, 1999a; Thelen, 1981). A critical review of 12 different studies (Symons, Sperry, Dropik, & Bodfish, 2005) reported that the onset of rhythmic movements was delayed in children at risk for developmental problems (including those with autism), but that their sequencing or developmental course was similarly predictable to typical development. Typical infant stereotypies appeared to be transient and associated with development of motor skills, neuromuscular development, and/or general neurological maturation, whereas in children with autism or other developmental delays, motor and object stereotypies may persist or change in their functions over time.

Well-controlled longitudinal studies of early motor features are lacking. Retrospective video analysis methods have analyzed motor features, predominantly in an effort for early diagnosis (Baranek, 1999a; Teitelbaum, Teitelbaum, Nye, Fryman, & Maurer, 1998). Baranek (1999a) reported in 9- to 12-month video footage that children with autism mouthed objects more than children with other developmental disabilities. Unusual motor posturing and visual object fixations were also noted in children with autism, at least more so than children developing typically, but other repetitive motor and object stereotypies did not differentiate the three groups. Teitelbaum et al. (1998) also reported movement differences very early in the development of children with autism as compared with typically developing children, although disability comparison groups were not studied.

A variety of abnormal involuntary movements, either idiopathic or medication-induced, may also occur in autism (Leary & Hill, 1996; Wing, 1997), but these features are reported less in studies with very young children. Detection of involuntary motor features is difficult because several discrete types of involuntary movements may co-occur, involve several body parts, show a variable course of expression over time, or become difficulty to differentiate from voluntary movement patterns (Lewis & Bodfish, 1998; Marsden, 1984). Case reports and empirical studies of persons with autism have reported the existence of tics, catatonia, dyskinesia, akathisia, bradykinesia, and gait/posture abnormalities (Bodfish, Symons, Parker, & Lewis, 2000; Damasio & Maurer, 1978; Realmuto & August, 1991; Wing & Shah, 2000). Gait and postural abnormalities have been observed via kinematic motion analysis (Kohen-Raz, Volkmar, & Cohen, 1992; Gepner & Mestre, 2002), but these studies are harder to conduct with very young children.

ASSESSMENT

Sensory–motor functions are but one aspect of development that may need to be considered in the assessment process for young children with autism. A variety of professionals, including occupational therapists, physical therapists, speech and language pathologists, teachers, psychologists and/or pediatricians, working together as a team may be involved. Based on recommended practices within the field of early intervention, the assessment of young children with disabilities, including those with autism, should be conducted using a family-centered approach, utilizing the expertise of parents about the strengths and needs of their children (Sandall, Hemmeter, Smith, & McLean, 2004). Ecological and transactional theories inform the multidisciplinary assessment process with a focus on the ability of the child to engage in everyday routines and activities in typical family and community environments (Wolery, Brashers, & Neitzel,

2002). Thus, sensory–motor functions are usually addressed within the broader context of how they impact on daily life.

The process of assessment for a young child with autism begins with parents and other significant caregivers (teachers, extended family members, etc.) as key informants about the contexts and activities in which the child is both successful and unsuccessful, and identifies their concerns and priorities as a guide for further assessment and intervention planning.

Case Vignette

Janelle, the mother of Aaron, a 2½-year-old boy with autism, relates during an interview assessment, "I've watched him on the playground out there—at his school. He either sits on the bench under the tree or walks around next to the fence. I think of him as loving to be outside, but . . . not there. He can't do it, for some reason. I would really like to see that change . . . see him having a good time out there on the school playground."

Analysis of the child's performance, conducted in the time, place, and social environment in which the activity or routine typically occurs, is an important aspect of the assessment process. (Occupational Therapy Practice Framework: Domain and Process, 2002). The analysis of this child/activity/context transaction provides the basis for more detailed evaluation, as breakdowns in functional performance and adaptive behaviors in everyday contexts are identified. In examining contextual issues, a therapist determines which qualities of the environment support the child's performance, and which inhibit it. These factors may include the physical environment, social milieu, cultural circumstances (e.g., values, family rituals, classroom routines), and temporal context (e.g., schedules, routines). In examining the activities with which the child has difficulty, as with contextual factors, the therapist determines which qualities of a task support the child's performance, and which inhibit it. Factors to be considered include the meaning of the task to the child or caregivers, as well as the various sensory, cognitive, social, communication, motor, and affective demands needed to complete the task. When examining the child's capacities, sensory–motor skills such as praxis, fine motor control, and sensory modulation abilities may be evaluated when it appears that these have a bearing on the child's functional performance. In the case example of Aaron (above), the therapist may interview the teacher and parents about the meaning of the playground activities and their expectations for performance, observe Aaron on the playground to gain a sense of his skills in the context of the physical and social environment, and conduct specific skills assessments.

Specific Sensory–Motor Assessments

There are several types of assessments that may be used to examine the specific sensory–motor capacities of a child with autism. The choice of an assessment tool is determined by the purpose of assessing. Such purposes include estimating the prevalence of sensory–motor features, systematically describing early sensory–motor development, assisting in detecting and quantifying deviations from typical trajectories, establishing a diagnosis, and providing guidelines for intervention and evaluating outcomes. Sensory–motor assessments can be broadly classified as screening and diagnostic assessments. Screenings are done for those infants who are at risk for developmental problems—for example, infants born prematurely, with low birth weight, or with other pre-, post-, or perinatal complications. Screenings are quick and provide information about the requirement for further in-depth evaluation, whereas diagnostic assessments are done for children who exhibit specific symptoms or concerns and thus require a more detailed assessment, the outcome of which can be a specific diagnosis or referral for services. Typically, such diagnostic evaluations use a combination of standardized assessments and clinical observations. Sensory–motor assessments are seldom used with young children with autism for the purpose of obtaining a clinical diagnosis of autism; however, many comprehensive developmental evaluations include an assessment of sensory–motor development. Consequentially, sensory–motor assessments may be used as a supplement to the diagnostic process for the purposes of further delineating the child's strengths and weakness as recommendations are made for intervention.

The next two sections present a variety of tools that are available and may be appropriate for the assessment of children ages birth through 3 years, including autism. Even though the assessments discussed below are standardized, norm-referenced to a typical sample or criterion-referenced to typical development, and possess acceptable psychometric properties, their use with children with autism in most instances is not validated. Therefore, clinicians planning to use these assessments with children with autism should be cautious when interpreting and comparing results to the published norm- and criterion-referenced criteria, especially if adaptations are made to standardized administration procedures.

Motor Assessments

Seven motor assessments with applicability to children ages birth through 3 years are summarized here. Given the decontextualized nature of the majority of standardized motor assessments, caution is advised when interpreting results, especially for intervention purposes. However, many of these assessments have validity for their intended purpose of classifying levels of delay in young children relative to the normative population, and some may be particularly useful in research contexts. Six of the seven assessments described utilize an observational format and, to be used validly, require some level of training in their administration and scoring. The *Ages and Stages Questionnaires* (ASQ; Squires, Potter, & Bricker, 1995) is the one exception that uses a parent-report format. It consists of 19 reproducible questionnaires that were designed to screen developmental delays and monitor the development of children from ages 4 to 60 months who may be at risk for developmental problems. Each form has 30 questions in five areas (i.e., communication, fine motor, gross motor, problem solving, personal social) that correspond to a specific age. Developmental quotients can be derived. This tool is most often used in pediatric practices or early intervention programs that conduct systematic screening and surveillance.

The *Alberta Infant Motor Scale* (AIMS; Piper & Darrah, 1994) is an observational screening tool that characterizes motor development of infants from 0 to 18 months. It consists of four subscales (i.e., Prone, Supine, Sitting, and Standing) that encompass movements typically observed in common body positions of young infants. It is often used by occupational or physical therapists working with young infants in high-risk settings. Raw scores, positional scores, and total scores can be calculated. The total scores are plotted to obtain a percentile ranking compared with a normative age-matched sample. This screener does not rely on verbal instruction and thus may have better applicability to children with autism, who often have difficulty in understanding verbal instructions.

The *Peabody Developmental Motor Scales–Second Edition* (PDMS-2; Folio & Fewell, 2000) were designed to assess motor development in young children with disabilities or developmental delays between the ages of birth and 6 years. This well-standardized tool consists of six subtests (Reflexes, Stationary, Locomotion, Object Manipulation, Grasping, Visual–motor Integration) that generate global indices of motor performance including Gross (GMQ), Fine (FMQ), and Total Motor Quotients (TMQ). Various quantitative scores (raw scores, norm-referenced standard scores, or age equivalents) can be obtained. The PDMS-2 has been evidenced to be sensitive to change and may be used as an outcome or evaluative measure (Kolobe, Palisano, & Stratford, 1998; Bayley, 1993; Goyen & Lui, 2002). Some items on the PDMS-2 require verbal instruction and/or imitation that may be difficult for some children with autism. This tool is often used by occupational and physical therapists in a variety of diagnostic and treatment settings, as well as by researchers studying motor development.

The *Gross Motor Function Measure* (GMFM; Russell, Rosenbaum, Avery, & Lane, 2002) was originally designed to assess gross motor skills in children with cerebral palsy or acute head injury. All items on the

GMFM can be completed by a typically developing 5-year-old child; thus, the test is most appropriate for children below 5 years or for those over 5 years with obvious movement impairments. Recent studies have validated its use with children with Down syndrome and other intellectual impairments (Kolobe et al., 1998; Palisano et al., 2001; Russell et al., 1998), and it has shown sensitivity to change in one study (Russell et al., 1993). Thus, this tool may be applicable to other similar populations evidencing quantitative or qualitative deficits in gross motor skills. Raw scores, criterion-referenced total percent scores, dimension percent scores, and motor growth scores can be calculated. The GMFM assesses skills in the context of five domains (i.e., Lying/rolling, Sitting, Crawling/kneeling, Standing, and Walking/running/jumping).

The *Toddler and Infant Motor Evaluation* (TIME; Miller & Roid, 1994) was designed to assess qualitative dimensions of motor abilities of children between 4 months and 3½ years of age and requires some clinical expertise to use skillfully. It consists of eight subtests (i.e., Mobility, Stability, Motor Organization, Functional Performance, Social/emotional Abilities, Component Analysis, Quality Rating, and Atypical Positions). Raw scores, standard scaled scores (except for quality rating and component analysis), and growth scores for motor organization can be calculated. All eight subtest scores have been evidenced to discriminate children with atypical development from those with typical development (Miller & Roid, 1994). The instructions and testing format are lengthy but allow much flexibility that is useful with infants across various settings. The TIME requires some pretend play in order to assess motor organization, a skill that is often a weakness for young children with autism.

The *Bayley Scales of Infant and Toddler Development, Third Edition* (Bayley-III; Bayley, 2006) is a well-validated and standardized observational assessment for children from birth to 42 months of age. The previous version of the Bayley has often been used in multidisciplinary clinical or research settings and has numerous validity studies showing its ability to discriminate between children with developmental delay and those who are typically developing (Bayley, 1993). The Bayley-III has a variety of developmental scales, including a Motor Scale that assesses fine and gross motor skills, and yields age-equivalent scores as well as a norm-referenced developmental index. A variety of professionals with expertise in motor development (e.g., occupational and physical therapists; early interventionists) are trained to validly administer this assessment and interpret the results.

The *Mullen Scales of Early Learning–AGS Edition* (MSEL; Mullen, 1995) is another well-validated, comprehensive observational assessment that is standardized for children from birth to 68 months. The MSEL is composed of gross motor, fine motor, visual reception, expressive language, and receptive language subscales and is widely used as a general measure of cognitive abilities in young children with autism in both clinical and research settings. Apart from obtaining an overall Early Learning Composite, standardized T-scores, percentiles, and age equivalents can be computed for each subscale, enabling the isolated use of the gross and fine motor subscales for diagnostic or tracking purposes by specialized professionals.

Sensory Processing Assessments

Five sensory processing assessments are reviewed here that may have applicability to very young children with autism and related disabilities, ages birth through 3 years. Three of these are parent-report instruments, and two are observational instruments. These tools are most often used by occupational therapists in either clinical or research settings, but are gaining popularity with other disciplines. Cautions about decontextualized assessments, similar to those presented in the discussion of motor assessments, are also warranted here. In addition, most of these sensory processing assessments are criterion-referenced and do not provide true norm-referenced scores, which are possible only with studies utilizing large representative samples.

The *Evaluation of Sensory Processing* (ESP; Parham & Ecker, 2002) is a 76 item caregiver questionnaire that assesses sensory processing difficulties in children from 2 to 12 years. It consists of six subscales: Auditory, Gustatory/Olfactory, Proprioception, Tactile, Vestibular, and Visual. The ESP has been shown to discriminate children with sensory dysfunction from typically developing children (Parham & Ecker, 2002; Johnson-Ecker & Parham, 2000), and studies with children with autism are in progress.

The *Infant/Toddler Sensory Profile* (Dunn, 2002) is a parent-report questionnaire designed to evaluate sensory processing patterns in infants and toddlers (0–3 years). Criterion-referenced cut-scores are obtained whereby the raw scores can be compared to the performance of typical children. For children 0–6 months the questionnaire consists of 36 items, from which four quadrant scores (i.e., low registration, sensation seeking, sensory sensitivity, and sensation avoiding) and one combined quadrant score (low threshold) can be calculated. For infants between 7 and 36 months the questionnaire consists of 48 items, from which five sensory processing section scores (auditory processing, visual processing, tactile processing, vestibular processing, and oral sensory processing), four quadrant scores, and one combined quadrant score can be obtained. Growth charts can also be constructed for sensation seeking, tactile processing, and oral sensory processing. One study indicated that the scores of children with autism and those with developmental delays were significantly different from those of typically developing children on this assessment (Rogers, Hepburn, & Wehner, 2003).

The *Sensory Experiences Questionnaire* (SEQ; Baranek, 1999b; Baranek et al., 2006) is a parent-report questionnaire consisting of 35 items in its current research version. It was specifically designed to screen young children with autism and developmental delays with mental ages between 6 and 72 months. The SEQ can be used as a supplement to traditional developmental assessments that do not typically include evaluation of sensory processing functions. Raw scores for the full scale, as well as subscales for Hypo/Hyper-responsiveness to Social/Nonsocial sensory stimuli and Sensory Modality Categories, can be derived and compared with the performance of typically developing children, children with developmental delays, and children with autism. Criterion-referenced cut-scores are provided. The SEQ has been evidenced to discriminate between children with autism and developmental delays, as well as between children with autism and typically developing children (Baranek et al., 2006).

The *Sensory Processing Assessment for Young Children* (SPA; Baranek, 1999c) was also designed specifically for infants and young children with autism and developmental delays from 9–62 months, as an observational companion to the SEQ. It is administered in a semistructured play format and consists of four parts: Approach/Avoidance and Action Strategies with Novel Sensory Toys, Sensory Orienting, Sensory Habituation (repeated stimuli), and Stereotyped Behaviors. It contains both exploratory tasks, during which the children interact with sensory toys, and specific probes, administered unexpectedly, to judge reactions to sensory stimuli. Raw scores and criterion-referenced scale scores are calculated, and validity studies are currently in progress.

The *Test of Sensory Function in Infants* (TSFI; DeGangi & Greenspan, 1989) is an observational measure for infants between 4 and 18 months with sensory integrative dysfunction, especially those at risk for later learning disability. The TSFI consists of fives subtests (i.e., Reactivity to Tactile Deep Pressure, Adaptive Motor Function, Visual-tactile Integration, Ocular-motor Control, Reactivity to Vestibular Stimulation) with items that utilize specific probes/stimuli to judge a behavioral response from the infant. Each subscale yields a criterion-referenced score specific for the four age groups (4–6, 7–9, 10–12, and 13–18 months). The subscales can be summed to calculate a total score. It is more stable in identifying infants with sensory processing dysfunction at 10–18 months than in the younger age groups.

Case Vignette

The preschool teacher is concerned that Aaron (introduced earlier in the chapter) does not engage in purposeful play on the playground. She notes that he tends to wander the fenced perimeter or sit on a bench under a tree. Aaron's parents report that he plays happily at their neighborhood playground, enjoying climbing up a short ladder and sliding down the slide. The therapist at Aaron's preschool is consulted to determine ways to engage him more fully in playground activities. She observes him in both environments and notes a variety of contextual differences potentially affecting his performance. Aaron's motor skills are adequate to climb simple structures, but the preschool playground is more complex. It has many different play spaces/climbing structures, is encircled by a wire fence, and is noisy because of a large number of children playing at once. The small neighborhood playground does not have the distraction of a wired fence, provides one simple play structure, and has few other children present. In both situations, the activity is outdoor play, but the physical and social environments of the two playgrounds afford vastly different levels of participation for Aaron. Given this assessment, the therapist is now better able to recommend a variety of appropriate and contextually relevant interventions. A standardized motor assessment was deemed unnecessary in this situation; however, the therapist chose to administer a parent-report sensory processing assessment to gain a better understanding of potential sensory problems that may be generalizing to the playground environment.

INTERVENTION

Guiding Principles

The multidisciplinary comprehensive assessment process ideally leads to the development of functional goals and meaningful outcomes for the child and family, as well as strategies for intervention. Family-centered practices acknowledge the expertise, priorities, routines, and goals of the family (Dunst, 2002) and recommend collaboration among all members of the intervention team. Though the intervention focus may at times be on supporting changes in the skills and performance of the child with sensory–motor deficits, consideration is given to the family's culture, values, and methods of orchestrating daily life. Ecological approaches support a perspective whereby the context in which an activity occurs is seen as both affecting and being affected by the child engaged in that activity. This interaction (between the child and the physical or social environment) may either support or hinder the child's performance (Thurman, 1977). Thus, an ecological perspective allows both intrinsic and external factors to be considered and supports the embedding of intervention strategies into daily life activities and natural environments to maximize the fit between child and environment, with a resultant enhancement of performance. As in the case of Aaron, discussed above, the therapist uses this ecological perspective, assessing a variety of child (e.g., sensory–motor or cognitive capabilities), task (e.g., climbing on play structures), and environmental (e.g., sensory distractions, social expectations) variables that are affecting Aaron's ability to succeed on the playground in order to recommend interventions that are likely to work in this specific context.

Theoretical Models Used to Address Sensory–Motor Issues

There are a number of theoretical models that may be used to think about and guide interventions for children experiencing sensory–motor difficulties. These ways of thinking may be used in combination with one another, but should be chosen on the basis of the individual characteristics of the child and contexts involved. Several of the most common theoretical models utilized by occupational and physical therapists for the treatment of sensory–motor issues with young children with autism are presented below, with brief explanations.

Transactional Theories

Transactional theory (see, e.g., Law et al., 1996) was alluded to in the section on assessment. This theory is consistent with the ecological perspective and emphasizes the ongoing dynamics between the child, the activity, and the environment to create optimal performance under well-matched conditions. The importance of transactional theory for sensory–motor issues lies in the opportunity to think broadly about the factors impacting the child's performance, and to provide intervention that may target changes in the task and/or changes to the context, rather than relying only on remediation strategies that seek to make changes in the child's sensory–motor functions directly.

Dynamic Systems

Dynamic systems theory (Smith & Thelen, 2003) similarly views the child as a highly complex organism in which self-organization and adaptation in all aspects of function are occurring constantly and simultaneously as a result of the demands of the environment and the organism's own effort to meet those demands. Application of this theory to young children with autism encourages a perspective in which the child is seen as capable of change, or learning, as a result of interactions with tasks and environments that provide an appropriate level of challenge.

Motor Learning Theory

Motor learning theory (Shumway-Cook & Woollacott, 2000) addresses the acquisition of and/or modification of movement and can be particularly useful in thinking about intervention for young children who have difficulty in the area of praxis (motor planning). With a desired outcome of increasing the child's ability to perform motor activities successfully and in a variety of environments, intervention based on motor learning theory includes frequent opportunities for practice in natural settings, provision of meaningful feedback (including enhanced sensory input), use of cognitive and/or language-based strategies, and a focus on generalization of skills.

Sensory Processing Theory

Sensory integration (SI) theory, originally developed in the 1960s by A. Jean Ayres, is based on assumptions that processing and organization of sensory input influences a child's motor functions, learning, and adaptive behavior. Classical sensory integration treatment utilizes prescribed sensory experiences (i.e., vestibular, proprioceptive, tactile) to enhance neural processing, with an assumption that this processing will lead to improved behaviors and learning. This model spurred the development of a variety of remedial sensory-based treatments that have been subject to controversy (see Baranek, 2002, for a review of research in autism). Newer sensory processing models stress the transactional effects of environmental affordances or challenges with the child's sensory processing style (Dunn, 1997, 2002) and provide treatment recommendations beyond remediation of deficits. Dunn (1997, 2002) identifies four patterns of sensory processing (i.e., low registration, sensory seeking, sensory sensitivity, and sensation avoiding) that are produced by the interaction of innate neurological thresholds (low and high) with the child's behavioral responses (passive and active) to those thresholds. Baranek and colleagues (2001) acknowledge the relevance of sensory thresholds (orientation and avoidance) to a child's ability to engage with the environment, but further suggest that an optimal level of engagement is also influenced by a variety of other intrinsic or extrinsic variables, besides sensory threshold. These newer conceptualizations are compatible with transactional and dynamic systems theories, allowing for individualized interventions that include environmental adaptations and tasks accommodating sensory preferences or avoidances to optimize performance in daily routines.

Coping Theory

Coping theory is based on a view of function that is defined as the ability to achieve emotional equilibrium after a new or challenging situation is encountered such that engagement in an activity can begin or continue (Olsen, 1999). Interventions based on coping theory seek to increase the child's ability to confront difficult situations in a positive way, simultaneously decreasing the amount of time a child spends withdrawing from or avoiding challenging situations. Application of this theory to young children with autism supports psychosocial interventions related to coping with sensory processing deficits or motor challenges and developing resiliency in the face of such challenges.

Models of Service Delivery

The ways in which interventions to address sensory–motor issues are put in place, and by whom, can vary greatly, depending on the setting in which the child is participating. Service delivery models that are congruent with the use of natural physical and social environments, accommodate daily activities and routines, and allow frequent opportunities for interventions to be implemented are typically considered best practice in early intervention (McWilliam, 1992). These integrated models of service delivery include the use of collaborative consultation and embedded intervention. However, more direct (one-on-one) approaches may also be useful at times. Figure 5.1 provides a summary of various service delivery models and how they may be used in addressing the various sensory–motor needs of young children with autism.

Intervention Strategies

Remediation, education, and modification are the three types of intervention most often used by therapists to support the participation of the young child with autism who may have specific sensory–motor deficits. Although the intended outcome of all of these types of intervention is to increase the fit between the child, his or her activities/routines, and environment, each type emphasizes a different focus of intervention. It is important to keep in mind that neurological maturation and repeated meaningful experiences play a role in successful adaptation to sensory–motor challenges for young children over the course of development, thus variability in outcomes is expected across individual children and at different points in development.

Remediation

Remediation strategies for sensory–motor deficits *seek to promote change in the child's performance* and typically include the provision of sensory–motor experiences to address deficits and/or the teaching of new sensory–motor skills. These interventions aim to effect relatively permanent changes in specific capacities targeted for intervention (e.g., fine motor coordination, praxis, tactile processing and discrimination, etc.) and, it is hoped, allow those capacities to generalize to appropriate contexts, activities, and routines. General teaching strategies may include modeling, prompting and time delay, feedback (including sensory input), practice/ repetition, peer mediation, chaining, and scaffolding. Although these strategies are supported by a body of empirical evidence (Wolery, 1994) in early childhood special education, more research about their efficacy for children with autism is warranted (Wolery, 2000). Studies utilizing these strategies specifically to address sensory–motor issues, particularly those that address a combination of techniques to support performance, are also needed. We return to the case of Aaron to exemplify remedial interventions for some of his newly emerging sensory–motor difficulties on the playground.

Case Vignette

Aaron, now 3 years old, is demonstrating difficulties with praxis, particularly in playground activities that require whole-body movement planning. For example, Aaron tries several unsuccessful methods of getting into a wagon to take a ride with his peers. His desire and intent are clear, but the planning and execution of this task are hindered by poor body scheme, difficulties in sequencing a series of movements, and lack of experience. The therapist tries some remediation strategies. First, she uses enhanced sensory feedback, holding Aaron's hips firmly and pressing toward the ground for the purpose of activating proprioceptors to improve body awareness. She taps loudly on the edge of the wagon, and then gently on the back of his hand, while providing simultaneous verbal prompts. Once this initial positioning is accomplished, she employs a brief time delay to see if Aaron can figure out what to do next with his body (i.e., motor plan). She feels his next attempt to move and realizes that it will move him in the wrong direction, so she continues to give enhanced sensory cues on his body and the wagon, simple verbal prompts, and opportunities for Aaron to initiate the next movement. The therapist continues to scaffold and chain a series of movements until he gets in the wagon successfully. After a ride around the track, she encourages Aaron to get out and give another child a turn, which creates both a visual model and an opportunity for requesting and practicing more rides in the wagon.

This example demonstrates a remediation approach utilizing several theoretical models and providing intervention in the context of the natural environment. Other types of remediation approaches, such as classical sensory integration treatment, may be conducted in clinical settings with specialized equipment (swings, therapy balls, etc.), whereby sensory input is controlled in terms of its type, frequency, duration, intensity, novelty, and complexity. Although there is substantial evidence of the existence of sensory processing difficulties in children with autism, sensory integra-

MODEL	DIRECT				EMBEDDED	CONSULTATIVE	
	Individual	Small group	One-on-one in natural environment	Group activity	Individual within regular activity or routine	Expert	Collaborative
SOCIAL CONTEXT	Therapist is primary adult. Teacher and/or parent typically not present, though may observe. Other children are not present.	Therapist is primary adult. Teacher and/or parent typically not present, though may suggest which peers/siblings should be included. Small group of children, to provide social context, modeling, opportunities for peer-mediated strategies.	Therapist directed or supported, with activity not necessarily related to current activity of others. Parent/teacher interacts with other children, may get/provide information later, may observe incidentally. Other children may be present in environment, but not interacting with target child.	Therapist directed or supported, but teacher/parent may help with planning and assist in conducting group. Other children participate in activity; may provide models for target child or use other methods of supporting intervention.	Teachers, parents, therapists share responsibility for developing and implementing intervention strategies. Other children are present and engaged in regular activities and routines with target child.	Adult in "expert" role provides information, suggestions, resources, and direction related to area of need identified by others. Others exchange information with the therapist, give and receive feedback. Other children may be present, if occurring in child environment, but they are not involved in process.	All members of intervention team exchange information and expertise and work together to plan future interventions. Other children may be present, if occurring in child environment, but they are not involved in process.
PHYSICAL CONTEXT	Isolated space in home, school, or clinic setting (e.g., therapy room) or space not in use by others.	Isolated space in home, school, or clinic setting (e.g., therapy room) or space not in use by others.	In classroom or other larger natural environment.	In classroom or other larger natural environment.	In classroom or other larger natural environment.	May occur in child environment, or separate meeting venue.	May occur in child environment, or separate meeting venue.

APPLICATION						
To assess performance capacities in controlled environment. To support initial skill acquisition. Use of this model should be purposeful, planned, and short-term.	To control social environment, teach peers modeling and other strategies, allow for practice in controlled environment before taking into larger social or physical environment. Use of this model should be purposeful, planned, and short-term.	To support child's presence in natural environment, but without immediate demand for engagement in same activity as others. To assess child's responses to specific environment when activity is motivating (e.g., child initiated). Use of this model should be purposeful, planned, and short-term.	To assess performance of child in natural social contexts. To support outcomes related to imitation, social interaction, communication, group membership and participation.	To support all aspects of participation, social interaction, and independence in natural environments with multiple opportunities for practice and feedback.	To broaden team perspectives, use pertinent resources, consider "second opinions," and develop increased knowledge for all team members, especially when confronted with difficult situations.	To support all aspects of participation, social interaction, and independence in natural environments with multiple opportunities for practice and feedback.

FIGURE 5.1. Models of service delivery for implementing sensory and motor intervention strategies for young children with autism.

tion treatments have been criticized for lacking empirical support and for inconsistencies with current understandings of neurological principles. A number of related intervention approaches have since evolved. Some therapists have prescribed a "sensory diet," based on the idea that an individually designed set of sensory activities integrated across the child's day can be helpful to meet the child's sensory needs. For example, trampoline jumping may be used to increase arousal prior to performing homework activities, or soft brushing of the skin surface may be used to decrease tactile defensiveness. Other sensory programs incorporate cognitive-behavioral and language-based strategies for older or higher-functioning children to further support self-regulatory behaviors. A variety of anecdotal data report that some families have found the various sensory integration-based treatments beneficial, at least for preschool-age children with autism and related conditions. However, it is unclear as to which aspects of the intervention (e.g., sensory input, play coaching, opportunities for enhanced social interaction, positive reinforcement, therapeutic relationship with families, etc.) may actually be responsible for the beneficial changes, inasmuch as good controlled studies are lacking (see Baranek, 2002, for a detailed review). Other controversial remediation methods are aimed at improving processing in a specific sensory modality such as audition, vision, or touch (e.g., Auditory Integration Therapy, Listening Approach, Prism Lenses, Hug Machine, weighted vests, etc.) for the purpose of effecting larger behavioral or developmental changes. Although the general principles of attending to sensory needs and preferences are salient for young children with autism and their families, it must be emphasized that there are no studies measuring the efficacy or safety of many of these alternative treatments with very young children with autism. Thus, therapeutic decisions need to be individualized and kept consistent with best clinical practice guidelines for early intervention.

Education

Educational approaches *seek to increase the knowledge and understanding of those around the child* (parents, teachers, siblings, classmates, etc.) regarding that child's particular sensory–motor needs and how those needs impact engagement and success in a variety of daily activities. Providing consultation, information, and resources to others involved with the child has at least two purposes: (1) to influence change in the expectations and behaviors of others, thus increasing the fit between the child and his or her social environment, and (2) to support the use of a collaborative model, as all those concerned about the needs of the child develop a common base of knowledge and can support one another in the implementation of intervention strategies.

Case Vignette

As the therapist collaborates with Aaron's teacher, she educates the teacher about sensory processing and its relationship to praxis, using examples of Aaron getting into his wagon. The teacher agrees to support Aaron's performance by using the same intervention strategies used by his therapist. Aaron gets much practice getting into the wagon and progressively decreases his need for sensory cues and prompting over the next few days. By the end of the week, Aaron is able to get into the wagon on his own. Remarkably, his mother reports that last night, for the first time, Aaron had the confidence to get into the bathtub on his own, showing generalization of the motor planning skills learned on the playground.

Modification

Approaches based on modification *seek to alter or adapt the context or the activity, or to provide compensatory mechanisms* that support the participation of the child. These strategies are many and varied and are often used because they lend themselves well to embedded models of service delivery in natural environments. Although some have empirical support for their use for children with autism, research literature related specifically to the use of modification strategies in addressing sensory–motor concerns for this population is scarce. Tasks and environments may be modified specifically to provide sensory input or motor affordances that match the child's particular needs. For instance, for a child with sensory-seeking behaviors, activities may be intensified in their sensory qualities (e.g., running errands, moving chairs, washing tables, etc.), and appropriate channels provided for needed stimulation (e.g., alternation of active and passive activities in daily routines). For a child with hyporesponsiveness, specific sensory stimuli (e.g., flashing a light, touching a hand) can be superimposed on existing activities to increase the likelihood that the child will orient initially or maintain engagement.

Task modifications may also include the use of priming techniques, visual supports, and social stories, among others. These strategies allow the child with autism to be prepared for, understand, and have an appropriate response to daily life events and the sensory–motor demands presented by those events. Priming (Dunn, Saiter, & Rinner, 2002) is a strategy used to familiarize the child with upcoming activities, without a demand for performance. Exposure, exploration, and accommodation are the goals of this strategy, and no attempts at "teaching" are made during priming. Although the whole task may not be modified, this method adapts the process of task initiation, thus providing greater predictability and time allowances. Empirical evidence for the use of priming to address sensory–motor issues is lacking, but several studies have shown the benefits of priming for decreasing problems behaviors and increasing pro-social behaviors in preschoolers with autism (Koegel, Koegel, Frea, & Green-Hopkins, 2003; Sawyer, Luiselli, Ricciardi, & Gower, 2005).

Case Vignette

Despite a general predisposition toward hyporesponsiveness to many sensory experiences, Aaron demonstrates hyperresponsiveness to certain auditory experiences, like exposure to noisy mechanical tools. Prior to a classroom cooking activity in which an electric hand mixer was to be used, the therapist and the teacher showed Aaron the mixer (not turned on), the bowl in which the batter would be mixed, and a picture of the muffins that would result. Aaron asked to hold the mixer, and he examined it carefully, including the on/off switch. The teacher prepared him for the sensory experience by telling him that the mixer would make noise when the switch was turned on. When the time came for the cooking activity, Aaron was permitted to choose where in the room he wanted to stand. Each child was given a turn with the mixer, counting to 10 before turning it off again. As each child took a turn, Aaron watched and came closer to the cook-ing table. When offered a turn, he held the mixer, turned it on him-self, and mixed batter to the count of 10.

Visual supports may include the use of several types of pictures (pho-tos, line drawings, etc.), as well as objects, to assist the child in the predic-tion, understanding, and response aspects of managing daily events (Bryan & Gast, 2000; Dunn et al., 2002). These methods may help gener-ate ideas for play activities, prepare for a sequence of events, make transi-tions easier, and provide more predictability and control over aversive fea-tures in the environment, thus providing supports for deficits in sensory processing as well as praxis in young children with autism. For example, in the case of Aaron, the teacher may design a book of "Fun Playground Ideas" to help him choose an activity each day and outline a picture sequence of how the task can be physically executed. Social stories were originally designed to support the social interactions of children with autism (Gray & Garand, 1993; Kuoch & Mirenda, 2003), but have been adapted to serve in a variety of situations (Baltazar & Bax, 2004; Brownell, 2002) and may have applicability to intervening with sensory–motor issues. In the case of Aaron, the therapist may construct a story (e.g., "Aaron and His Friends Ride in the Wagon"), describing events in detail to help him understand what will or should happen, what his role is, and how to respond or enact that role. These stories assist in the preparation of managing daily life events (e.g., stressful situations with loud mechani-cal noises) and are read with the child prior to the actual event.

Modifications that specifically target the environment (as opposed to the task) may include setting up a "home base" (i.e., a location apart from the child's routine environment that allows him or her to plan, regroup, or recover) (Dunn et al., 2002). The emphasis in using a home base should be on the positive aspects of recovering from stressful situations, rather than on more punitive concepts of "time-out" or providing a place for the child to avoid participation. In addition, arranging aspects of the built and natural environment to support various types of sensory–motor experiences, engineering the proximity of peers and adults, and attending to the temporal aspects of performance, including routines, schedules, and habitual behaviors, may be useful in home or early intervention settings. The general arrangement of the physical environment can be planned to make materials and tools more or less available, create paths, or invite particular activities, for example. Few studies target arrangement of the physical environment as the primary intervention strategy, but one study (Duker & Rasing, 1989) found that redesigning a classroom environment increased on-task behaviors and decreased the incidence of self-stimulation and inactivity for three adolescent/young adult males with autism. The social contexts can also influence a child's sensory experiences, and thus adult- or peer-mediated strategies may be helpful in addressing specific sensory–motor issues and increasing overall participation in meaningful activities. For example, a child with sensory hyporesponsiveness may be assigned several partners to dance with to music at the beginning of circle time in order to increase her arousal level and general responsiveness and provide role models for this sensory–motor activity. In contrast, the child with hyperresponsiveness may need a reduction in the number of peers (and therefore the likelihood of noise and unexpected touch) while playing in the block area of the classroom. For a child with praxis difficulties, peers and adults can be used as "sources of information" to help the child generate ideas for new activities. Adaptations to the temporal context may be orchestrated when a child's patterns of sensory processing and circadian rhythms (e.g., eating, sleeping, waking cycles) do not fit neatly with existing routines and expectations. While promoting flexibility coping mechanisms, caregivers may find that changing the order in which some daily events occur also increases the ability of the child to participate in those events.

Case Vignette

Benjamin, a 2-year-old boy with hyperresponsiveness to tactile sensation, wakes up hungry. He fights his parent's attempts to change his diaper and dress him (activities that involve high levels of tactile input), which are part of his usual routine. Benjamin runs from the room in search of breakfast bars that he knows are in the pantry downstairs. Benjamin's parents, discontented with the amount of effort needed to accomplish the morning routine, consult with his early interventionist, who suggests altering the temporal order of morning activities to better fit with his physiological state—Benjamin is allowed to get a breakfast bar prior to beginning the more stressful grooming activities. The interventionist also consults on adaptations to the grooming routine (e.g., use firm pressure when applying lotion in smooth, even strokes) to make it more tolerable for Benjamin and his parents.

CONCLUSION

A knowledge of sensory–motor features, their prevalence, and developmental trajectories in young children with autism is critical to clinical assessment and effective early intervention. Meaningful and repeated sensory–motor experiences during the early infant and toddler years are among the important building blocks for later development and learning. Although more research is needed, studies have confirmed the presence of a variety of sensory processing difficulties, qualitative movement differences, and repetitive motor behaviors that manifest very early in children with autism and create challenges for teachers and families. It is not clear as to which of these features are specific to autism and which may be more related to developmental disorders in general. Professionals working with young children with autism must consider the individualized nature of sensory–motor experiences and the transaction of the child's intrinsic capacities with the task and environmental features in both the assessment and intervention processes. Best practices in early intervention suggest providing interventions in the context of naturalistic environments and with multiple opportunities. Such practices also utilize a collaborative team approach, whereby teachers, therapists, and families are all viewed as contributing important expertise to the child's intervention plan. Studies on the efficacy of various sensory–motor interventions with very young children with autism are needed, although a variety of sound theoretical approaches and empirically validated strategies are available in the general early intervention literature that may be applied to this population. A variety of models (e.g., sensory processing, motor learning, cognitive-behavioral, psychosocial, and coping) and strategies (e.g., remediation, education, and task and environmental modification) are considered when formulating individualized goals and outcomes for a young child experiencing sensory–motor difficulties that interfere with daily routines and social participation.

ACKNOWLEDGMENTS

We thank the staff, children, and families who participated in our clinical practices and research programs and contributed to examples used in this chapter. All names in the case examples and interviews were de-identified and fictionalized to preserve confidentiality. Informed consent was obtained for the use of quotes. We also acknowledge partial funding from the National Institute of Child Health and Human Development (Grant No. R01-HD42168) to the Sensory Experiences Project at the University of North Carolina at Chapel Hill that enabled the compilation of literature and data for this chapter.

REFERENCES

Adams, L. (1998). Oral–motor and motor–speech characteristics of children with autism. *Focus on Autism and Other Developmental Disabilities, 13*(2), 108–112.

Adrien, J. L., Lenoir, P., Martineau, J., Perrot, A., Hameury, L., Larmande, C., et al. (1993). Blind ratings of early symptoms of autism based upon family home movies. *Journal of the American Academy of Child and Adolescent Psychiatry, 32*(3), 617–626.

Ayres, A. J. (1985). *Developmental dyspraxia and adult onset apraxia.* Torrance, CA: Sensory Integration International.

Baltazar, A., & Bax, B. E. (2004). Writing social stories for the child with sensory integration dysfunction: An introductory resource and guide for therapists, teachers, and parents. *Sensory Integration Special Interest Section Quarterly, 27,* 1–3.

Baranek, G. T. (1999a). Autism during infancy: A retrospective video analysis of sensory–motor and social behaviors at 9–12 months of age. *Journal of Autism and Developmental Disorders, 29*(3), 213–224.

Baranek, G. T. (1999b). *Sensory Experiences Questionnaire (SEQ).* Unpublished manuscript, University of North Carolina at Chapel Hill.

Baranek, G. T. (1999c). *Sensory Processing Assessment for Young Children (SPA).* Unpublished manuscript, University of North Carolina at Chapel Hill.

Baranek, G. T. (2002). Efficacy of sensory–motor interventions for children with autism. *Journal of Autism and Developmental Disorders, 32*(5), 397–422.

Baranek, G. T., Boyd, B. A., Poe, M. D., David, F. J., & Watson, L. R. (2007). Hyperresponsive sensory patterns in young children with autism, developmental delay, and typical development. *American Journal of Mental Retardation, 112*(4), 233–245.

Baranek, G. T., David, F. J., Poe, M. D., Stone, W. L., & Watson, L. R. (2006). The Sensory Experiences Questionnaire: Discriminating response patterns in young children with autism, developmental delays, and typical development. *Journal of Child Psychology and Psychiatry, 47*(6), 591–601.

Baranek, G. T., Foster, L. G., & Berkson, G. (1997). Tactile defensiveness and stereotyped behaviors. *American Journal of Occupational Therapy, 51*(2), 91–95.

Baranek, G. T., Parham, D. L., & Bodfish, J. W. (2005). Sensory and motor features in autism: Assessment and intervention. In F. Volkmar, A. Klin, & R. Paul (Eds.), *Handbook of autism and pervasive developmental disorders* (3rd ed., pp. 831–857). Hoboken, NJ: Wiley.

Baranek, G. T., Reinhartsen, D., & Wannamaker, S. (2001). Play: Engaging children with autism. In R. Heubner (Ed.), *Sensorimotor interventions in autism* (pp. 311–351). Philadelphia: Davis.

Baron-Cohen, S. (2000). Theory of mind and autism: A review. In L. M. Glidden (Ed.), *International review of research in mental retardation* (Vol. 23, pp. 169–184). San Diego: Academic Press.

Bayley, N. (1993). Bayley Scales of Infant Development–Second Edition (BSID-II). San Antonio, TX: Psychological Corporation.

Bayley, N. (2006). *Bayley Scales of Infant and Toddler Development, Third Edition.* San Antonio, TX: Harcourt Assessment.

Bodfish, J. W., Symons, F. J., Parker, D. E., & Lewis, M. H. (2000). Varieties of repetitive behavior in autism: Comparisons to mental retardation. *Journal of Autism and Developmental Disorders, 30,* 237–243.

Brownell, M. D. (2002). Musically adapted social stories to modify behaviors in students with autism: Four case studies. *Journal of Music Therapy, 39*(2), 117–144.

Bryan, L. C., & Gast, D. L. (2000). Teaching on-task and on-schedule behaviors to high-functioning children with autism via picture activity schedules. *Journal of Autism and Developmental Disorders, 30*(6), 553–567.

Charman, T., Swettenham, J., Baron-Cohen, S., Cox, A., Baird, G., & Drew, A. (1997). Infants with autism: An investigation of empathy, pretend play, joint attention, and imitation. *Developmental Psychology, 33*(5), 781–789.

Cox, A., Klein, K., Charman, T., Baird, G., Baron-Cohen, S., Swettenham, J., et al. (1999). Autism spectrum disorders at 20 and 42 months of age: Stability of clinical and ADI-R diagnosis. *Journal of Child Psychology and Psychiatry, 40*(5), 719–732.

Cytowic, R. E. (2002). *Synesthesia: A union of the senses* (2nd ed.). Cambridge, MA: MIT Press.

Damasio, A., & Maurer, R. (1978). A neurological model for childhood autism. *Archives of Neurology, 35,* 777–786.

David, F. J., Baranek, G. T., Giuliani, C. A., Mercer, V. S., Poe, M. D., & Thorpe, D. E. (2007). *A pilot study: Coordination of precision grip in children and adolescents with high functioning autism.* Manuscript submitted for publication.

Dawson, G., Osterling, J., Meltzoff, A. N., & Kuhl, P. (2000). Case study of the development of an infant with autism from birth to two years of age. *Journal of Applied Developmental Psychology, 21,* 299–313.

Dawson, G., & Watling, R. (2000). Interventions to facilitate auditory, visual, and motor integration in autism: A review of the evidence. *Journal of Autism and Developmental Disorders, 30*(5), 415–421.

DeGangi, G. A., & Greenspan, S. (1989). *Test of Sensory Functions in Infants.* Los Angeles: Western Psychological.

DeMyer, M. K., Barton, S., & Norton, J. A. (1972). A comparison of adaptive, verbal, and motor profiles of psychotic and non-psychotic subnormal children. *Journal of Autism and Childhood Schizophrenia, 2*(4), 359–377.

Duker, P. C., & Rasing, E. (1989). Effects of redesigning the physical environment on self-stimulation and on-task behavior in three autistic-type developmentally disabled individuals. *Journal of Autism and Developmental Disorders, 19*(3), 449–460.

Dunn, W. (1997). Impact of sensory processing on the daily lives of young children and their families: A conceptual model. *Infants and Young Children, 9*(4), 23–35.

Dunn, W. (2002). *Infant/Toddler Sensory Profile*. San Antonio, TX: Psychological Corporation.

Dunn, W., Saiter, J., & Rinner, L. (2002). Asperger syndrome and sensory processing: A conceptual model and guidance for intervention planning. *Focus on Autism and Other Developmental Disabilities, 17*(3), 172–185.

Dunst, C. J. (2002). Family-centered practices: Birth through high school. *Journal of Special Education, 36*(3), 139–147.

Fellows, S. J., Ernst, J., Schwarz, M., Topper, R., & Noth, J. (2001). Precision grip deficits in cerebellar disorders in man. *Clinical Neurophysiology, 112*(10), 1793–1802.

Fogassi, L., & Gallese, V. (2004). Action as a binding key to multisensory integration. In G. G. Calvert, C. Spence, & Stein B. E. (Eds.), *The handbook of multisensory processes* (pp. 425–441). Cambridge, MA: MIT Press.

Folio, M. R., & Fewell, R. R. (2000). *Peabody Developmental Motor Scales–Second Edition*. Itasca, IL: Riverside.

Frankland, P. W., Wang, Y., Rosner, B., Shimizu, T., Balleine, B. W., Dykens, E. M., et al. (2004). Sensorimotor gating abnormalities in young males with fragile X syndrome and Fmr1-knockout mice. *Molecular Psychiatry, 9*(4), 417–425.

Gepner, B., & Mestre, D. R. (2002). Brief report: Postural reactivity to fast visual motion differentiates autistic from children with Asperger syndrome. *Journal of Autism and Developmental Disorders, 32*(3), 231–238.

Gesell, A., & Thompson, H. (1943). Learning and maturation in identical infant twins. In R. G. Barker, J. S. Kounin, & H. F. Wright (Eds.), *Child behavior and development: A course of representative studies* (pp. 209–227). New York: McGraw-Hill.

Ghaziuddin, M., & Butler, E. (1998). Clumsiness in autism and Asperger syndrome: A further report. *Journal of Intellectual Disability Research, 42*(1), 43–48.

Gilotty, L., Kenworthy, L., Sirian, L., Black, D. O., & Wagner, A. E. (2002). Adaptive skills and executive function in autism spectrum disorders. *Neuropsychology Development and Cognition: C. Child Neuropsychology, 8*(4), 241–248.

Goyen, T. A., & Lui, K. (2002). Longitudinal motor development of "apparently normal" high-risk infants at 18 months, 3 and 5 years. *Early Human Development, 70*(1–2), 103–115.

Grandin, T. (1996). *Thinking in pictures and other reports from my life with autism*. New York: Vintage Books.

Gray, C. A., & Garand, J. D. (1993). Social stories: Improving responses of students with autism with accurate social information. *Focus on Autistic Behavior, 8*(1), 1–10.

Greenspan, S., & Wieder, S. (1997). Developmental patterns and outcomes in infants and children with disorders in relating and communicating: A chart review of 200 cases of children with autistic spectrum diagnoses. *Journal of Developmental and Learning Disorders, 1*(1), 87–141.

Happe, F. G. (1994). Annotation: Current psychological theories of autism: The "theory of mind" account and rival theories. *Journal of Child Psychology and Psychiatry, 35*(2), 215–229.

Happe, F. G., & Frith, U. (1995). Theory of mind in autism. In E. Schopler & G. B. Mesibov (Eds.), *Learning and cognition in autism*. New York: Plenum Press.

Hazlett, H. C., Poe, M., Gerig, G., Smith, R. G., Provenzale, J., Ross, A., et al. (2005). Magnetic resonance imaging and head circumference study of brain size in autism: Birth through age 2 years. *Archives of General Psychiatry, 62*(12), 1366–1376.

Hirstein, W., Iversen, P., & Ramachandran, V. S. (2001). Autonomic responses of autistic children to people and objects. *Proceedings of the Royal Society of London: B. Biological Sciences, 268*(1479), 1883–1888.

Hobson, R. P., & Lee, A. (1999). Imitation and identification in autism. *Journal of Child Psychology and Psychiatry, 40*(4), 649–659.

Hoshino, Y., Kumashiro, H., Yashima, Y., Tachibana, R., Watanabe, M., & Furukawa, H. (1982). Early symptoms of autistic children and its diagnostic significance. *Folia Psychiatrica et Neurologica Japonica, 36*(4), 367–374.

Hughes, C., & Russell, J. (1993). Autistic children's difficulty with mental disengagement from an object: Its implications for theories of autism. *Developmental Psychology, 29*, 498–510.

Johnson, M. H., Siddons, F., Frith, U., & Morton, J. (1992). Can autism be predicted on the basis of infant screening tests? *Developmental Medicine and Child Neurology, 34*(4), 316–320.

Johnson-Ecker, C. L., & Parham, L. D. (2000). The evaluation of sensory processing: A validity study using contrasting groups. *American Journal of Occupational Therapy, 54*(5), 494–503.

Jones, R. S. P., Quigney, C., & Huws, J. C. (2003). First hand accounts of sensory perceptual experiences in autism: A qualitative analysis. *Journal of Intellectual and Developmental Disability, 28*, 112–121.

Kemner, C., Oranje, B., Verbaten, M. N., & Van Engeland, H. (2002). Normal P50 gating in children with autism. *Journal of Clinical Psychiatry, 63*(3), 214–217.

Kientz, M. A., & Dunn, W. (1997). A comparison of the performance of children with and without autism on the Sensory Profile. *American Journal of Occupational Therapy, 51*(7), 530–537.

Koegel, L. K., Koegel, R. L., Frea, W., & Green-Hopkins, I. (2003). Priming as a method of coordinating educational services for students with autism. *Language, Speech, and Hearing Services in Schools, 34*(3), 228–235.

Kohen-Raz, R., Volkmar, F. R., & Cohen, D. (1992). Postural control in children with autism. *Journal of Autism and Developmental Disorders, 22*, 419–432.

Kolobe, T. H., Palisano, R. J., & Stratford, P. W. (1998). Comparison of two outcome measures for infants with cerebral palsy and infants with motor delays. *Physical Therapy, 78*(10), 1062–1072.

Kuoch, H., & Mirenda, P. (2003). Social story interventions for young children with autism spectrum disorders. *Focus on Autism and Other Developmental Disabilities, 18*(4), 219–227.

Lainhart, J. E., Piven, J., Wzorek, M., Landa, R., Santangelo, S. L., Coon, H., et al. (1997). Macrocephaly in children and adults with autism. *Journal of the American Academy of Child and Adolescent Psychiatry, 36*(2), 282–290.

Law, M., Cooper, B., Strong, S., Stewart, D., Rigby, P., & Letts, L. (1996). The Person-Environment-Occupation Model: A transactive approach to occupational performance. *Canadian Journal of Occupational Therapy, 63*, 9–23.

Leary, M. R., & Hill, D. A. (1996). Moving on: Autism and movement disturbance. *Mental Retardation, 34*, 39–53.

Lewis, M. H., & Bodfish, J. W. (1998). Repetitive behavior disorders in autism. *Mental Retardation and Developmental Disabilities Research Reviews, 4,* 80–89.

Lewkowicz, D. J. (2002). Heterogeneity and heterochrony in the development of intersensory perception. *Cognitive Brain Research, 14*(1), 41–63.

Lord, C. (1995). Follow-up of two-year-olds referred for possible autism. *Journal of Child Psychology and Psychiatry, 36*(8), 1365–1382.

Manjiviona, J., & Prior, M. (1995). Comparison of Asperger syndrome and high-functioning autistic children on a test of motor impairment. *Journal of Autism and Developmental Disorders, 25,* 23–29.

Mari, M., Castiello, U., Marks, D., Marraffa, C., & Prior, M. (2003). The reach-to-grasp movement in children with autism spectrum disorder. *Philosophical Transactions of the Royal Society of London: B. Biological Sciences, 358*(1430), 393–403.

Marsden, D. D. (1984). Motor disorders in basal ganglia disease. *Human Neurobiology, 2,* 245–250.

McAlonan, G. M., Daly, E., Kumari, V., Critchley, H. D., van Amelsvoort, T., Suckling, J., et al. (2002). Brain anatomy and sensorimotor gating in Asperger's syndrome. *Brain, 125*(Pt. 7), 1594–1606.

McWilliam, R. A. (1992). *Family-centered intervention planning: A routines-based approach.* Tucson, AZ: Communication Skill Builders.

Miller, L. J., Reisman, J. E., McIntosh, D. N., & Simon, J. (2001). An ecological model of sensory modulation: Performance of children with fragile X syndrome, autistic disorder, attention-deficit/hyperactivity disorder, and sensory modulation dysfunction. In S. Smith-Roley, E. I. Blanche, & R. C. Schaaf (Eds.), *Understanding the nature of sensory integration with diverse populations* (pp. 57–88). San Antonio, TX: Therapy Skill Builders.

Miller, L. J., & Roid, G. H. (1994). *The T.I.M.E.: Toddler and Infant Motor Evaluation.* San Antonio, TX: Therapy Skill Builders.

Miyahara, M., Tsujii, M., Hori, M., Nakanishi, K., Kageyama, H., & Sugiyama, T. (1997). Brief report: Motor incoordination in children with Asperger syndrome and learning disabilities. *Journal of Autism and Developmental Disorders, 27*(5), 595–603.

Mullen, E. M. (1995). *Mullen Scales of Early Learning (AGS Edition).* Los Angeles: Western Psychological.

Occupational Therapy Practice Framework: Domain and process. (2002). *American Journal of Occupational Therapy, 56*(6), 609–639.

Ohta, M., Nagai, Y., Hara, H., & Sasaki, M. (1987). Parental perception of behavioral symptoms in Japanese autistic children. *Journal of Autism and Developmental Disorders, 17*(4), 549–563.

Olsen, L. J. (1999). Psychosocial frame of reference. In P. Kramer & J. Hinojosa (Eds), *Frames of reference in pediatric occupational therapy* (2nd ed., pp. 323–350). Baltimore: Lippincott, Williams & Wilkins.

Ornitz, E. M., Guthrie, D., & Farley, A. H. (1977). The early development of autistic children. *Journal of Autism and Childhood Schizophrenia, 7*(3), 207–229.

Ornitz, E. M., & Ritvo, E. R. (1968). Perceptual inconstancy in early infantile autism: The syndrome of early infant autism and its variants including certain cases of childhood schizophrenia. *Archives of General Psychiatry, 18*(1), 76–98.

Page, J., & Boucher, J. (1998). Motor impairments in children with autistic disorder. *Child Language Teaching and Therapy, 14*, 233–259.

Palisano, R. J., Walter, S. D., Russell, D. J., Rosenbaum, P. L., Gemus, M., Galuppi, B. E., et al. (2001). Gross motor function of children with Down syndrome: Creation of motor growth curves. *Archives of Physical Medicine and Rehabilitation, 82*(4), 494–500.

Parham, L. D., & Ecker, C. (2002). Evaluation of sensory processing. In A. Bundy, S. Lane, & E. Murray (Eds.), *Sensory integration: Theory and practice* (2nd ed., pp. 194–196). Philadelphia: Davis.

Parham, L. D., Mailloux, Z., & Roley, S. (2000). *Sensory processing and praxis in high functioning children with autism.* Paper presented at the Research 2000 Conference of the Pediatric Therapy Network, Redondo Beach, CA.

Pierce, K., & Courchesne, E. (2001). Evidence for a cerebellar role in reduced exploration and stereotyped behavior in autism. *Biological Psychiatry, 49*, 655–664.

Piper, M. C., & Darrah, D. (1994). *Motor assessment of the developing infant.* Philadelphia: Saunders.

Realmuto, G. M., & August, G. (1991). Catatonia in autistic disorder: A sign of comorbidity or variable expression? *Journal of Autism and Developmental Disorders, 21*, 517–528.

Redcay, E., & Courchesne, E. (2005). When is the brain enlarged in autism?: A meta-analysis of all brain size reports. *Biological Psychiatry, 58*(1), 1–9.

Rinehart, N. J., Bradshaw, J. L., Brereton, A. V., & Tonge, B. J. (2001). Movement preparation in high-functioning autism and Asperger disorder: A serial choice reaction time task involving motor reprogramming. *Journal of Autism and Developmental Disorders, 31*(1), 79–88.

Rizzolatti, G., & Craighero, L. (2004). The mirror-neuron system. *Annual Review of Neuroscience, 27*, 169–192.

Rogers, S., & Bennetto, L. (2000). Intersubjectivity in autism: The roles of imitation and executive function. In A. Wetherby & B. Prizant (Eds.), *Autism spectrum disorders: A transactional developmental perspective.* (pp. 79–107). Baltimore: Brookes.

Rogers, S. J., Bennetto, L., McEvoy, R., & Pennington, B. F. (1996). Imitation and pantomime in high-functioning adolescents with autism spectrum disorders. *Child Development, 67*(5), 2060–2073.

Rogers, S. J., Hepburn, S. L., Stackhouse, T., & Wehner, E. (2003). Imitation performance in toddlers with autism and those with other developmental disorders. *Journal of Child Psychology and Psychiatry, 44*(5), 763–781.

Rogers, S. J., Hepburn, S., & Wehner, E. (2003). Parent reports of sensory symptoms in toddlers with autism and those with other developmental disorders. *Journal of Autism and Developmental Disorders, 33*(6), 631–642.

Rogers, S. J., & Pennington, B. F. (1991). A theoretical approach to deficits in infantile autism. *Development and Psychopathology, 3*, 137–162.

Russell, D., Palisano, R., Walter, S., Rosenbaum, P., Gemus, M., Gowland, C., et al. (1998). Evaluating motor function in children with Down syndrome: Validity of the GMFM. *Developmental Medicine and Child Neurology, 40*(10), 693–701.

Russell, D., Rosenbaum, P., Avery, L., & Lane, M. (2002). *The Gross Motor Function Measure (GMFM-66 & GMFM-88) user's manual.* London: MacKeith Press.

Sandall, S., Hemmeter, M. L., Smith, B., & McLean, M. E. (2004). *DEC recommended practices: A comprehensive guide for practical application in early intervention/early childhood special education.* Longmont, CO: Sopris West.

Sawyer, L. M., Luiselli, J. K., Ricciardi, J. N., & Gower, J. L. (2005). Teaching a child with autism to share among peers in an integrated preschool classroom: Acquisition, maintenance, and social validation. *Education and Treatment of Children, 28*(1), 1–10.

Schmitz, C., Martineau, J., Barthelemy, C., & Assaiante, C. (2003). Motor control and children with autism: Deficit of anticipatory function? *Neuroscience Letters, 348*(1), 17–20.

Seal, B. C., & Bonvillian, J. D. (1997). Sign language and motor functioning in students with autistic disorder. *Journal of Autism and Developmental Disorders, 27,* 437–466.

Shumway-Cook, A., & Woollacott, M. (2000). *Motor control: Theory and practical applications* (2nd ed.). Baltimore: Lippincott Williams & Wilkins.

Sigman, M., & Ungerer, J. A. (1984). Cognitive and language skills in autistic, mentally retarded, and normal children. *Developmental Psychology, 20,* 293–302.

Smith, A. M., Roux, S., Naidoo, N. T., & Venter, D. J. (2005). Food choice of tactile defensive children. *Nutrition, 21*(1), 14–19.

Smith, I. M., & Bryson, S. E. (1994). Imitation and action in autism: A critical review. *Psychological Bulletin, 116*(2), 259–273.

Smith, L. B., & Thelen, E. (2003). Development as a dynamic system. *Trends in Cognitive Science, 7*(8), 343–348.

Squires, J., Potter, L., & Bricker, D. (1995). *Ages and Stages Questionnaires (ASQ).* Baltimore: Brookes.

Stone, W. L., Ousley, O. Y., Hepburn, S. L., Hogan, K. L., & Brown, C. S. (1999). Patterns of adaptive behavior in very young children with autism. *American Journal of Mental Retardation, 104*(2), 187–199.

Stone, W. L., Ousley, O. Y., & Littleford, C. D. (1997). Motor imitation in young children with autism: What's the object? *Journal of Abnormal Child Psychology, 25*(6), 475–485.

Sweeney, J. A., Takarae, Y., Macmillan, C., Luna, B., & Minshew, N. J. (2004). Eye movements in neurodevelopmental disorders. *Current Opinions in Neurology, 17*(1), 37–42.

Symons, F. J., Sperry, L. A., Dropik, P. L., & Bodfish, J. W. (2005). The early development of stereotypy and self-injury: A review of research methods. *Journal of Intellectual Disability Research, 49*(2), 144–158.

Takarae, Y., Minshew, N. J., Luna, B., Krisky, C. M., & Sweeney, J. A. (2004). Pursuit eye movement deficits in autism. *Brain, 127*(12), 2584–2594.

Talay-Ongan, A., & Wood, K. (2000). Unusual sensory sensitivities in autism: A possible crossroads. *International Journal of Disability, Development and Education, 47*(2), 201–212.

Tecchio, F., Benassi, F., Zappasodi, F., Gialloreti, L. E., Palermo, M., Seri, S., et al. (2003). Auditory sensory processing in autism: A magnetoencephalographic study. *Biological Psychiatry, 54*(6), 647–654.

Teitelbaum, P., Teitelbaum, O., Nye, J., Fryman, J., & Maurer, R. (1998). Movement analysis in infancy may be useful for early diagnosis of autism. *Proceedings of the National Academy of Sciences USA, 95*(23), 13982–13987.

Thelen, E. (1981). Kicking, rocking, and waving: Contextual analysis of rhythmical stereotypies in normal human infants. *Animal Behavior, 29*(1), 3–11.

Thelen, E., & Smith, L. (1994). *A dynamic systems approach to the development of cognition and action.* Cambridge, MA: MIT Press.

Thurman, S. K. (1977). Congruence of behavioral ecologies: A model for special education programming. *Journal of Special Education, 11*(3), 329–333.

Trecker, A. (2001). Play and praxis in children with autism: Observations and intervention strategies. In H. Miller-Kuhaneck (Ed.), *Autism: A comprehensive occupational therapy approach* (pp. 133–151). Bethesda, MD: American Occupational Therapy Association.

Wallace, M. T. (2004). The development of multisensory integration. In G. G. Calvert, C. Spence, & B. E. Stein (Eds.), *Handbook of multisensory processes* (pp. 625–642). Cambridge, MA: MIT Press.

Watling, R. L., Deitz, J., & White, O. (2001). comparison of sensory profile scores of young children with and without autism spectrum disorders. *American Journal of Occupational Therapy, 55*(4), 416–423.

Werner, E., Dawson, G., Osterling, J., & Dinno, N. (2000). Brief report: Recognition of autism spectrum disorder before one year of age: A retrospective study based on home videotapes. *Journal of Autism and Developmental Disorders, 30*(2), 157–162.

Wetherby, A. M., Woods, J., Allen, L., Cleary, J., Dickinson, H., & Lord, C. (2004). Early indicators of autism spectrum disorders in the second year of life. *Journal of Autism and Developmental Disorders, 34*(5), 473–493.

Wing, L. (1981). Asperger's syndrome: A clinical account. *Psychological Medicine, 11*(1), 115–129.

Wing, L. (1997). Syndromes of autism and atypical development. In D. J. Cohen & F. R. Volkmar (Eds.), *Handbook of autism and pervasive developmental disorders* (2nd ed., pp. 148–170). New York: Wiley.

Wing, L., & Shah, A. (2000). Catatonia in autistic spectrum disorders. *British Journal of Psychiatry, 176,* 357–362.

Wolery, M. (1994). Instructional strategies for teaching young children with special needs. In M. Wolery & J. S. Wilkers (Eds.), *Including children with special needs in early childhood programs* (pp. 119–149). Washington, DC: National Association for the Education of Young Children.

Wolery, M. (2000). Commentary: The environment as a source of variability: Implications for research with individuals who have autism. *Journal of Autism and Developmental Disorders, 30*(5), 379–381.

Wolery, M., Brashers, M. S., & Neitzel, J. C. (2002). Ecological congruence assessment for classroom activities and routines: Identifying goals and intervention practices in childcare. *Topics in Early Childhood Special Education, 22*(3), 131–142.

Zwaigenbaum, L., Bryson, S., Rogers, T., Roberts, W., Brian, J., & Szatmari, P. (2005). Behavioral manifestations of autism in the first year of life. *International Journal of Developmental Neuroscience, 23,* 143–152.

CHAPTER 6

Case Studies of Infants First Evaluated in the Second Year of Life

AMI KLIN
CELINE SAULNIER
KATARZYNA CHAWARSKA
FRED R. VOLKMAR

Only 20 years ago, centers specializing in autism spectrum disorders (ASD) rarely evaluated children under the age of 4 years (Siegel, Piner, Eschler, & Elliott, 1988). Nowadays, referrals in the second year of life are commonplace (Chawarska et al., 2007), and knowledge resulting from direct observations of infants subsequently found to have ASD is accruing at a fast pace (Zwaigenbaum et al., 2005). Longitudinal studies of children with ASD first seen in the second and third years of life have begun to clarify issues of developmental trajectories (Lord, 1995; Lord et al., 2006), and promising early predictors of outcome have been identified (Charman et al., 2005). And yet the extreme variability in syndrome manifestation and developmental course continues to be among the most challenging factors in autism research (Volkmar, Lord, Bailey, Schultz, & Klin, 2004).

Nowhere is this challenge more clearly illustrated than in individual cases of infants with ASD followed prospectively during their preschool years. Anxious parents invariably ask examiners what to expect from the future. Experienced clinicians are aware of the limitations of current knowledge to predict the developmental course of individual children. They have to temper any predictions based on group studies, as they have seen multiple permutations of concerning and promising profiles in infants turn into different levels of ability and disability when these children reach school age. And given the premium associated with early intervention in maximizing outcome (National Research Council, 2001), it is still very disappointing that treatments cannot be tailored to individual profiles on the basis of solid knowledge, prescribing the best way of advancing social, communicative, and adaptive skills for one child at a time.

The purpose of this chapter is to present three rather different cases of children with ASD first seen in the second year of life and then followed up until the age of 4 years. Each one was assessed three times and all completed very similar comprehensive developmental disabilities evaluations. We summarize the trajectory of their developmental, speech-language, adaptive, and diagnostic profiles in each one of these evaluations. Developmental status was measured with the *Mullen Scales of Early Learning* (MSEL; Mullen, 1995); speech-language assessments included parent reports such as the *MacArthur–Bates Communicative Development Inventory* (Fenson, 1989) and direct measures such as the *Communication and Symbolic Behavior Scales–Developmental Profile* (CSBS-DP; Wetherby & Prizant, 1993) and the *Reynell Developmental Language Scales–III* (Edwards et al., 1999); adaptive functioning was assessed with the *Vineland Adaptive Behavior Scales, Expanded Edition* (VABS; Sparrow, Balla, & Cicchetti, 1984); and diagnostic assessment included a parent interview—the Autism Diagnostic Interview—Revised (Rutter, LeCouteur, & Lord, 2003), direct observation—the Autism Diagnostic Observation Schedule–Generic, Modules 1 and 2 (ADOS-G; Lord, Rutter, DiLavore, & Risi, 1999), and a consensual diagnosis formulated by at least two experienced clinicians.

These three cases illustrate, among other things, (1) how profiles of development in infants that share many similarities may result in exceedingly different outcomes; (2) how the abrupt emergence of language may dramatically change rate of progress; (3) how language by itself does not guarantee successful social and communicative adaptation; and (4) how little we could predict about these children on the basis of knowledge of their first years of life, or even on the basis of their first comprehensive assessments carried out at 15, 18, and 20 months, respectively, for the three children. The names used in these cases are fictitious.

THE CASE OF "HELEN"

Helen was evaluated at the ages of 15, 34, and 50 months. A more comprehensive description of her early profile is provided elsewhere (Klin et al., 2004). From the time of her initial evaluation, she presented with severe language and social communication deficits that persisted throughout her early childhood. In contrast, her nonverbal cognitive and fine motor skills were at age level at 15 months, but slowed considerably over time, resulting in intellectual impairment by the age of 50 months (and severe intellectual disability as she grew older). Scores on diagnostic instrumentation and clinical diagnosis were consistent with autism in all three evaluations. Neither her parents nor her attentive pediatrician had concerns about her development in the first year of life.

Early Developmental History

Helen was born after a pregnancy complicated by thyroid disease. After delivery, she was kept in a newborn special care unit for a short period of time because of low blood sugar, but she did well after discharge. Milestones were grossly on time. She smiled at 3 weeks of age, sat at 4 months, crawled at 6 months, and walked at 12 months. By parental report, at 12 months she was saying words such as "hi," "baby," "mommy," and "daddy." Helen's pediatrician followed her closely because her older brother had been diagnosed with autism by our group. Shortly after 12 months, Helen stopped vocalizing and became increasingly less socially engaged. At 15 months, she developed an aversion to bright lights and loud noises. Concerned about what was perceived as her deteriorating development, her parents sought a developmental disabilities evaluation.

Family and Medical History

As noted, Helen's brother had been diagnosed with a prototypical form of autism a short time before her birth. Otherwise, there was no family history of autism or developmental or psychiatric disability in the immediate or extended family. Medically, with the exception of four ear infections within a span of 2 or 3 months between 12 and 15 months, she had been entirely healthy. Her parents had initially associated her loss of skills to the ear infections. In genetic and neurological examination, Helen was found to be macrocephalic, but this was a family trait. And yet Helen's head circumference went from the 50th percentile at 6 months to above the 95th percentile at 9 months, stabilizing thereafter. Genetic screening and neuroimaging tests were noncontributory to the diagnostic process.

Intervention History

At about 16 months, Helen began to receive speech–language therapy for 1 hour three times per week and occupational therapy for 1 hour per week. She also received close to 8 hours per week of therapy based on applied behavior analysis (ABA) and attended a play group for about 1 hour twice per week. All of these services were gradually increased in intensity and were maintained after she transitioned to the school system. At 50 months, her program included an ABA setting for a full morning five times per week, a mainstream preschool environment in the afternoon that included "pull-out" occupational therapy and speech–language services, and work with an educational specialist at home after school for about 2 hours four to five times per week.

Assessment

At all three time points, Helen was administered the MSEL, the VABS, the ADI-R, and the ADOS-G (Module 1 for the three assessments).

Developmental Profile

During her initial evaluation at 15 months, Helen's scores were at age level on nonverbal problem-solving skills ("visual reception"; e.g., functional use of objects, object permanence, emerging shape discrimination skills) and fine and gross motor skills (e.g., eye–hand coordination, scribbling in imitation, running, throwing a ball). In contrast, she had severe deficits in language development, with delays of 6–8 months in receptive and expressive skills, respectively. At 34 months she had made steady but slow progress in nonverbal cognitive and fine motor skills, resulting in delays of 12–14 months. She continued to have severe language deficits, with delays of 21–23 months. By the third evaluation, there was progress in language but slowing down of nonverbal reasoning and fine motor skills. At 50 months, she continued to show delays in development, ranging from 19 to 29 months, with the most severe deficits in expressive language. Figure 6.1 ("Helen") illustrates her rate of progress from 15 to 50 months of age.

Speech, Language, and Communication Profile

At 15 months, Helen displayed no conventional or communicative gestures. She at times pulled the examiner's hand to execute a desired action. If left by herself, Helen was extremely isolated. She could seek her parents' contact when distressed, but not often. She could respond to verbal directions only in the presence of exaggerated visual cues, or following predictable routines. Her vocalizations consisted of primarily nonword sounds, and they were not directed at another person. At 34 months, her presentation was virtually unchanged. She did not orient spontaneously to unfamiliar adults, but at times she sought the proximity of her parents. Her vocalizations, smiles, and gestures occurred primarily when she was watching herself in a mirror. It was very difficult to engage her in imitative games, but she liked singing to herself. All communication functions

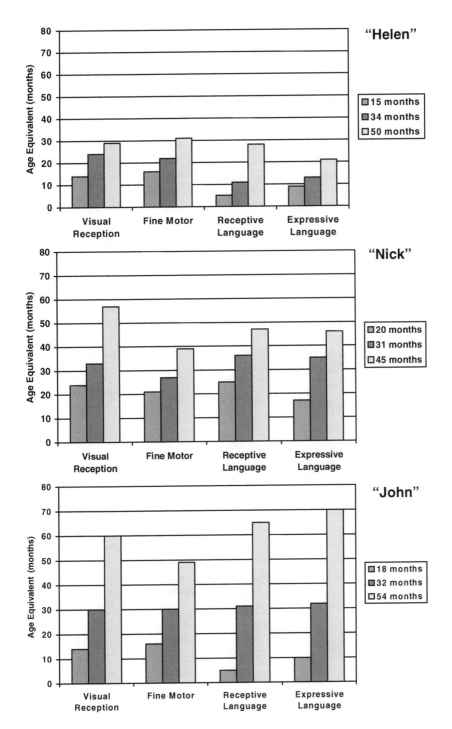

FIGURE 6.1. Age-equivalent scores on the Mullen Scales of Early Learning achieved by "Helen," "Nick," and "John" during their successive visits at the clinic.

were severely impaired, including nonverbal gestures, shared attention, visual engagement, and eye contact. She imitated some sounds but only a handful of words, although she could sing a nursery rhyme from beginning to end. Attention to language in general was extremely limited.

At 50 months, Helen had learned many words, but she was much more likely to label objects or figures than to use them in communicative contexts (e.g., making a request from an adult). She could follow simple directions containing two attributes (e.g., "show me the red car"), but could not understand sentences that contained order or causation (e.g., "the baby pushes the mommy"). When a word was presented to her in the context of a sentence, she was much less likely to understand it than when the word was given to her in isolation (e.g., a single word paired to an object, action, or figure). In fact, her ability to label pictures in isolation was close to age level. But she often had nonmeaningful associations that made it difficult for others to understand her (e.g., "thumb" for "fingers" more generally; "couch" for "chair"). She could use a handful of simple signs for requests (e.g., for "more" or "stop"). In summary, with the exception of some isolated areas of strength such as a single-word vocabulary, Helen made steady but very slow progress in speech and language, and particularly in communication development.

Adaptive Functioning

At 15 months, Helen showed severe delays in socialization and expressive language skills, with relative strengths in receptive language and motor skills. Over the next 35 months, her rate of progress in language, interpersonal, and play skills was extremely slow, and by 50 months she had profound delays in her ability to use language and social skills consistently in real-life settings. Motor skills showed slow but steady progress, but by 50 months they were also lagging age expectations by some 16 months. Interestingly, beginning sometime before her second evaluation, Helen became fascinated with letters and numbers. This is reflected in her "written" score (knowledge of letters and numbers, and "readiness" or preacademic skills). And by the time she was 50 months old, her reading abilities in fact exceeded her chronological age by more than 20 months. In other words, she was reading (i.e., decoding graphemes) almost like a 6-year-old despite her severe cognitive and language deficits. Her understanding, however, was very limited. Figure 6.2 ("Helen") illustrates her rates of growth in adaptive functioning from 15 to 50 months.

Diagnostic Presentation

At 15 months, Helen was extremely self-isolated. If left to her own devices, she perseverated in exploration of cause–effect toys (e.g., blocks, pop-up

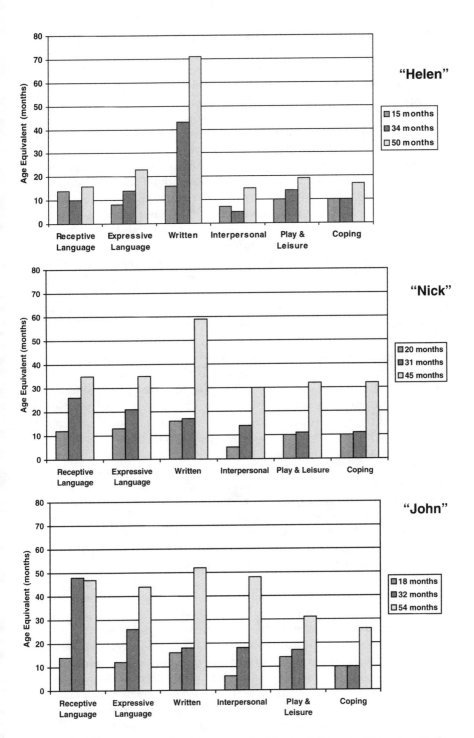

FIGURE 6.2. Age-equivalent scores on the Vineland Adaptive Behaviors Scales achieved by "Helen," "Nick," and "John" during their successive visits at the clinic.

toys) and objects with special textures, ignoring others' bids for engagement. Eye contact was infrequent and could not be elicited in a predictable manner. Her smiles were mostly in response to her own actions (e.g., flicking a doll's eye) or in response to sensory experiences (e.g., with lights, shiny objects). She could not be engaged in anticipatory games (e.g., "peek-a-boo"). If an adult intruded upon her field of vision, she typically focused on the periphery (e.g., hair, chin) of the approaching adult's head or overfixated on the adult's mouth. She did not show any interest in miniatures or representational toys. When frustrated, she made high-pitched sounds that were self-stimulatory rather than communicative. She did not use unfamiliar adults or her parents to get things she wanted, and she was not sensitive to or use pointing or other gestures. She exhibited a number of stereotypic behaviors, including hand flapping and posturing of her fingers. She was acutely aware of visual details in the environment (e.g., finding a piece of candy some 5 feet away) and was easily frightened by noises or novel events (e.g., the noise of a balloon being inflated).

Helen's presentation at 34 months was virtually unchanged. Her vocalizations consisted primarily of high-pitched sounds and cries. She had no words or word approximations. The intonation of her vocalizations had a self-stimulatory quality (e.g., singsong sounds made to herself rather than as part of communication with others). She liked to verbally label objects, but did not use any words to request, protest, or otherwise share an experience. She was best engaged by her parents in the context of "rough-and-tumble" routines, when she would smile and enjoy the movement. Her facial expressions, however, were rarely directed at others, reflecting instead her sense of contentment during the exploration of an object, when looking at herself in the mirror, or when otherwise engaged in self-stimulatory behaviors. Her sensory-seeking behaviors and motor mannerisms increased markedly between the first and second evaluations.

By 50 months, Helen's presentation had changed somewhat. She was now much more able to follow activities that were imposed by the examiner, was less likely to shift attention fleetingly from object to object, and could tolerate working with an adult for longer periods of time. Self-injurious behaviors shown previously when demands were placed on her had diminished considerably. She began to use words for the purpose of making familiar requests and could pair them with pointing. These abilities had been the focus of much of her therapy by then. Verbal utterances were primarily limited to single words, and many of them involved stereotypic language or self-talk. Intonation was very flat, and she now exhibited immediate echolalia. In less structured, predictable, or familiar routines, however, Helen's social and communication presentation still reflected a marked degree of self-isolation and independence. She was not likely to seek contact with others, appeared confused when approached by others in verbal or nonverbal ways if this was not part of her learned repertoire, and continued to be drawn to object manipulation or cause–effect routines rather than representational toys or symbolic play with others.

Summary

Helen may have developed well until about 12 months of age, although we were unable to confirm this directly (e.g., using videotapes made during her first year of life). By the time of her first evaluation, however, she had a prototypical autistic presentation that remained stable. And although most areas of social and communicative development were already severely impaired at 15 months, her nonverbal cognitive and fine motor skills were close to age level. By the time of her third evaluation, she exhibited marked developmental delays in all domains, which were particularly severe in the areas of socialization and communication skills. Despite a great deal of treatment and intervention, her gains were only modest. In contrast to exhibiting these severe disabilities, she developed a fascination with letters and numbers, and by 50 months of age she had reading decoding skills that exceeded her chronological age by almost 1½ years.

THE CASE OF "NICK"

Nick was evaluated at the ages of 20, 31, and 45 months. From the time of his initial evaluation, and consistently through his early childhood, Nick presented with a profile of strong developmental skills accompanied by significant deficits in social reciprocity and communication. Scores on diagnostic instrumentation and clinical diagnosis were consistent with autism in all three evaluations.

Early Developmental History

Nick was born after a pregnancy complicated by severe viral or flu-like illness and severe nausea. Concern about a low level of amniotic fluid resulted in an emergency C-section. Birth weight was 7 pounds 13 ounces, and Apgar scores were 4 and 9. He was noted to have somewhat low tonus at birth. His mother felt that he did not like to be held. He was hard to feed and seemed unresponsive at first. Other concerns emerged within days of his birth and remained throughout his first year of life. He did not seem to be interested in looking at other people and did not startle to loud sounds. He had staring spells and could not seem to nestle when held. By 9 months of age, he was able to sit up if held and soon started to crawl. He began to walk at about the age of 15 months. Nick liked fans and other spinning objects and was also interested in bright lights. As a toddler, Nick's response to others was variable. He could discriminate between his parents and other people, but only rarely imitated simple adult movements. He was only rarely interested in other children. He was unresponsive when his name was called, and eye contact was inconsistent.

Family and Medical History

Nick's family history was positive for a first cousin with autism, and his father had a seizure disorder. Nick has never had signs or symptoms of seizures, although, as noted, he had an early history of long staring spells. Results of electroencephalographic (EEG) studies, brain magnetic resonance imaging (MRI), and cytogenetic testing were noncontributory to the diagnostic process. Nick was evaluated by a neuropsychologist at the age of 11 months. Results revealed mild delays in cognitive and fine motor skills and more significant delays in gross motor and language skills. The most significant delays were noted in social communication and social relatedness. Diagnostic impressions at that time were consistent with an autism spectrum disorder, and Nick was then referred to the Yale Developmental Disabilities Clinics.

Intervention History

Nick began receiving early intervention services when he was 9 months of age. By the time he was first evaluated in our Clinics at the age of 20 months, he was receiving occupational therapy, physical therapy, speech–language services, and 3 hours a week of applied behavior analysis (ABA). Services continued when Nick entered the school system at age 3, with a marked increase of 20 hours per week of in-home ABA services. His parents attended numerous workshops and support groups for parents of children with developmental disabilities.

Assessment

At all three time points, Nick was administered the MSEL, the VABS, the ADI-R, and the ADOS-G (Module 1 for the first two assessments, and Module 2 for the third assessment).

Developmental Profile

During his initial evaluation at the age of 20 months, Nick's developmental profile was quite strong, with scores ranging from average to above average as compared with same-age peers. Receptive language was his strongest ability, with an age-equivalent score falling at the 25-month level. Expressive language was less well developed, falling at the 17-month level.

Nonverbal problem solving was at the 24-month level, and fine motor skills were at the 21-month level.

Figure 6.1 ("Nick") illustrates the variable rate of progress that Nick made between his first and third evaluations. At 31 months, nonverbal cognitive and receptive language skills developed at a pace consistent with chronological growth. There was tremendous growth in expressive language, going from age equivalents of 17 months to 35 months from the first to the second evaluation, indicating a growth of 18 months within an 11-month period. In contrast, he showed a progress of only 6 months in fine motor skills within the same time span. At 45 months, a different pattern was obtained. Nick showed remarkable growth in nonverbal cognitive skills, with a gain of 24 months within a 14-month period. His score in this domain was in the superior range, 12 months above his chronological age. Rates of receptive and expressive language skills slowed a little, but overall levels were commensurate with his chronological age. Fine motor skills continued to be somewhat delayed.

Speech, Language, and Communication Profile

At 20 months, Nick's speech was limited to approximately 20 single-word approximations, which was commensurate with the 13- to 17-month developmental level. He showed a reduced frequency of spontaneous and intentional communication, little use of communicative gaze to direct his communication, and a reduced capacity to respond to or establish joint attention. Conventional gestures were limited to a "give" gesture, touch, and a head shake. By 31 months, Nick's speech had improved sufficiently to make possible an administration of the Reynell Developmental Language Scales, which resulted in comprehension and expression scores in the lower portion of the normative range (thus lower than his language scores on the MSEL). The average mean length of utterance (MLU) was 2.08 words, which fell at the 26-month age level. Despite these gains, Nick's repertoire of two- and three-word combinations and simple sentence structures was still limited. He relied heavily on verbal prompting and exhibited immediate echolalia. At 45 months, language comprehension and expression, as measured with the Reynell, continued to improve and now fell in the upper portion of the normative range. The MLU was 3.81, falling within expected levels. Nevertheless, conversation patterns were dominated by his strong interests (e.g., cameras and fans), and his speech continued to have a repetitious quality.

Adaptive Functioning

At 20 months, with the exception of (fine and gross) motor skills, Nick's adaptive behavior profile was significantly delayed across all areas, relative to both his chronological and his developmental age, with extreme delays in the area of interpersonal skills (at the 5-month level). Figure 6.2 ("Nick") illustrates the variable rate of progress that Nick made between his first and third evaluations. At 31 months, receptive and expressive skills improved, although they were still below chronological and developmental levels, and motor skills appeared to be slowing relative to chronological growth. There was improvement in interpersonal skills but almost none in play skills, and both areas of socialization remained significantly delayed. At 45 months, there was continued growth in receptive and language skills, marked improvement in interpersonal and, particularly, play skills, although all of these domains were still significantly delayed relative to his age and developmental level. There was remarkable growth in "readiness" or preacademic skills, with his "written" skills reaching the 59-month level when he was still 45 months of age. This was a reflection of Nick's affinity for numbers and letters. This score inflated his overall score in the communication domain (which by then fell in the lower portion of the normative range), which combines receptive, expressive, and written skills, thus misrepresenting his true language abilities if subdomain scores were not considered separately. Overall, he made the largest gains between his second and third evaluations, but as seen in Figure 6.2, this growth was selective and highly variable across domains. Overall, at 45 months he was still about 1 year below chronological and developmental level. Also of concern were Nick's functional motor skills, which showed no growth between 31 and 45 months, resulting in substantial delays. This was consistent with scores on the MSEL, which showed that fine motor skills became progressively more impaired over time relative to chronological growth.

Diagnostic Presentation

On the ADOS-G, Module 1 at 20 months, when the supports inherent in the format of structured developmental and speech testing were removed, Nick presented as a self-directed and self-absorbed little boy. Social-communicative skills acquired during structured one-to-one teaching situations had not generalized to more naturalistic settings. Although he was fairly interested in a number of presented materials, he was not likely to show them to others or to ask for help in operating some of the toys. His first "line of defense" was to try and get things done or to "fix" things independently. If this failed, he was likely to lose interest in the toy or activity rather than to ask for help. His play was limited to cause-and-effect toys, construction materials, and manipulation of little cars. Although he was aware of the function of many objects and was able to use them appropriately, he was drawn to extraneous characteristics of objects, such as shiny details, car wheels, doll's eyes, and edges of books. The diagnostic impression was consistent with autism.

On the ADOS-G, Module 1 at 31 months, progress in social communication was evident but much vulnerability remained. Nick had become more responsive to others and more likely to make attempts to involve other people in his activities (e.g., by holding up objects for show). Yet the quality and frequency of his spontaneous bids for interaction were limited. For instance, he was less likely to monitor the behavior of others or to use eye contact for communicative purposes, and when left to his own devices entirely, he engaged in self-stimulatory and repetitive behaviors (e.g., making things spin, examining edges and surfaces through the corners of his eyes). His play was still dominated by cause-and-effect toys. Yet with intrusive prompting and scaffolding, he could be engaged in simple one-step pretend-play episodes with figurines (e.g., feeding the dolls or placing them in furniture). Overall, his presentation was still very much consistent with autism.

On the ADOS-G, Module 2 at 45 months, Nick's social and communicative gains were much more pronounced. By then he used complex sentences to describe his activities, provided a narrative in play, recounted past events, shared attention and made requests. He was more interested in novel adults and could follow and participate in social exchanges, but only if these were highly structured and supported by the examiner. If these supports were removed, however, Nick again gravitated toward his strong interests, which mainly involved self-stimulatory behaviors (e.g., spinning things) and cause–effect play. Interestingly, he began to "intellectualize" some of these stereotypic behaviors by adding narration to them in an attempt to make them appear more appropriate. For instance, when spinning a disc, he stated that it might be a "CD"; he would then begin to hum a tune while covering his ears with his hands. His perseverative interests more generally, however, began to pervade his social interactions and play. For example, he moved his hands like a fan or windshield wipers. And despite his significant growth in language, his speech was still echolalic and repetitive and his voice was often high-pitched. Thus, his many gains notwithstanding, his presentation was still consistent with autism.

Summary

In contrast to Helen, whose first year of life appeared not to be of concern to her parents and pediatrician, Nick had a first year filled with serious worries for his parents. And yet Helen's outcome was much more compromised than Nick's. Despite apparent developmental delays at 11 months, at his first evaluation at 20 months he was already showing skills at close to age expectations, but these contrasted with severe limitations in language and communication beyond labeling of objects. His social impairment and repetitive and stereotypic patterns of behavior were prototypically autistic, with severe delays in social adaptation. In the next 25 months he made remarkable developmental gains, first in expressive language and then in nonverbal cognitive skills. At 45 months his nonverbal functioning was 12 months above expected age level, language was within the average range, and fine motor skills were delayed. But he was unable to translate this potential into real-life skills, with moderate delays in language use, socialization, and what appeared to be a plateau in motor skills. A remarkable jump in reading (decoding) skills resulted in levels that were 14 months above his chronological age. Diagnostically, Nick's speech and language were marked by echolalia and rigidities; imagination was impoverished and communication was disrupted by circumscribed interests; and he had a wide range of stereotypic behaviors. Overall, his behavioral presentation was consistent with prototypical autism, but he had strong skills, albeit quite variable across domains.

THE CASE OF "JOHN"

John was evaluated at the ages of 18, 32, and 54 months. His early presentation was consistent with autism and global developmental delays. In his subsequent developmental trajectory, however, he showed remarkable progress in language. Delays in social reciprocity and communication remained, although by the age of 54 months these could be described as "residual" and more consistent with a diagnosis of Pervasive Developmental Disorder-Not Otherwise Specified (PDD-NOS) rather than autism. We raised the possibility that future evaluators might "move" him out of the autism spectrum if his developmental history was not considered. In many ways, his presentation was more complex than Nick's.

Early Developmental History

John was the youngest of three children, with two older typical siblings. Delivery was performed at 36 weeks of gestation via C-section because of placenta accreta. John weighed 6 pounds, 7.5 ounces, at birth. He was described as an easy, placid infant who was not as demanding as his two older brothers. Initial developmental milestones were on time with subsequent delays. He smiled by 2–3 months, sat without support at 6 months, and crawled by 9 months. His first words emerged at 15–16 months (e.g., "Hi," "mama," "dada"), but were not followed by the acquisition of new words. He did not start walking until 18 months.

John's parents became concerned about his development when he was approximately 15 months of age. They noticed that his eye contact was very limited, particularly with less familiar people, and he was unlikely to respond to his name or to approach a family member other than parents. In addition, his speech and motor development were not progressing as expected. By the age of 18 months, John had about three words, which he used infrequently and indiscriminately. He had difficulties in walking by himself. He developed an aversion to forms of sensory stimulation, and he would cover his ears or eyes in response to sound or light. He also avoided being touched and would bang his head against hard surfaces. Although he could usually tell the difference between his parents and other people, he responded to others very inconsistently. He had almost no interest in other children, although he would, occasionally, play very simple interaction games. He rarely imitated simple adult movements or sounds.

John began speaking in two-word phrases at the age of 30 months, and by 54 moths he was speaking in full sentences. Nevertheless, his parents remained concerned about a range of behaviors. He showed an interest in looking at spinning objects and sought out activities that involved body spinning, twirling, or running in circles. His parents described him as "very high maintenance" and not easy to care for, as he seemed to get upset and frustrated very easily and frequently. When upset, he would hit himself on the head and scream rather than use his words to express his frustration or to otherwise attain what he wanted. On a few occasions when upset, he talked about wanting to kill himself and others. He remained sensitive to sensations in his environment, like temperature and sound.

Family and Medical History

There was no reported history of autism or developmental disabilities in John's extended family. John was generally a healthy baby, except for one ear infection and suspected respiratory syncytial virus (RSV) infection at 9 months. Behavioral audiometry at 18 months was within normal limits. As per the advice of a homeopathic doctor, he was placed on a gluten-, casein-, and soy-free diet, although a regular diet was introduced by the time he was 4 years of age.

Intervention History

After John's initial diagnosis, he began to receive early intervention services consisting of speech–language therapy for 1 hour ten times per week, 1 hour of occupational therapy four times per week, and play therapy 1 hour six times per week. John had "therapeutic listening" for 1 hour per day, as well as applied behavior analysis (ABA) therapy for 4 hours per week. He also attended a preschool program 3 days per week, 2 hours per day, where an aide accompanied him.

Assessment

At all three time points, Nick was administered the MSEL, the VABS, the ADI-R, and the ADOS-G (Module 1 for the first assessment and Module 2 for the second and third assessments).

Developmental Profile

At 18 months, John was exhibiting global developmental delays, with moderate delays in his nonverbal reasoning skills and, to a lesser extent, fine motor skills and very severe delays in his language abilities. At 32 months, he had made marked progress in all areas of development, in fact catching up with expectations on the basis of chronological age. Figure 6.1 ("John") illustrates these gains, with the most significant progress noted in his receptive and expressive language. John's language skills continued to improve at a striking rate, with receptive and expressive language scores falling significantly above age expectations (by 11–16 months) at the time of his third evaluation at 54 months. Nonverbal reasoning also evidenced marked improvement; fine motor skills improved but still lagged behind age expectations. To highlight his rate of progress in language: From the second to the third evaluation, he made a 32- to 38-month gain within the period of 22 months.

Speech, Language, and Communication Profile

At 18 months, John's speech, language, and communication were extremely delayed. He had no words, and very little in terms of spontaneous and intentional communication, communicative gaze, and joint attention. Nonverbal and verbal forms of communication (e.g., gestures, vocalizations, word approximations) were commensurate with the 8- to 9-month developmental level, and his comprehension of words and simple directions was commensurate with the 10- to 12-month developmental level. At 32 months, there was remarkable growth. He used an appropriate range of word classes, with a mean length of utterance (MLU) of 3.44 morphemes, which was at age level. He varied volume, inflection, and pitch in a communicative way, especially when he wanted to convey intense emotion and when asking questions. John's comprehension of language also improved markedly. His understanding of both routine phrases and commands and novel sentence structures was age appropriate. He could use gestures and words to regulate others' behavior (e.g., requesting objects and actions and protesting), to draw others' attention to environmental stimuli of interest to him (e.g., verbal commenting, pointing, asking for information), to clarify information, to respond to others' greetings, to request comfort, and, on one occasion, to show off. Although he was adept at selecting appropriate words and gestures to achieve these goals, John's communication often lacked persistence and intentionality. For example, he might comment on an interesting picture, but would not look to see if others were paying attention or otherwise insist that they should. Overall, he was less likely than other children his age to use communication to attract another person's attention to himself and to engage in social interaction.

At 54 months, John was administered the Reynell test, and his scores in both comprehension and expression tasks fell within the average range. On the receptive portion, he was able to do all items on the test, except those that required the ability to draw inferences from a picture in answer to specific questions. Although this difficulty was not atypical for 4-year-olds, John was unable to use the information he had to even make a guess. He seemed quite baffled by the nonliteral questions. On the expressive portion of this test, John had difficulty in imitating sentences and correcting incorrect forms ("He drive the car"). Again, these difficulties were not indicative of a significant delay, but suggested that John needed extra practice in holding linguistic information in mind and in using it to make decisions.

Adaptive Functioning

John's profile of adaptive skills is quite interesting. At 18 months, he had very severe delays in interpersonal skills and moderate impairments in all other areas of adaptive functioning. These delays were consistent with cognitive and speech–language testing. By 32 months, he had made great but variable progress, with remarkable gains in receptive language (a jump of 34 months within a 14-month period), significant progress in expressive language and fine motor skills (although he remained delayed relative to his age), and more modest gains in socialization. Interestingly, his receptive language score on the VABS (an age-equivalent score of 48 months at the chronological age of 32 months) was in fact higher than the receptive language score on the MSEL and in direct speech–language testing. In other words, he could understand more language and communication in a real-world environment than one would predict on the basis of his language potential (e.g., size of vocabulary, syntactic forms, response to standardized directions). As discussed subsequently, this is an anomaly in individuals with ASD, whose almost universal profile indicates higher scores on direct testing (i.e., potential) relative to consistent use of skill to meet the demands of everyday life (i.e., competence), which is what the VABS measures. And yet this contrasted with his adaptive skills in expressive language, which lagged behind relative to his testing scores and relative to age expectations. As noted, socialization skills lagged behind even farther. Figure 6.2 ("John") illustrates the variability in gains by domain of adaptive behavior from the first to the third evaluation results.

At 54 months, John had made marked progress in all areas of adaptive functioning, with levels getting close to age expectations though still somewhat lagging behind (the lack of change in receptive skills reflects the low ceiling levels in this subdomain of communication on the VABS). There were two important exceptions, in opposite directions: His play skills were still very significantly delayed (besides having some limitations in imagination, disruptive behaviors were now affecting his ability to play with peers); in contrast, "written" or preacademic skills showed the largest improvement and were now at age level. These various gains notwithstanding, John's adaptive scores were much lower than one would expect on the basis of his cognitive and language potential as tested directly (e.g., a gap of 26 months in expressive language if comparing MSEL with VABS results). Thus, he could perform much better on testing than he could avail himself of these skills when trying to meet the communication demands in real life (e.g., with peers). That is, a sizable portion of his progress was still not translating into competence (e.g., generalizing to new settings and functional contexts).

Diagnostic Presentation

At 18 months, John explored new environments in a very isolated fashion, neither seeking nor responding to his parents' bids. He failed to spontaneously acknowledge the presence of unfamiliar people and, in fact, it was quite difficult to attract his attention or establish eye contact with him at all. Although he vocalized a great deal, words or word approximations were not heard during the diagnostic session. He also displayed a number of unusual sensory-related behaviors, particularly in the realm of visual stimulation (e.g., inspecting objects closely). On the ADOS-G algorithm, he obtained a combined score of 20, which fell solidly above the threshold for autism. Clinician-assigned diagnosis was consistent with autism.

At 32 months, John was already speaking in full sentences for both requesting desired objects and commenting about the environment. However, he still exhibited immediate echolalia. And despite his impressive language and communicative gains, John typically failed to integrate eye contact with verbal requests. Very significant limitations in pretend or symbolic play persisted. On the ADOS-G, despite a lower score on the communication cluster (i.e., less impairment), his scores continued to be above the autism threshold. At 54 months, language and communication vulnerabilities were much less apparent, and yet impairments in reciprocal social interaction and in symbolic play behaviors persisted. The "prototypicality" of his autistic behaviors had disappeared, and his vulnerabilities were more confined to social situations in which contingency and reciprocity were critical, and when play activities involved a key pretend component for joint play to take place (e.g., developing an imaginary sequence or plot, sharing the pretend scheme introduced by the other person). His scores on the ADOS-G were no longer above the threshold for autism, but still met the criteria for ASD (or PDD-NOS).

Summary

In many ways, John's presentation at the age of 18 months was almost as troubling as that of Helen's. And yet their eventual outcomes were extremely different. Helen became severely intellectually disabled and prototypically autistic, whereas John's developmental skills reached average levels and his social and communication presentation was more of a "residual" quality, with clear vulnerabilities, but these were noticeable only in more demanding social and communicative situations. Besides his initial severe social impairments and self-stimulatory behaviors, he had delayed motor development, beginning to walk only at about the age of 18 months. His language progressed rapidly, and eventually echolalic utterances faded and his ability to use language for the purpose of communication improved greatly. Reading decoding skills were a relative strength by 4½ years. Yet despite this extremely positive outcome, there was a wide range of highly concerning behaviors. These included poor self-regulation, low frustration levels associated with self-injury, persistent sensory sensitivities, and deep despondency. It seemed that as his social disability improved, his behavioral and emotional presentation became increasingly more concerning. Emerging social awareness and frustration with persistent difficulties appeared to fuel his dissatisfaction and maladaptive, as well as aggressive, reactions.

DISCUSSION

The notion that there is no autism, but "autisms," is gaining some popularity among researchers frustrated by the vast heterogeneity of both phenotype and genotype in ASD. Etiology is likely to be multifactorial and complex, evidenced already in discoveries of genes associated with autism (Gupta & State, 2007), which come with warnings of strong epigenetic effects. And yet the older notion that autism represents a syndrome that results from a "common pathway" to social disability is still tenable. After all, the main stage of social and communication development is the earliest iterative experiences of reciprocal social engagement (Klin, Jones, Schultz, & Volkmar, 2003). Disruptions of this pathway were already hypothesized to be at the root of autism by Kanner in his original description of the syndrome (1943). But social and communicative development is also impacted by an assortment of other developmental skills. Language is critical, but it may at times grow as if outside the realm of social interaction. A large vocabulary is not a guarantee of competence in communication (Paul, 2005). Intelligence is highly correlated with language development, but it may leave it behind as nonverbal problem-solving skills forge ahead, creating disconnections between verbal and nonverbal intelligence (Klin, Saulnier, Tsatsanis, & Volkmar, 2005). Motor skills are critical not only in inquisitive exploration of the environment, but also in tactile intersubjectivity in the life of the infant. Most small children can be at times overwhelmed by sensations and sensory stimulation, but children with ASD may have extreme though variable responses to both environment and social stimuli, erecting an additional barrier to exploratory learning and to social intimacy. Thus, the notion of a single "final common pathway" is challenged by varied permutations of all of these factors and how they might interrelate to yield developmental profiles in individual children.

Nowhere are we as challenged as when attempting to predict outcome in infants with ASD. There were serious developmental concerns in Nick's and in John's first years of life, and apparently none in Helen's case. And yet she had the worst outcome. At their first evaluations in the second year of life, Helen and John presented with serious developmental delays; yet John's autism could be characterized as "residual" by the third evaluation, whereas Helen's could be characterized as "prototypical." Nick's initial developmental profile was the strongest of the three, and yet, despite his marked gains, his autism was still much more pronounced at the third evaluation than John's.

These challenges notwithstanding, there are a number of lines of conceptual convergence suggested by these three cases, which have clinical and research implications, as explored in the following paragraphs.

How Low Can We Measure Sociability?

All three children had severe social adaptive disabilities at their first assessments. At 15 months, 20 months, and 18 months, Helen, Nick and John, respectively, had age-equivalent scores on the interpersonal subdomain of the VABS at 7, 5, and 6 months. However, detailed diagnostic observations by experienced clinicians discerned the most socially disconnected and isolated picture in Helen's case (see Klin et al., 2004, for a detailed description). Unfortunately, standardized instrumentation available to clinicians may not be sufficient to truly quantify levels of sociability covering accomplishments taking place in the full first year of life. And yet the amount of social and communicative growth from 1 to 12 months is truly astounding. Developmental psychologists should challenge the notion that someone with her profile can be characterized with social adaptive skills at the 7th month level. After all, anyone who has interacted sufficiently with 7-month-old babies knows how profoundly social and reciprocal they are.

In Helen's case, she failed to exhibit skills such as preferential attention to speech sounds, orientation to socially revealing aspects of the face such as the eye region, reactions to the presence and intrusion of another person, and differentiated behaviors resulting from exaggerated facial and bodily gestures as well as playful voice inflections, all of which are fully online in the first months if not weeks of life of typically developing babies (Klin et al., 2003). As clinicians, we questioned what were Helen's perceptual and mental experiences of another person, and considered how we could capture what appeared to be profound unrelatedness.

To address this concern, we performed two experiments intended to answer the following questions (Klin & Jones, 2007): (1) Is Helen capable of imparting social meaning to what she sees? In other words, can she think about people? And (2) does Helen visually inspect approaching people in ways that reveal her understanding of a complex visual configuration as a person? In other words, can she see people? To answer the first question, we used point-light animations emulating social experiences in infancy. The capacity for recognizing point-light displays of this nature as exemplars of "biological motion" (e.g., distinguishing moving dots depicting a walking person from dots moving randomly) has been shown in 3-month-old infants (Fox & McDaniel, 1982). Helen's looking behavior in response to such displays was entirely random, indicating an inability to impose mental templates of human action onto these displays. But an exception occurred when we inadvertently created a contingency that involved physical causation (points "colliding" and making a sound in the act of playing "pat-a-cake'). She was acutely aware of this phenomenon. Thus, she was unable to appreciate the motion contingencies of human action but could fully appreciate the physical contingencies of points colliding and making sounds.

Following these observations, and to address the second question, we explored whether Helen's sensitivities to physically contingent versus socially contingent stimuli might also result in atypical visual fixation patterns when she looked at people. Typical infants prefer to focus on the eye region of the face from at least the age of 3 months (Haith, Bergman, & Moore, 1977), consistent with the idea that the eyes convey the most social-affective information (Emery, 2000). In contrast, Helen's sensitivity to information that was physically synchronous in the point-light animations, together with the cross-modal physical contingency of speech sounds and lip movements, predicted that when looking at videos of a caregiver, Helen would preferentially fixate on the mouth region of the face. We compared her visual fixation patterns to those of two typically developing infants matched to her on nonverbal and verbal mental age, respectively. As shown in Figure 6.3, Helen spent most of her viewing time focused on caregivers' mouth regions. These fixation patterns contrasted markedly with those of the two other infants. Based on these

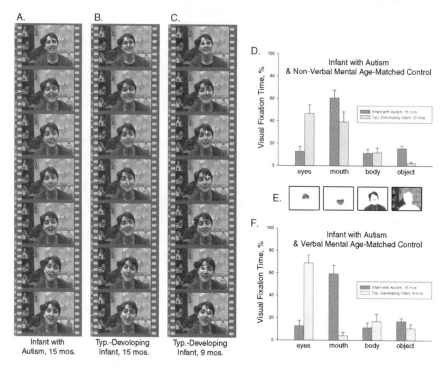

FIGURE 6.3. Visual fixation while watching scenes of a caregiver. (A) Screenshots of data from infant with autism (age 15 months). (B) Screenshots of data from typically developing control matched on nonverbal mental age (age 15 months). (C) Screenshots of data from typically developing control matched on verbal mental age (age 9 months). (D) Percentage of visual fixation time on eyes, mouth, body, and object regions for infant with autism and nonverbal mental age-matched control. (E) Example coding regions for one frame of video. (F) Percentage of visual fixation time on eyes, mouth, body, and object regions for infant with autism and verbal mental age-matched control. Bar graphs are percentage of total fixation time, with *SEM* error bars. From Klin and Jones (2007). Copyright 2007 by Blackwell Publishing. Reprinted by permission.

results, we hypothesized that this pattern of looking would suggest seeing the world, and even people, as a collection of physical contingencies, unmoored from their social context or adaptive relevance. Living in such a world would likely have a profound impact on the development of the social mind and on the organization of the social brain (Johnson 2001).

There is no doubt that Helen's developmental trajectory reflected a complex interplay between her genetic and neurobiological makeup and experiential factors. However, her social disability limited significantly the range of experiences typically available to nonaffected infants and toddlers. Helen tended to isolate herself and responded with active avoidance to purely social overtures. Her extremely limited motor and vocal imitation skills severely restricted her ability to learn through observation. Over time, her tendency to explore novel toys declined and her attention became more fleeting. Her spontaneous activities consisted frequently of seemingly aimless wandering, climbing, mouthing objects, or engaging with toys producing immediate effects (e.g., pushing buttons). She appeared more restless and more perturbed by changes in the environment and the demands placed on her. Her self-stimulatory and repetitive behaviors intensified, and the range of her interests became much narrower. In light of this developmental course, we would not rule out the possibility that her eventual severe intellectual impairment resulted from, rather than simply contributed to, her profound social impairments.

To advance the field in this domain, however, there is a dire need for more sensitive, more quantified, and more encompassing measurements of sociability that span all levels of development from the first weeks of life. At present, our standardized measurements of social functioning are blunt instruments that may in fact blur important differences among similarly impaired infants. The importance of such measurements lies in the fact that more traditional predictors of outcome such as nonverbal intelligence and even language, as measured in infants, are not predictive of outcome, as illustrated in the three cases described here. The use of the word *spectrum* to denote different levels of affectedness implies that one or more factors or dimensions are generating this spectrum, either alone or in complex combinations. Sociability is a likely candidate, particularly given that subsequent and related social-cognitive accomplishments, such as aspects of joint-attention skills, have been shown to be powerful predictors of language use, communication, and symbolic development in ASD (Mundy & Burnette, 2005).

Variability in Outcome: Is It the Result of Interplay between Available Skills and Social Adaptation?

If Helen embodies profound social disability and disconnectedness with the social experience, Nick and John illustrate the challenge of understanding the developmental trajectories of more successful outcomes. In both cases there were substantial gains in nonverbal intelligence and in language. Yet their adaptive skill profiles indicate the marked differences in their ability to translate this potential into tools of adaptation to meet the demands of everyday life. Nick's severe deficits in adaptive behavior was consistent with his more prototypical autistic presentation, whereas John's milder adaptive behavior delays were consistent with a more residual autistic presentation. But what could have accounted for the divergence in their developmental pathways?

A more detailed account of their diagnostic presentation, even during the first assessment in their second years of life, pointed to some variability in John's social and communicative disabilities. Some emerging relatedness skills were noted, but these were highly inconsistent and situational. In contrast, Nick's social and communicative disabilities were more stable and rigid. John began to exhibit self-regulation problems and escalating maladaptive behaviors associated with frustration. These often related to people around him and their demands. They implied a sense of social awareness, albeit as a source of discomfort and confusion. Nick appeared to be increasingly more immersed in the inanimate world, developing circumscribed interests associated with self-stimulatory habits. John's language and nonverbal intelligence flourished in concert, whereas Nick's nonverbal intelligence grew at a much faster pace than his language abilities. This is particularly so if language use and communication are used for the comparison rather than if a comparison is made using their formal language skills as measured with the MSEL. Nick did not acquire severe maladaptive behaviors, whereas John had tantrums, self-injurious behaviors, and despondent affect.

Given these profiles, it is tempting to speculate that their outcomes may have resulted from the interplay of their developmental skills and what appeared to be their different adaptive tasks. In John's case, he appeared to be playing the "social game" without knowing how, as it were. His task was social adaptation, but he was ill equipped for it. His emerging awareness of the complex demands of others, as well as the discrepancy between desired and real outcome in social contacts, all enveloped by a sense of confusion and an inability to make sense of them, or seek sense from others, could have unleashed what his parents described as a "high-maintenance" child. His progress in social relatedness appeared to go hand in hand with his challenging behaviors and sense of despair. In Nick's case, the adaptive task appeared to be primarily confined to the inanimate world, touching briefly on the world of others only when they impinged on his isolated activities. Thus, he had very few maladaptive behaviors associated with social demands or experiences.

What is of interest is that in the cases of the three children, despite their variable levels of language and intelligence, there was a fascination with letters and numbers, reflected in acquisition of reading decoding skills. In Helen's case, this was devoid of comprehension. In Nick's case, reading was associated with some accumulation of facts but quite dissociated from social or emotional experiences. And in John's case, reading appeared to be more tied to and related to his everyday activities and thus imbued with some self-referenced content. It may appear that, challenged by the changeable nature of the social world, children with ASD gravitate to the unchangeable nature of symbols and rules inherent in the alphabet and numbers, and subsequently in the decoding of graphemes and fluent reading (Klin et al., 2003).

Although the phenomenon of "hyperlexia" (which encompasses precocious reading decoding skills and typically denotes reading decoding without reading comprehension; Grigorenko, Klin, & Volkmar, 2003) has been studied primarily from the standpoint of reading skill (e.g., Grigorenko et al., 2002), the fact that this occurs much more frequently in individuals with ASD than in individuals with any other developmental or psychiatric condition suggests a connection with social disability. In a sense, it would be adaptive for a socially disabled child to gravitate to an activity that is predicated on explicit, rote, rule-governed, and unchangeable contingencies, when the alternative is a (social) world that is implicit, conceptual, intuitive, and constantly changing. In a recent study of higher-functioning children and adolescents with ASD (Klin, Danovitch, Merz, Dohrmann, & Volkmar, 2007), more than 80% of a group of close to 100 individuals had an intense circumscribed interest manifested in terms of verbal learning and memorization. A large proportion of this group had demonstrated intense interests in letters, numbers, and reading during their preschool years.

Standardized Instrumentation: Obvious Limitations and Discontinuities

One of the more immediate conclusions drawn from these case studies is that different instruments measuring a given concept may not in fact measure the same concept. For example, the receptive and expressive scales of the MSEL are very different from the scales focused on the same concepts in the Reynell, which, again, are very different from what is meant by *receptive and expressive skills* in the VABS. Although obvious to the experienced clinician in the field of developmental disabilities, this is hardly self-evident to other professionals who are used to the high intercorrelation of all of these measures in typical populations. As evident in each of the profiles of the three children, MSEL scores in the language domains tend to be higher than in the equivalent scales on the Reynell, which tend to be higher than the equivalent scales on the VABS. As the MSEL focuses primarily on the labeling of objects and on response to single-world utterances, the typical associative nature of language learning in infants and young children with ASD frequently results in peak performance on such tasks. In contrast, the Reynell embeds testing in language that is used to understand a task, to relate objects to one another, to differentiate or to group them, and to formulate word combinations as phrases that make sense relative to a given task. In other words, the Reynell's concept of "language" is much closer to language use than the concept of "language" in the MSEL. VABS results typically indicate more significant developmental delays than both of these, because here the concept of "language" means a child's ability to use language to meet the communicative demands in real life, where there is no scaffolding or structure provided by an examiner, and where the context for a given task needs to be created by the child him- or herself as the child understands a particular social situation. From a practical standpoint, different measures of language provide different information about a given concept. They can all contribute to a more comprehensive picture of a child's language abilities. But given the typical profiles found in children with ASD (Paul, 2005), it is apparent that we can easily misrepresent a child's skills on the basis of our choice of instrument to be used.

Similarly, the fact that a given testing domain is provided in an instrument for ages extending from infancy to late childhood does not guarantee, and in fact is very unlikely to accomplish, continuity in that concept. For example, most wide-ranging cognitive tests intended for infants and preschoolers use increasingly more challenging tasks to measure problem-solving skills (Klin et al., 2005). Thus, one may progress from object permanence, to simple identical matching tasks (e.g., on the basis of color, shape, number), to conceptual matching tasks (e.g., on the basis of class of objects, meanings, patterns), to problem-solving tasks (e.g., transforming information, integrating information, reasoning). Given that children with ASD are much more likely to display a nonverbal reasoning style marked by associative and rote learning, and that they typically have deficits in integrative and conceptual learning, it is no surprise that one may often see a slowing in the rate of progress in these children. For example, a child may perform within the normative range at younger ages and display significant deficits later on, not necessarily because his or her learning is slowing down but simply because the sections of the same test for older children involve tasks that they have difficulty with. Thus, one may see dropping scores on the same instrument over two testing periods simply because of the nature of the test. For this reason, tests of nonverbal cognition in infants and toddlers with ASD appear to hold little predictive power for subsequent IQ tests. It is not surprising, therefore, that scores on nonverbal problem-solving skills on the MSEL (called "visual reception") obtained during the first evaluation could hardly be considered predictive of these children's cognitive outcomes.

Regression at 12 Months: What Does It Mean?

Helen's very early referral to a specialized clinic (at 15 months, relative to the epidemiological mean age of 40 months for a diagnosis of autism; Chakrabarti & Fombonne, 2001) was the result of her pediatrician's alertness and the fact that her parents were sensitized (and anxious) about increased genetic liability following the diagnosis of Helen's older brother. Yet despite the pediatric follow-up that Helen had during the first year of life, it is still unclear as to the extent to which she suffered a very meaningful regression at the age of 12–14 months, or conversely, whether detectable social symptomatology could have been identified in the first year of life (using methods that are not practical in routine pediatric visits). It is unequivocal, however, that she lost some words that she previously had. There are several possibilities that could account for this regression: (1) A meaningful regressive phase characterizes the onset of autism in a group of children, not unlike what is observed in children with Childhood Disintegrative Disorder but earlier in life (Richler et al., 2006); (2) the perception of "regression" is an artifact of parental perception, given that the disability becomes more "visible" in the second year of life (i.e., earlier development is seen as "normal") because environmental demands and expectations are greater (e.g., one expects toddlers to begin to talk; Richler et al., 2006); and (3) a "pseudo-regressive phase" takes place (e.g., a child loses some words), but this process is part of the natural course of autism (i.e., onset of the condition does not coincide with the "regression" phase but precedes it, and words lost are results of a maturational process of speech acquisition that is not an integral part of the development of communication), and therefore is not reinforced by the typical natural predisposition to seek and communicate with others. This is a process not unlike the emergence of babbling in congenitally deaf children, which subsequently fades away (Lenneberg, 1967). The issue of regression in autism is far from resolved, despite an ongoing concerted effort to elucidate it (Lord, Shulman, & DiLavore, 2004).

CONCLUSION

The ultimate challenge of research focused on infants with ASD is to predict developmental trajectories of individual children. Its validity and utility depends to a great extent on our ability to answer parents' questions about the future of their children. This includes knowledge in the prescription of specific regimens, modalities, and foci of treatment that are individualized to the findings of quantifiable skills and disabilities revealed during comprehensive assessments. The case studies described in this chapter highlight some of the limitations of the current concepts and instruments used in the assessment of infants and toddlers. This is not surprising, given the difficulties inherent in capturing highly heterogeneous phenotypes changing at fast rates, and the short length of time that the research enterprise has focused on very young children with ASD. We suggest that core concepts, such as sociability, are still poorly understood and measured and that novel experimental paradigms are needed in order to more fully understand factors that mediate outcome. In other fields of science, the word *spectrum* often means a range of possibilities created by fairly discrete dimensions and their interrelationships (e.g., light, pitch). If so, we are not quite ready to use this word in the context of autism.

REFERENCES

Chakrabarti, S., & Fombonne, E. (2001). Pervasive developmental disorders in preschool children. *Journal of the American Medical Association, 285*(24), 3093–3099.

Charman, T., Taylor, E., Drew, A., Cockerill, H., Brown, J. A., & Baird, G. (2005). Outcome at 7 years of children diagnosed with autism at age 2: Predictive validity of assessments conducted at 2 and 3 years of age and pattern of symptom change over time. *Journal of Child Psychology and Psychiatry, 46*(5), 500–513.

Chawarska, K., Paul, R., Klin, A., Hannigen, S., Dichtel, L. E., & Volkmar, F. R. (2007). Parental recognition of developmental problems in toddlers with autism spectrum disorders. *Journal of Autism and Developmental Disorders, 37*(1), 62–72.

Edwards, S., Fletcher, P., Garman, M., Hughes, A., Letts, C., & Sinka, I. (1999). *Reynell Developmental Language Scales–III*. Windsor, UK: NFER-Nelson.

Emery, N. J. (2000). The eyes have it: The neuroethology, function and evolution of social gaze. *Neuroscience and Biobehavioral Reviews, 24*, 581–604.

Fenson, L. (1989). *The MacArthur Communicative Development Inventory: Infant and Toddler Versions*. San Diego: San Diego State University.

Fox, R., & McDaniel, C. (1982). The perception of biological motion by human infants. *Science, 218*, 486–487.

Grigorenko, E. L., Klin, A., Pauls, D. L., Senft, R., Hooper, C., & Volkmar, F. R. (2002). A descriptive study of hyperlexia in a clinically referred sample of children with developmental delays. *Journal of Autism and Developmental Disorders, 32*(1), 3–12.

Grigorenko, E. L., Klin, A., & Volkmar, F. R. (2003). Annotation: Hyperlexia: Disability or superability? *Journal of Child Psychology and Psychiatry, 44*(8), 1079–1091.

Gupta, A. R., & State, M. W. (2007). Recent advances in the genetics of autism. *Biological Psychiatry, 61*(4), 429–437.

Haith, M. M., Bergman, T., & Moore, M. (1977). Eye contact and face scanning in early infancy. *Science, 218*, 179–181.

Johnson, M. (2001). Functional brain development in humans. *Nature Reviews Neuroscience, 2*, 475–483.

Kanner, L. (1943). Autistic disturbances of affective contact. *Nervous Child, 2*, 217–250.

Klin, A., Chawarska, K., Paul, R., Rubin, E., Morgan, T., Weisner, L., et al. (2004). Clinical case conference: Autism in a 15-month-old child. *American Journal of Psychiatry, 161*(11), 1–8.

Klin, A., Danovitch, J. H., Merz, A. B., Dohrmann, E. H., & Volkmar, F. R. (2007). Circumscribed interests in higher-functioning individuals with autism spectrum disorders: An exploratory study. *Research and Practice for Persons with Severe Disabilities, 32*(3), 89–100.

Klin, A., & Jones, W. (2007). Altered face scanning and impaired recognition of biological motion in a 15 month-old infant with autism. *Developmental Science.* Available online at doi.10.1111/j.1467-7687.200700608.x

Klin, A., Jones, W., Schultz, R. T., & Volkmar, F. R. (2003). The enactive mind–

from actions to cognition: Lessons from autism. *Philosophical Transactions of the Royal Society: Biological Sciences, 358,* 345–360.

Klin, A., Saulnier, C., Tsatsanis, K., & Volkmar, F. R. (2005). Clinical evaluation in autism spectrum disorders: Psychological assessment within a transdisciplinary framework. In F. R. Volkmar, R. Paul, A. Klin, & D. J. Cohen (Eds.), *Handbook of autism and pervasive developmental disorders* (3rd ed., pp. 772–798). New York: Wiley.

Lenneberg, E. H. (1967). *Biological foundations of language.* New York: Wiley.

Lord, C. (1995). Follow-up of two year-olds referred for possible autism. *Journal of Child Psychology and Psychiatry, 36,* 1365–1382.

Lord, C., Risi, S., DiLavore, P. S., Shulman, C., Thurm, A., & Pickles, A. (2006). Autism from 2 to 9 years of age. *Archives of General Psychiatry, 63*(6), 694–701.

Lord, C., Rutter, M. J. DiLavore, P., & Risi, S. (1999). *Autism diagnostic observation schedule.* Los Angeles: Western Psychological Services.

Lord, C., Shulman, C., & DiLavore, P. (2004). Regression and word loss in autism spectrum disorders. *Journal of Child Psychology and Psychiatry, 45,* 1–21.

Mullen, E. M. (1995). *Mullen Scales of Early Learning: AGS Edition.* Circle Pines, MN: American Guidance Service.

Mundy, P., & Burnette, C. (2005). Joint attention and neurodevelopmental models of autism. In F. R. Volkmar, R. Paul, A. Klin, & D. J. Cohen (Eds.), *Handbook of autism and pervasive developmental disorders* (3rd ed., pp. 650–682). New York: Wiley.

National Research Council. (2001). *Educating children with autism.* Washington, DC: National Academy Press.

Paul, R. (2005). Assessing communication in autism. In F. R. Volkmar, R. Paul, A. Klin, & D. J. Cohen (Eds.), *Handbook of autism and pervasive developmental disorders* (3rd ed., pp. 799–816). New York: Wiley.

Richler, J., Luyster, R., Risi, S., Wan-Ling, H., Dawson, G., Bernier, R., et al. (2006). Is there a regressive "phenotype" of autism spectrum disorder associated with the measles-mumps-rubella vaccine?: A CPEA study. *Journal of Autism and Developmental Disorders, 36*(3), 299–316.

Rutter, M., LeCouteur, A., & Lord, C. (2003). *Autism Diagnostic Interview–Revised.* Los Angeles: Western Psychological Services.

Siegel, B., Piner, C., Eschler, J., & Elliott, G. R. (1988). How children with autism are diagnosed: Difficulties in identification of children with multiple developmental delays. *Journal of Developmental and Behavioral Pediatrics, 9*(4), 199–204.

Sparrow, S. S., Balla, D., & Cicchetti, D. (1984). *Vineland Adaptive Behavior Scales, Expanded Edition.* Circle Pines, MN: American Guidance Service.

Volkmar, F. R., Lord, C., Bailey, A., Schultz, R. T., & Klin, A. (2004). Autism and pervasive developmental disorders. *Journal of Child Psychology and Psychiatry, 45,* 135–170.

Wetherby, A., & Prizant, B. (1993). *Communication and Symbolic Behavior Scales–Developmental Profile (CSBS-DP).* Baltimore: Brookes.

Zwaigenbaum, L., Bryson, S., Rogers, T., Roberts, W., Brian, J., & Szatmari, P. (2005). Behavioral manifestations of autism in the first year of life. *International Journal of Developmental Neuroscience, 23*(2–3), 143–152.

CHAPTER 7

——•——

Developmental Approaches
to Treatment

Amy M. Wetherby
Juliann Woods

Major advances have been made over the past two decades in early detection and diagnosis of autism spectrum disorders (ASD). With the increased number of infants and toddlers identified with ASD, there is a pressing need for interventions that are appropriate and effective for very young children with ASD and their families. There are a growing number of treatment studies documenting the effectiveness of interventions using developmental approaches with young children with ASD. This chapter begins with a brief synopsis of the core social communication deficits of very young children with ASD to provide a framework for considering the contributions of developmental treatment approaches. Next, we delineate the core features and guiding principles of developmental treatment approaches for very young children with ASD and how these are similar to and contrast with behavioral interventions. We attempt to identify "active ingredients" or intervention components that are used in developmental interventions and review empirical studies of their efficacy. The chapter highlights how developmental approaches may contribute to ameliorating core deficits in ASD and suggests directions for future research.

CORE SOCIAL COMMUNICATION DEFICITS
IN CHILDREN WITH ASD

There is a large body of research defining core social communication deficits of toddlers and preschool children with ASD. A deficit is considered to be core if it distinguishes children with ASD from other children with developmental delays (DD) and children with typical development (TD; Sigman, Dijamco, Gratier, & Rozga, 2004). Two core social communication deficits have been found to distinguish young children with ASD: (1) a deficit in joint attention, which is reflected in difficulty in coordinating attention between people and objects, and (2) a deficit in symbol use, which is evident in difficulty in learning conventional meanings through gestures, words, and actions in play (Charman et al., 1997; Dawson et al., 2004; Loveland & Landry, 1986; Mundy, Sigman, & Kasari, 1990; Sigman, Mundy, Sherman, & Ungerer, 1986; Stone, Ousley, Yoder, Hogan, & Hepburn, 1997; Wetherby, Prizant, & Hutchinson,1998). A number of longitudinal studies provide evidence of a relationship between early social communication skills and language outcomes. Mundy et al. (1990) found that responding to and initiating gestural joint attention at a mean age of 3 years 9 months were significant predictors of language development 13 months later for children with ASD, whereas none of the other nonverbal measures, initial language scores, mental age, chronological age, or IQ were significant predictors. These findings were further substantiated in a long-term follow-up study demonstrating that initial joint attention skills of 51 children with autism at a mean age of 3 years 11 months predicted gains in expressive language at a mean age of 12 years 10 months (Sigman & Ruskin, 1999).

Most children identified as having ASD are reported by their caregivers to demonstrate symptoms within the first 2 years of life, based on retrospective accounts (Short & Schopler, 1988; Wimpory, Hobson, Williams & Nash, 2000). Furthermore, most family members initially express concern to their pediatrician by the time their child is 18 months old (Howlin & Moore, 1997; Siegel, Pliner, Eschler, & Elliot, 1988). Observational studies of social communication skills in children under 2 years of age with ASD are emerging from two different sources of information, retrospective analyses of home videotapes and prospective longitudinal designs. The largest cohort of retrospective analyses are based on home videotapes from first birthday parties of children later diagnosed with ASD. Osterling and colleagues (Osterling & Dawson, 1994; Osterling, Dawson, & Munson, 2002) found that children with ASD could be distinguished at their first birthday parties with four features—lack of pointing, showing, looking at faces, and orienting to name; however, children with DD also showed the first two features.

One line of research employing prospective longitudinal designs has been to screen general pediatric samples in order to identify very young children at risk for ASD and then study the differences between these children and matched groups of children with DD and TD. A series of studies involving two prospective cohorts identified before 2 years of age from a general pediatric screen have been published. The first cohort consisted of children identified using the CHecklist for Autism in Toddlers (CHAT; Baron-Cohen et al., 1996; Charman et al., 1997; Swettenham et al., 1998). The second cohort consisted of children identified using the Communication and Symbolic Behavior Scales–Developmental Profile (CSBS-DP; Wetherby et al., 2004; Wetherby, Watt, Morgan, & Shumway, 2007). Findings from these studies indicate that core deficits in shifting gaze between people and objects, responding to and initiating joint attention, using conventional gestures, and rate of communicating (i.e., number of communicative behaviors per unit of time) distinguish children with ASD from those with DD or TD by 18 months of age. Charman et al. (2003) found that measures of joint attention late in the second year predicted language at 3 years of age. Wetherby et al. (2007) examined a larger set of predictive measures and found that many measures, including joint attention, predicted language outcome at 3, but that understanding of language in the second year was the strongest predictor. In addition to social communication deficits, Wetherby et al. (2004) found red flags in repetitive movements with objects and body that distinguished children with ASD in the second year.

A second line of ongoing research is the prospective study of younger siblings of children with ASD, inasmuch as they represent a high genetic risk for ASD. Several very recent publications reporting on studies of infant siblings have documented that delays in social communication begin to be evident by 12–14 months of age in younger siblings who later receive a diagnosis of ASD (Landa & Garrett-Mayer, 2006; Mitchell et al., 2006; Yirmiya et al., 2006; Zwaigenbaum et al., 2005).

Collectively, these findings indicate that children with ASD can be distinguished from those with DD or TD in the second year, based on a combination of lack of typical behaviors and presence of atypical behaviors, and underscore the importance of social communication along with repetitive behaviors in earlier identification of ASD and as targets for early intervention. This growing body of research on early red flags makes it more possible to identify children with ASD when they are toddlers, which emphasizes the pressing need for interventions that are appropriate and effective for very young children with ASD and their families.

INTERACTION OF CORE DEFICITS OF ASD, BRAIN DEVELOPMENT, AND THE LEARNING ENVIRONMENT

Although it is known that ASD is a neurobiological disorder, current theories emphasize the interaction of abnormal brain development, the child's profile, and the learning environment. Mundy and Burnette (2005) suggested that an initial neurological deficit in infants with autism leads to an early impairment in social orienting and joint attention, which contributes to subsequent neurodevelopmental pathology by an attenuation of social input. This transactional process can lead to a cumulative spiraling that may compromise subsequent neurological and behavioral development, or may possibly be ameliorated through early intervention. The core deficits in social communication and repetitive behavior that have been identified in the second year of life may attenuate the quality of the social input that children with ASD are exposed to very early in life, and through a transactional process, have a cascading effect on later developmental outcome and autism symptoms (Wetherby et al., 2007). In other words, the symptoms of ASD may further disrupt brain development and this disruption may be cumulative. Because of the transactional and cumulative detrimental impact on brain development, these core deficits may be critical targets for early intervention in order to enhance social communication skills that are likely to impact the social environment and thus lead to better outcomes for children with ASD. Very early intervention may be viewed as a mechanism to prevent the full unfolding of symptoms of ASD by minimizing the associated secondary abnormalities in brain development.

A caregiver may be able to compensate for a child's deficits in joint attention by ensuring a common focus of attention when modeling language. In a longitudinal study of 25 children with ASD, Siller and Sigman (2002) investigated whether caregivers followed the child's focus of attention and toy engagement during play and the extent to which this predicted language outcomes. Play samples were initially gathered when the children with ASD were a mean age of 50 months. The caregivers of children with ASD synchronized their behaviors to their children's attention and activities as much as caregivers of typically developing children matched on language abilities. However, the children with ASD whose caregivers showed higher levels of synchronization during initial play samples developed better joint attention skills 1 year later and better language outcomes 10 and 16 years later, as compared with children of caregivers who showed lower levels of synchronization initially. The strongest predictor of a child's increase in initiating joint attention was the caregiver's initiation of joint attention that was synchronized to the child's attentional focus. The strongest predictor of gain in language was caregiver utterances that followed the child's attentional focus and allowed the child to continue the ongoing toy engagement. These findings have important implications for targeting joint attention skills in intervention by enhancing the child's skills, as well as the partner's ability to support shared attention, and for intervening early to establish or enhance synchronization by caregivers as soon as possible.

Wimpory, Hobson, and Nash (2007) provide further evidence of the association between adult behavior and active social engagement in young children with ASD. They examined clinician behavior during naturalistic play samples immediately prior to episodes of social engagement in 22 children with ASD from 2 to 4 years of age. They operationalized social engagement as the child's being communicatively available by looking at the adult and making a gesture or other communicative expression. They found that social engagement occurred significantly more often when the adult's verbal or nonverbal behavior followed the child's lead or allowed the child to continue his or her attentional focus, as compared with when the adult redirected the child's action or focus of attention, was silently attentive to the child, or ignored the child. They examined the scaffolding that the adult provided and found that episodes of social engagement occurred significantly more often when the adult supported social routines, imitated the child and adult repetitions of verbal or nonverbal behavior within a turn. These findings provide observational evidence of temporal contingencies between the quality of adult turns and child social engagement. The authors point out that it may seem *paradoxical* that the adult behaviors associated with social engagement in young children with ASD are essentially those that have been found to support development in typical children. These findings suggest that a developmental framework may have important implications for designing interventions for young children with ASD.

MEANINGFUL INTERVENTION OUTCOME MEASURES FOR INFANTS AND TODDLERS WITH ASD

A critical issue in determining if a treatment is effective is the outcome measure used to study treatment efficacy. Although there are a large number of observational studies delineating the core social communication deficits associated with ASD, there are very few studies that have documented intervention effects on these core deficits. The most widely used outcome measures in intervention research for children with ASD have been changes in IQ and proportion of children placed in a regular classroom after intervention (National Research Council [NRC], 2001). Such outcome measures are problematic, because they may reflect increased compliance or parent preference in placement, rather than meaningful changes. Furthermore, these measures are not applicable with infants and toddlers. Further research is needed to document meaningful changes that reflect core social communication deficits in young children with ASD.

The available research suggests that multiple aspects of joint attention and symbol use should be measured both to describe the participants and to indicate possible treatment outcomes. Even the most effective treatment studies of children with ASD show variable outcomes (NRC, 2001), and a child's social communication skills before treatment may influence the response to treatment. Bono, Daley, and Sigman (2004) found that the relation between amount of intervention and gain in language for children with ASD depended on their ability to respond to joint attention as well as their initial language skills. Systematic measurement of social communication can contribute to our understanding of the interactions between treatment and child characteristics. For example, treatments that use adult-directed teaching strategies may be more effective for children with better skills in responding to joint attention or language comprehension. Treatments in which the adult synchronizes with the child's attentional focus may be more effective than more directive approaches for children with limited skills in responding to or initiating joint attention. Documenting change in social communication skills is even more critical for younger children, because these skills form the underpinnings of social competence and enable children to participate more successfully in a variety of learning contexts.

THE IMPORTANCE OF EVIDENCE-BASED INTERVENTION FOR YOUNG CHILDREN WITH ASD

The NRC (2001) conducted a systematic review of research on educational interventions for children with ASD from birth through 8 years of age. The NRC concluded that a large body of research has demonstrated significant progress in response to intervention with a substantial proportion of children with ASD, using a range of techniques. However, few well-controlled studies with random assignment are available, and therefore it is not yet known whether particular intervention approaches are more effective than others. Furthermore, children's outcomes are variable, with some making substantial progress and others showing slow gains. The committee concluded that there is a convergence of evidence that the following characteristics are essential active ingredients of effective interventions for children with ASD:

1. Entry into intervention programs as soon as ASD is suspected.
2. Active engagement in intensive instruction for a minimum of 5 hours per day, 5 days a week.
3. Use of repeated planned teaching opportunities that are structured over brief periods of time.
4. Sufficient individualized adult attention on a daily basis.
5. Inclusion of a family component, including parent training.

6. Mechanisms for ongoing assessment with corresponding adjustments in programming.
7. Priority for instruction in (a) functional, spontaneous communication, (b) social instruction across settings, (c) play skills, with a focus on peer interaction, (d) new skill maintenance and generalization in natural contexts, and (e) functional assessment and positive behavior support to address problem behaviors.

Most studies reviewed by the NRC included children 3–5 years of age. Stone and Yoder (2001) found a strong positive association between the number of hours of speech therapy received between the ages of 2 and 3 and language skills at age 4 in 35 toddlers with ASD. These findings suggest that beginning intervention before 3 years of age may have a greater impact than beginning later. Because most children with ASD are not identified until close to 3 years of age, there is little research on intervention with infants and toddlers at risk for ASD. Evidence-based practice with preschoolers with ASD, as delineated in the report of the NRC (2001), offers the best available guidelines for providing services for younger children until intervention research with infants and toddlers is available.

Building on the efforts of the NRC committee, a working group supported by the National Institute of Mental Health from 2002 to 2004 developed guidelines for designing research studies of psychosocial interventions for children with ASD (Smith et al., 2007). The working group delineated the following steps for developing, validating, and disseminating interventions: (1) formulation and systematic application of new intervention through initial efficacy studies using singe-subject design or quasi-experimental group designs, (2) manualization and protocol development with feasibility testing, (3) efficacy studies with large-scale randomized clinical trials (RCTs) and effects demonstrated across sites, and (4) community effectiveness studies with RCTs conducted by clinicians in the community implementing the treatment. The next section of this chapter first defines developmental interventions in terms of the key features. Next, it examines the evidence available on developmental interventions for young children with ASD in relation to the steps delineated by Smith et al. (2007).

CONTINUUM OF INTERVENTION APPROACHES FROM BEHAVIORAL TO DEVELOPMENTAL

Although there is consensus on the importance of enhancing social communication abilities for children with ASD, intervention approaches vary greatly and even appear diametrically opposed in regard to the specific methods advocated. In order to examine the critical elements of treatment approaches that impact social communication of children with ASD, it is useful to characterize the key elements of treatment approaches along a continuum ranging from traditional discrete trials, to more contemporary behavioral approaches that utilize naturalistic language teaching techniques, to developmental approaches (Prizant & Wetherby, 1998). The earliest research efforts at teaching speech and language to children with autism used massed discrete trial methods to teach verbal behavior. Lovaas (1977, 1981) provided the most detailed account of the procedures for language training using traditional discrete trial behavioral approaches. Outcomes of discrete trial approaches have included improvements in IQ and improvements in communication domains of broader measures, such as the Vineland Adaptive Behavior Scales (VABS; McEachin, Smith, & Lovaas, 1993). A major limitation of a discrete trial approach in language acquisition is the lack of spontaneity and generalization (NRC, 2001). Lovaas (1977) stated that "the training regime . . . its use of 'unnatural' reinforcers, and the like may have been responsible for producing the very situation-specific, restricted verbal output which we observed in many of our children" (p. 170). In a review of research on discrete trial approaches, it was noted by Koegel (1995) that "not only did language fail to be exhibited or generalized to other environments, but most behaviors taught in this highly controlled environment also failed to generalize" (p. 23).

The limitations of the traditional behavioral approaches stimulated the advent of both behavioral and developmental approaches that incorporate more naturalistic strategies. There is now a large body of empirical support for more contemporary behavioral approaches using naturalistic teaching methods that demonstrate efficacy for teaching not only speech and language, but also communication (Hepting & Goldstein, 1996). Examples of naturalistic behavioral approaches include the use of natural language paradigm (Koegel, O'Dell, & Koegel, 1987), incidental teaching (Hart, 1985; McGee, Krantz, & McClannahan, 1985; McGee, Morrier, & Daly, 1999), time delay and milieu intervention (Charlop, Schreibman, & Thibodeau, 1985; Charlop & Trasowech, 1991; Kaiser, 1993; Kaiser, Yoder, & Keetz, 1992), and pivotal response training (Koegel, 1995; Koegel, Camarata, Koegel, Ben-Tall, & Smith, 1998). These approaches use systematic teaching trials that have the following key features: (1) initiated by the child and focusing on the child's interest, (2) interspersed and embedded in functional activities, and (3) using natural reinforcers that follow what the child is trying to communicate. There are only a few studies, all using single-subject design, that have compared traditional discrete trials with naturalistic behavioral approaches. These studies have reported that naturalistic approaches are more effective at leading to generalization of language gains to natural contexts (Koegel et al., 1998; Koegel, Koegel, & Surratt, 1992; McGee et al., 1985).

There are numerous developmental intervention approaches that are described in the literature (e.g., Greenspan & Weider, 1997; Klinger & Dawson, 1992; Prizant, Wetherby, & Rydell, 2000; Rogers & Lewis, 1989). A common feature of developmental approaches is that they are child-directed. The environment is arranged to provide opportunities for communication; the child initiates the interaction or teaching episode, and the adult follows the child's lead by being responsive to the child's intentions and imitating or expanding on the child's behavior. Developmental approaches share many common key features with contemporary naturalistic behavioral approaches and are compatible along many, if not most, dimensions (Prizant & Wetherby, 1998), thus muddying the distinctions between them. The following section delineates the key features of developmental approaches.

KEY FEATURES
OF DEVELOPMENTAL APPROACHES

Just exactly what constitutes a developmental approach to treatment is elusive in the literature on children with ASD. Here we attempt to delineate the key features that are associated with a developmental perspective and incorporated into most developmental approaches. Because there is no agreement on how many of these features are required for an approach to be considered developmental, and because some of these features are shared with contemporary behavioral approaches, it is more useful to think of a continuum of approaches, with traditional behavioral on one end, which would likely not incorporate any of these features; contemporary behavioral in the middle, which would incorporate some of these features; and developmental on the other end, which would incorporate most if not all of these features (Prizant & Wetherby, 2005). Those contemporary behavioral approaches that incorporate many of these features would fall closer to the developmental end of the continuum. Many of these features are consistent with the recommendations of the NRC (2001) and compatible with contemporary behavioral approaches.

DEVELOPMENTAL FRAMEWORK
FOR TARGETING SOCIAL COMMUNICATION
GOALS AND STRATEGIES

A hallmark of developmental approaches is the use of a developmental framework to prioritize individualized goals and objectives. The expansive literature on typical development provides a rich theoretical and empirical basis for both understanding core social communication deficits in ASD and guiding developmentally appropriate interventions. In their pioneering work, Bates and colleagues (Bates, 1976; Bates, Camaioni, & Volterra, 1975) provided a developmental pragmatics framework to describe the emergence of communication and language from *intentional* to *symbolic* to *linguistic communication*. This work was monumental in going beyond the models of Piaget and Vygotsky to influence our understanding of how children proceed through these transitions in typical development and to offer a road map to guide clinicians (Bates, O'Connell, & Shore, 1987). Developmental theories view language learning as an active process in which children "construct" or build knowledge and shared meanings based on emotions and interactions with people and experiences in their environment (Bates, 1979; Bloom, 1993; Tronick, 1989). The work of Stern (1985) has also been influential in our understanding of the core deficits of ASD. Stern described three achievements that contribute to a child's sense of self and capacity to use language to share experiences about events and things, and thus provide the foundation for social communication development—sharing the focus of attention ("interattentionality"), sharing of intentions ("interintentionality"), and sharing of affective states ("interaffectivity"). These three achievements lead to the capacity of "intersubjective relatedness" as the infant discovers that he or she has a mind, that other people have minds, and that inner subjective experiences can be shared. From a developmental perspective, the language deficits of children with ASD reflect core deficits in these social underpinnings—shared attention, shared affect, and shared intentions—leading to difficulties in sharing experiences (i.e., intersubjective relatedness).

Pragmatic/social interactive theories have placed great emphasis on the context of social interaction in language development (Bates, 1976; Bloom & Lahey, 1978; McLean & Snyder-McLean, 1978; Sameroff, 1987). Children are viewed as active participants who learn to affect the behavior and attitudes of others through active signaling and gradually learn to use more sophisticated and conventional means to communicate through caregivers' contingent social responsiveness (Dunst, Lowe, & Bartholomew, 1990; Sameroff, 1987). Proponents of developmental pragmatic theory believe that child development can be understood only by analysis of the interactive context, not simply by focusing solely on the child or the caregivers, because successful communication involves reciprocity and mutual negotiation (Bates, 1976; Bruner, 1978, 1981). Reflecting the theory of Vygotsky (1986), that the acquisition of communicative symbols is a social enterprise, Tomasello, Kruger, and Ratner (1993) suggested that two components are essential for a child to develop language—development within a cultural context that structures events for the child, and the child's special capacity to learn from this cultural structuring. The structuring for language acquisition entails routine cultural activities that employ coordinated attention and delineated roles. The child's capacity requires the social-cognitive skills of being able to attribute intentions to others and to see an event from another's perspective.

Wetherby, Schuler, and Prizant (1997) identified three significant principles drawn from the developmental literature that are critical for children with ASD and should be incorporated into a developmental intervention. First, social communication development involves continuity from preverbal to verbal communication. That is, the development of preverbal communication is a necessary precursor to the development of the intentional use of language to communicate. For children with ASD who are not yet talking, emphasis should be placed on developing preverbal social communication skills and words should be mapped onto preverbal communication skills. Second, being a competent communicator is the outcome of a developmental interaction of the child's cognitive, social-emotional, and language capacities and the language learning environment. A child's developmental profile across these domains should provide the basis for decision making for communication enhancement. Third, in a developmental framework, all behavior should be viewed in reference to the child's relative level of functioning across developmental domains. For example, many of the challenging behaviors used by children with ASD can be understood as attempts to communicate if such behavior is interpreted relative to developmental discrepancies, and as coping strategies in the face of significant communicative limitations.

These rich developmental theories, and the research that they have generated, offer a framework for understanding a child's developing competencies in relationship to the social context and how these patterns change over developmental transitions, and this framework is woven into developmental interventions. Many patterns and sequences of development in children with ASD are similar to those in typical development, although the timing of acquisition is different, and therefore the combination of skills (i.e., discrepancies in skill level across social, cognitive, and linguistic domains) that a child with ASD has at any one point in time is unlikely to be seen in typical development. Too rigid an interpretation of a developmental model has resulted in "readiness models" that require that a certain level of ability must be reached before working on subsequent skills (Wetherby et al., 1997). Working within a developmental model does not imply teaching to a developmental checklist. Rather than merely offering a guideline for sequencing communication objectives, developmental information provides a frame of reference for understanding a child's behavioral competencies and for individualizing appropriate, developmentally sensible goals and objectives. Furthermore, a developmental framework offers strategies used by caregivers of typically developing children to support communication and language development.

FOCUS ON THE CORE DEFICITS
ASSOCIATED WITH AUTISM

The core deficits of ASD affect many aspects of social communication and learning. Developmental approaches focus on the core deficits of children with ASD, such as expanding the use of gestures, initiating verbal and nonverbal communication, understanding and using words with referential meaning, initiating and responding to joint attention, and reciprocity in interaction, because these skills predict later cognitive, social, and language outcomes in children with ASD. Developmental approaches usually advocate the use of nonspeech communication systems (e.g., sign language or picture communication) to jump-start the speech system and boost cognitive and social underpinnings. When social communication difficulties are present, parents face significant challenges in learning to modify their interaction style and the environment in order to ensure successful communication exchanges. Therefore, developmental interventions focus not only on targeting goals to address directly the core deficits of the child, but also on targeting strategies for parents to use to support social communication development.

A FAMILY-CENTERED APPROACH
TO MEET THE FAMILY'S NEEDS, CONCERNS,
AND PRIORITIES

A family-centered approach holds the notion that parents and caregivers are the most knowledgeable source of information about the child and are partners in the assessment and intervention process (McWilliam, 1992). Respecting family members' perceptions, priorities, and preferences, planning for active participation of family members, sharing in decision making, and building unity are key components of an effective family-centered program (Dunst, Trivette, & Deal, 1988; Woods & Wetherby, 2003). In a developmental intervention the child is recognized as part of a larger family system. It is this larger system that is the focus of assessment and intervention efforts. Cultural and family values are considered throughout the process. Families tend to be more involved in the achievement of goals if they have been stakeholders in selecting them. Research has shown that parents recognize that working together toward a common goal has a positive impact on their child (Sperry, Whaley, Shaw, & Brame, 1999). The review of research by the NRC (2001) identified family involvement as a key component of effective interventions for children with ASD.

Families are maximally involved in the services for infants and toddlers with ASD because of the simple fact of the child's age and reliance on parents for nurturance. Although the amount and type of participation by parents in the intervention process varies significantly—a parent's role may range from primary teacher to observer and informant—two results are clear. First, evidence of the effectiveness of parent-implemented intervention for children with varying types of developmental delays, and specifically for children with ASD, has been consistently documented across a wide range of adaptive, behavioral, social, and communication child outcomes (Koegel, Bimbela, & Schreibman, 1996; McClannahan, Krantz, & McGee, 1982; Schreibman, Kaneko, & Koegel, 1991; Seifer, Clark, & Sameroff, 1991). Second, parents are able to learn a variety of broad and specific intervention strategies to teach their children functional and meaningful outcomes (Kaiser, Hancock, & Nietfeld, 2000). Training parents to implement intervention strategies during everyday activities is a logical method to achieve the intensity of active engagement needed for young children with ASD.

Parent-implemented intervention that results in optimal learning requires planning and problem solving with the parents to ensure that sufficient instructional opportunities are attached to specific routines and activities (Strain, McGee, & Kohler, 2001). Interventionists providing interactive toys, visual supports, or social games that they might use in a clinician-directed session must provide adequate demonstration and guided practice to the parent on what, how, when, and how often to use the specific strategies with the child. For example, simply providing or arranging an environment that supports communication, play, and social interaction has not produced adequate effects (Strain et al., 2001). McGee and Morrier (2005) recommend that caregivers be instructed on how to "market" new toys or materials to the child. Research conducted on the effectiveness of parent-implemented interventions far exceeds research on methods of training parents to implement interventions. Developmental approaches incorporate the existing research that supports the use of adult learning strategies that encompass the adult's experiences and interests, demonstration and specific feedback, problem-solving strategies to increase independent decision making and generalized use of information, self-assessment on effectiveness, and sequential instruction (Buysse & Wesley, 2005; McGee & Morrier, 2005).

The key element of family-centered practice that is incorporated into developmental interventions is individualization for each family based on the family's priorities, concerns, and interests (Allen & Petr, 1996; Sandall, McLean, & Smith, 2000). Developmental interventions are designed so that family members, as well as the child, benefit from involvement. Interventionists must recognize that time spent by parents working with their child can enhance their confidence and competence to interact with their child, increase the child's independence in family activities, and improve the quality of the family's life (Turnbull & Ruef, 1997).

PROVIDING INTERVENTION
IN NATURAL ENVIRONMENTS

In developmental approaches, it is recognized that most learning in childhood takes place in the social context of daily activities and experiences. Efforts to support a child's development occur with caregivers and familiar partners in everyday activities in a variety of social situations, and not primarily by working with a child in isolation. Natural environments are the everyday routines, activities, and places that are typical or natural for the family and usually include locations such as the home, child care facility, homes of extended family and friends, and other community locations such as a park or church. Daily routines such as dressing, mealtime, and play provide excellent opportunities to embed teaching of objectives that are functional and meaningful and therefore naturally support acquisition and generalization of learning (Woods & Wetherby, 2003). Most young children spend a majority of their waking hours engaged in frequently occurring play and caregiving routines that can have a joint focus of attention, a logical and predictable sequence, turn taking, and repetition, when carefully analyzed for maximal teaching opportunities and supportive instructional strategies. Developmental approaches embed intervention into everyday routines, activities, and places and require interventionist and parent consideration of the sequence, ease of strategy use, and frequency of opportunity within various routines (Strain et al., 2001; Woods Cripe & Venn, 1997). A variety of naturalistic language intervention strategies (e.g., Goldstein, 2002; Hwang & Hughes, 2000; Kaiser et al., 2000) can be used as appropriate. It is well documented that generalization of child and family outcomes is enhanced by embedding intervention in family-preferred routines and contexts (Dunst, Hamby, Trivette, Raab, & Bruder, 2000; Woods, Kashinath & Goldstein, 2004). Furthermore, incorporating intervention into existing family routines provides a context for the family and clinician to develop an active, mutually respectful partnership.

The philosophy of intervention in natural environments encompasses more than just the location of services and includes the utilization of naturalistic interventions. Interventions in the natural environment are approaches that maximize teaching and learning throughout the day, using routines, materials, and people common to the family and the child (Dunst et al., 2000; Woods Cripe & Venn, 1997). They include the caregiver(s), with the child, undertaking the activities, events, and chores of daily life as defined by the family's values and choices. The basic tenets of intervention in natural environments include the following: (1) children learn functional and meaningful skills, (2) learning occurs within daily caregiving, play, and social interactions, and (3) caregivers mediate the teaching and learning process for the child as it occurs. This philosophy is compatible with many of the contemporary behavioral and developmental approaches used for children with ASD (Dunlap & Fox, 1999; McGee et al., 1999; Prizant et al., 2000), but is difficult to reconcile with traditional discrete trial interventions (e.g., Lovaas, 1981). The NRC (2001) recommended that children with ASD be given functional and meaningful opportunities for learning in their natural environments to promote generalization. The embedding of intervention within typical daily routines and community activities focuses on the generalization of skills for the child while reducing the stress of specialized training activities irrelevant to the child's challenging behaviors for families (Dunlap & Fox, 1999; Horner, O'Neill, & Flannery, 1993).

Providing intervention of adequate intensity for very young children with ASD is challenging for the health care and education systems. Services delivered by professionals within Part C of the Individuals with Disabilities Education Improvement Act of 2004 (IDEA; Public Law 108-446; U.S. Department of Education, 2004) average 2–3 hours per week. In only a few states that have designated intensive services for children with ASD, services may be provided for as much as 20+ hours per week. Although the intensity of intervention needed for optimal outcomes is not yet determined for infants and toddlers with ASD, it has been shown that the amount of time spent in active and productive engagement impacts the outcomes for preschoolers, with a critical minimum threshold of at least 5 hours per day, 5 days per week (NRC, 2001). Children with ASD participating in activities with other children would not be expected to learn simply by being there. Inclusive opportunities must have adequate support for a child with ASD to learn from engagement with the materials, activities, and other children (Strain et al., 2001). Providing intervention in the natural environment is a way to maximize learning throughout the day and thus achieve the intensity of active engagement that is critical for children with ASD.

NATURALISTIC TEACHING STRATEGIES

Both developmental and contemporary behavioral approaches have emphasized the importance of teaching strategies that encourage children with communication impairments to initiate communication and language use. In the developmental literature, the pragmatics movement has led to strategies that *follow the child's lead* to develop communication and conversational abilities (MacDonald & Carroll, 1992; Yoder, Warren,

McCathren, & Leew, 1998). The developmental literature emphasizes the importance of caregiver responsivity to enhance communication and language and the shift in the balance of power or control to the child (see MacDonald, 1989; Prizant & Wetherby, 1998). If there is not a balance of power or shared control in interactions with a child, the child may become a passive partner or use challenging behavior to claim power (MacDonald, 1989).

The contemporary behavioral literature has described "incidental language teaching" as a method of achieving a more naturalistic approach to language training. In contrast to a discrete trial format in which the trainer controls the interaction, an incidental teaching episode is initiated by the child. The adult waits for the child to initiate a communicative behavior (i.e., gesture, vocalization), focuses attention on the child and the child's topic, asks for a language elaboration or models a verbal response for the child to imitate, and then indicates the correctness of the child's language or gives the child what is asked for. Incidental teaching has been found to enhance generalization in teaching language to children with severe disabilities, including ASD (see Hart, 1985, and Kaiser, 1993, for reviews).

Numerous strategies are described in the literature for designing the environment to encourage the initiation of communication (Prizant & Wetherby, 1993). The developmental literature has emphasized the importance of "engineering" or arranging the environment to provide opportunities and reasons for the child to initiate communication. The contemporary behavioral literature has described specific strategies to occasion language use, such as to delay at critical moments in natural routines and to interrupt chains of behavior by removing an object needed to complete a task (Kaiser, 1993; Rowland & Schweigert, 1993). By making the initiation of communication a priority, natural opportunities for communicating can be capitalized on in all settings.

WHAT IS THE EVIDENCE BASE
FOR DEVELOPMENTAL INTERVENTIONS
FOR YOUNG CHILDREN WITH ASD?

Using the framework of Smith et al. (2007), empirical research studies on developmental interventions are summarized in Table 7.1, with the developmental features incorporated in each study indicated. We have restricted this review to research studies meeting the following criteria: (1) published in a peer-reviewed journal, (2) used an experimental research design, (3) included children 3 years of age or younger, and (4) reported at least one social communication outcome measure. We have organized the research into the following levels of experiment research design, with true experimental design being the highest level of evidence:

TABLE 7.1. Level of Research Evidence for Studies Implementing Developmental Intervention Approaches

	Child outcome measures	n for ASD treatment group	Age in months at entry	Developmental features				
				Developmental framework	Core deficits	Family guided	Natural environments	Naturalistic strategies
True experimental group designs								
Aldred, Green, & Adams (2004)	Autism symptoms, parent synchrony, and communication rate	14	M = 48	×	×	×	×	×
Drew et al. (2002)	Parent-report measures of language with CDI	12	M = 23	×	×	×	×	×
Kasari, Freeman, & Paparella (2006)	Autism symptoms, Early Social Communication Scales (ESCS), play, and caregiver–child interaction	41	M = 43	×	×			×
McConachie, Randle, Hammal, & LeCouteur (2005)	Autism symptoms, language with CDI, and parent outcomes	26	M = 38		×	×	×	×
Yoder & Stone (2006)	Object exchange turn taking, requesting, initiating joint attention	36	M = 31	×	×			×
Quasi-Experimental Group Designs								
Boulware, Schwartz, Sandall, & McBride (2006)	Developmental level, social communication with CSBS	8	M = 25	×	×	×	×	×

Study	Outcomes	N	Age (months)					
Mahoney & Perales (2005)	Parent interaction and child pivotal behavior	20	$M = 32$	X		X	X	X
McGee, Morrier, & Daly (1999)	Generalized use of language and time spent in proximity with peers	28	$M = 29$	X	X	X	X	X
Rogers & DiLalla (1991)	Developmental level, language measures	49	$M = 46$	X		X	X	X
Wetherby & Woods (2006)	Social communication measured with CSBS	17	$M = 18$	X	X	X	X	X
Single-subject experimental designs								
Hancock & Kaiser (2002)	Rate and spontaneous use of language targets	4	35–54	X			X	X
Hwang & Hughes (2000)	Eye contact, joint attention, and motor imitation	3	32–43	X			X	X
Ingersoll, Dvortcsak, Whalen, & Sikora (2005)	Rate of spontaneous use of language	3	32–46	X			X	X
Kaiser, Hancock, & Nietfeld (2000)	Rate and spontaneous use of language targets	6	35–54	X		X	X	X
Kashinath, Woods, & Goldstein (2006)	Rate of communicative gestures, sounds, or words	5	33–65	X	X	X	X	X
Rogers et al. (2006)	Spontaneous speech, social communication with ADOS-G	10	20–65	X		X	X	X

1. Single-subject experimental treatment designs to examine specific intervention strategies that are incorporated in developmental interventions.
2. Quasi-experimental group treatment designs to demonstrate the feasibility of implementing the model and document group treatment effects.
3. True experimental group treatment designs with randomized clinical trials to document group treatment effects under controlled conditions.

Single-Subject Experimental Designs

Single-subject designs are intended to demonstrate causal relations between specific treatment conditions and dependent variables measured at baseline and during different phases of treatment (Kazdin, 2003). This experimental design does not lend itself easily to developmental approaches that implement a package of intervention strategies. However, there have been six recent single-subject design studies that have incorporated some developmental features and add to the evidence base of developmental approaches for young children with ASD.

Hwang and Hughes (2000) evaluated the effects of a social interactive training on nonverbal social communication skills of three preschoolers with ASD. The social interactive training, adapted from that described by Klinger and Dawson (1992), was implemented by a clinician and consisted of four strategies: (1) environmental arrangement, (2) natural reinforcers, (3) a 5-second wait with an expectant look, and (4) contingent imitation. A multiple-baseline design across participants demonstrated increases in outcome measures of eye contact, joint attention, and motor imitation. Generalization was found with eye contact and motor imitation, but not with joint attention. Measures of social validation supported the fact that positive changes in child behavior had occurred.

Two different single-subject design studies have been conducted by Kaiser and colleagues (Hancock & Kaiser, 2002; Kaiser et al., 2000) to demonstrate the effectiveness of enhanced milieu teaching (EMT) on social communication of children with ASD. EMT is a hybrid approach that blends contemporary behavioral and developmental strategies and consists of three components: (1) environmental arrangement to promote child engagement with activities and partners, (2) responsive interaction techniques to build social interaction with new language forms, and (3) milieu teaching procedures including modeling, mand-model, time delay, and incidental teaching. Kaiser et al. (2000) demonstrated the effects of training six parents of children with ASD to use the naturalistic language intervention strategies during training sessions and maintain the use at follow-up sessions 6 months later. Child effects generalized and were maintained for four of the six children. Hancock and Kaiser (2002) demonstrated the effects of EMT delivered by interventionists to four children with ASD. All four children increased specific language targets and maintained these increases at 6-month follow-up observations. Collectively, these findings suggest that the components of EMT as a package were effective for these children with ASD.

Ingersoll, Dvortcsak, Whalen, and Sikora (2005) implemented a single-subject, multiple-baseline design across participants to examine the effectiveness of a developmental social-pragmatic (DSP) language intervention for three children with ASD. The DSP intervention was implemented by a clinician for 90 minutes per week for 10 weeks and included the following components: (1) following the child's lead, (2) environmental arrangement, (3) responding to all of the child's communicative attempts, (4) emphasizing appropriate affect, and (5) modeling language without elicitation. The authors demonstrated increases in use of spontaneous speech in all three children (although for one child the baseline was not stable) and generalization to parent–child play samples. They suggested that these findings provide preliminary support for the conclusion that direct elicitation is not necessary for increases in rate of spontaneous language.

Although it is broadly accepted that parent-implemented interventions can have positive effects on child communication, there is limited research on parents implementing intervention outside a clinical setting. Preliminary research on embedding intervention within daily routines has shown limited generalization of effects. Kashinath, Woods, and Goldstein (2006) examined the effects of facilitating generalized use of naturalistic teaching strategies by parents of five preschool children with ASD. Using a multiple-baseline design across teaching strategies, they taught each parent three of the following six strategies: environmental arrangement, natural reinforcement, time delay, contingent imitation, modeling, and gestural/visual cues. The programming of generalization occurred by systematic selection of routines and by embedding intervention in multiple routines. Parents learned to use two teaching strategies in target routines to synchronize with their children's attentional focus and address individualized communication objectives. Routines were categorized into one of six classes: play routines, outdoor activities or recreation, caregiving routines, household chores, community activities, and other disability-related routines. For example, playing with puzzles, blocks, ball, bubbles, and music toys were exemplars of indoor play routines. Diapering, hand washing, bath, and mealtime were caregiving routines. No consistent differences were noted in the frequency of strategy use across routines from the same routine class and from a different routine class. Generalization data were collected by measuring strategy use in untrained routines both within the same routine class and across classes of routines. All five parents demonstrated proficient use of teaching strategies and generalized their use across routines both in the same class and across classes of routines. The intervention had positive effects on communication outcomes for four of the five children. All five parents perceived the intervention to be useful in facilitating the child's communication.

Rogers and colleagues (2006) conducted a single-subject design study to compare the Denver Model, which is a blend of contemporary behavioral and developmental approaches, with Prompts for Restructuring Oral Muscular Phonetic Targets (PROMPT), which is a developmental approach focused on speech production disorders. Ten nonverbal children with ASD were matched in pairs and randomly assigned to one of these two treatments. The outcome measures included spontaneous speech samples, as well as social communication behaviors measured by the Autism Diagnostic Observation Schedule–Generic (ADOS-G; Lord, Rutter, DiLavore, & Risi, 1999) and the Social Communication Questionnaire (SCQ; Rutter, Bailey, Berument, Lord, & Pickles, 2001). The treatments were implemented in 12 one-hour weekly therapy sessions. Eight of the 10 children used five or more functional words spontaneously after treatment, and there were no differences in acquired language skills between treatments. Collateral gains in early social communication behaviors were observed in both treatments. More children in the Denver Model showed gains in imitation, and more children in the PROMPT treatment demonstrated gains in functional play. Children who were the best responders to treatment had mild to moderate symptoms of autism, better motor imitation skills, and emerging joint attention skills.

Collectively, these single-subject design studies suggest that components of developmental interventions as a package were effective for these children with ASD. The findings of these studies offer important preliminary data for developmental interventions by providing (1) evidence that naturalistic teaching strategies lead to improvements in core social communication deficits in children with ASD, (2) evidence that parents of children with ASD can learn multiple strategies to synchronize with the child's attentional focus and generalize use of these strategies across routines in natural environments, and (3) evidence of the impact of parent-implemented strategies on communication outcomes for children with ASD.

Quasi-Experimental Group Designs

Many developmental interventions have completed the process of manualization, meaning that a detailed treatment manual that specifies the treatment protocol has been developed for each of them. Examples include the Denver Model (Rogers & DiLalla, 1991; Rogers & Lewis, 1989; Rogers,

Hall, Osaki, Reaven, & Herbison, 2000), Floortime or Developmental, Individual-Difference, Relationship-Based Model (DIR; Greenspan, 1992; Greenspan & Wieder, 1997, 1998, 2000), the Walden Program (McGee et al., 1999), More than Words (Sussman, 1999), Social Communication, Emotional Regulation, Transaction Supports Model (SCERTS; Prizant, Wetherby, Rubin, Laurent, & Rydell, 2006; Prizant et al., 2000), Do–Watch–Listen–Say (Quill, 2000), Relationship Development Intervention (RDI; Gutstein & Sheely, 2002), and Responsive Teaching (RT; Mahoney & Perales, 2005). However, quasi-experimental studies that document the efficacy of these developmental interventions have been published for only a small subset of these approaches.

Two studies have reported on the effectiveness of center-based developmental interventions with young children with ASD. Rogers and DiLalla (1991) were the first to report outcomes using a developmentally based curriculum for preschool children with ASD. They reported the results for 49 children, with a mean age of 46 months, who received 22.5 hours per week of a center-based program for at least 6 months, as compared with children with DD or other psychiatric disorders. The children with ASD made more significant gains than the comparison group in their developmental profiles and on language measures. McGee, Morrier, and Daly (1999) described the curriculum for the Walden Toddler Program, which used incidental teaching in a child care center and a home-based component. Goals were selected by an interdisciplinary team. The intervention components included environmental arrangement and incidental teaching procedures, including vigorous speech shaping, active social instruction, wait–ask–say–show–do, and promotion of engagement. In a project evaluation, which was a weak pretest–posttest quasi-experimental design, McGee et al. reported good verbal outcomes for 28 toddlers with ASD who had entered the center-based incidental teaching program at the Walden Toddler Program at Emory University at a mean age of 29 months. At the time of exit after 6 months in the Walden Program, 82% of the toddlers used meaningful words, an increase from 36% at program entry. On a measure of the amount of time the children spent in proximity to other children, 71% of the children with ASD showed improvement. Because there was no control group, it is not possible to sort out treatment effects from maturation and other confounding variables or to determine whether this sample of children with ASD is representative.

Boulware, Schwartz, Sandall, and McBride (2006) developed Project DATA (Developmentally Appropriate Treatment for Autism) to bridge the features of developmental and behavioral programs for children with ASD under 3 years of age. The primary components of Project DATA included a high-quality inclusive early childhood program, extended instructional time, and family support, totaling 16 hours per week. The focus was on embedding social communication learning opportunities using naturalistic teaching strategies. The authors reported pretest and posttest results for eight children ranging from 18 to 29 months at program entry, with an average of 13.5 months in the program. Six of the eight children demonstrated increases in developmental level, and five of seven children given the CSBS showed substantial improvements. Four of seven families contacted the following year indicated that the child with ASD was placed full-time in a regular education classroom. This study is weak in terms of the research design and small sample size but demonstrates the feasibility of implementing an inclusive educational program for toddlers with ASD.

Mahoney and Perales (2005) compared the effects of a relationship-focused (RF) intervention with a group of 20 children with ASD and a control group of 30 children with DD. The RF intervention consisted of teaching parents a set of responsive interaction strategies designed to enhance the following pivotal developmental behaviors in their children: attention, persistence, interest, initiation, cooperation, joint attention, and affect, in 1-hour weekly sessions for a year. The groups were matched on all measures of demographic or developmental characteristics except age, as the ASD group was significantly older. Both groups made significant increases, with moderate to large effect sizes in cognitive, communication, and socioemotional functioning based on a play-based assessment and parent-report measures. Furthermore, children's improvements were related to increases in both parents' responsiveness and the children's gains in pivotal behaviors. Although the effects of maturation or other treatments cannot be ruled out with this research design, the findings of this study are intriguing in light of the modest amount of time that professionals spent with parents.

Early Social Interaction (ESI) was designed to extend the recommendations of the NRC (2001) to toddlers with ASD using a parent-implemented intervention embedding naturalistic teaching strategies in everyday routines compatible with IDEA, Part C. Wetherby and Woods (2006) reported on a pre–posttest quasi-experimental study as a preliminary effort to evaluate the effects of ESI on social communication outcomes in a group of 17 children with ASD who entered ESI in the second year of life. Parents were taught naturalistic teaching strategies in two weekly sessions in natural environments over the course of a year. Intervention goals were individualized and selected from a developmental framework targeting social interaction, joint attention, communication, imitation, play, and emotional regulation (Prizant et al., 2000). Results indicated significant improvement, with large effect sizes in 11 of 13 social communication outcomes measured with the CSBS (Wetherby & Prizant, 2002). It is particularly noteworthy that significant changes were demonstrated in initiating and responding to joint attention, because few studies have demonstrated significant changes on these measures.

In an effort to strengthen this design, the ESI group was compared with a no-treatment contrast group of 18 children with ASD who entered early intervention during the third year of life. Social communication measures were collected from the contrast group at the same age as the ESI group at posttest and compared to those of the ESI group. Thus, the contrast group provides some information about the possible effects of maturation without treatment. However, pretest measures are not available for the contrast group, because these children were not identified at a younger age, and therefore it cannot be determined whether the groups were comparable at pretest. The contrast group was comparable to the ESI postintervention group on communicative means and play but had significantly poorer performance, with moderate to large effect size on all other measures of social communication. At a mean age of 31 months, 77% of the children in the ESI group were using words, as compared with 56% of those in the contrast group. A weakness of the study was that it was not possible to determine that the groups were matched in the second year of life because children in the contrast group had not been identified and tested at a younger age. These findings offer promise for the use of parent-implemented intervention to impact social communication in toddlers with ASD.

Collectively, these quasi-experimental design studies offer preliminary evidence of the feasibility of implementing developmental interventions and demonstrating changes in core social communication deficits with treatment. Several studies document the feasibility of teaching parents responsive interaction strategies in a few hours per week of professional time and producing meaningful changes in child social communication outcomes. The magnitude of the pre–posttreatment effects in two studies were moderate to large on core social communication deficits that have not been well documented in previous research. Because of the nature of the quasi-experimental designs, these studies have inherent weaknesses due to threats to internal validity, limiting the causal conclusions that can be drawn.

True Experimental Designs

There have been a number of randomized-group design studies that have focused on teaching parents to implement naturalistic strategies with their children with ASD. Drew et al. (2002) reported on a pilot randomized control trial (RCT) administered with 12 families of children with ASD. The parent training program focused on teaching parents how to support social communication within joint action routines within everyday activities. The training consisted of home visits by speech–language therapists once every 6 weeks for 3 hours, with telephone support in between, over the course of a year. The parent training group was compared with a group of children receiving only local services and was found to have made slightly more gains on the language measure. In spite of randomization, the nonverbal developmental level of children in the parent training group was significantly higher than that of children in the local services group, which is a serious internal threat to the validity of this study. A further limitation of this study is that the outcome measure was exclusively via parent reports, using the MacAurthur–Bates Communicative Development Inventory (CDI; Fenson et al., 1993). Although this study had serious methodological flaws, the authors used the difficulties encountered to make recommendations for planning future well-designed RCTs.

In a more successful randomized-group design study, Aldred, Green, and Adams (2004) implemented a monthly parent training program for 14 preschool children in their treatment group and compared the outcomes with those for 14 children in a community treatment control group. Aldred et al. found significantly lower scores with a large effect size on the ADOS-G—which indicated that there were fewer autism symptoms in the treatment group—and significantly better outcomes with a large effect size for parental positive synchronous communication and a moderate effect size for rate of child communicative acts. However, they found no significant difference between the two groups in number of episodes in which the parent and child shared attentional focus. These results suggest that significant gains with moderate to large effect sizes in some aspects of social communication can be achieved by teaching parents how to enhance their children's communication in a cost-effective treatment, but that gains in joint attention may require a more intensive or different approach to intervention.

McConachie, Randle, Hammal, and LeCouteur (2005) implemented an RCT with 26 parents of children with ASD and 25 control families. The groups were not significantly different in adaptive behavior at the beginning of treatment. The parent training used the More than Words Program (Sussman, 1999), administered in 20 hours of weekly group instruction and three home visits for individual discussion and feedback. Although this program is broadly based on a developmental framework, goals were not individualized on the basis of the children's developmental profiles. Measures at pretest and posttest 7 months later included child outcomes based on the MacArthur–Bates Communicative Development Inventory (CDI) as a parent-report measure of language, social communication skills based on the ADOS-G, and a set of parent outcome measures of the parent's use of facilitation strategies, family resources and stress, and adaptation to the child. A significant advantage was found for the parent training group, with moderate effect sizes in the parents' use of facilitative strategies and the children's vocabulary size, but no significant group differences were found on the social communication algorithm of the ADOS-G.

Two additional RCTs were recently published that compared two treatments for preschool children with ASD. Kasari, Freeman, and Paparella (2006) randomly assigned participants to one of three treatments: 20 to a joint attention treatment, 21 to a symbolic play treatment, and 17 to a no-treatment control. The treatment involved a blend of contemporary behavioral and developmental procedures of responsive and facilitative interactive methods and was implemented 30 minutes daily for 5–6 weeks. Both treatment groups showed significant improvement, with large effect sizes in relation to the control group. Children in the joint attention treatment group initiated significantly more showing and responding to joint attention. There were no significant group differences in initiation of joint attention. The play treatment group showed more diversity in symbolic play action schemes and higher play levels, both during play assessments with clinicians and in interactions with their mothers. The children were able to generalize learned skills from treatment sessions with clinicians to playing with their caregivers. These findings provide promising data regarding the specificity of treatment effects and show that these children generalized their treatment effects to new contexts and people.

Yoder & Stone (2006) conducted an RCT to compare the efficacy of two communication interventions: (1) Responsive Education and Prelinguistic Milieu Teaching (RPMT) and the Picture Exchange Communication System (PECS; Bondy & Frost, 1994). There is a large empirical base supporting the efficacy of RPMT with children with DD; however, this was the first study to examine its effect on turn-taking skills of children with ASD. RPMT uses procedures similar to those of EMT, with a focus on prelinguistic skills combined with an education program for parents on responsive interaction, because previous research demonstrated that maternal responsivity was a treatment mediator (Yoder & Warren, 1999, 2002). RPMT is a developmental intervention that incorporates naturalistic behavioral teaching strategies. PECS is a contemporary behavioral treatment program that teaches requesting and commenting behaviors through the exchange of pictures, using natural reinforcers and building to picture–symbol combinations. Both treatments were implemented by clinicians three times a week in 20-minute sessions for 6 months. The results indicated that RPMT was significantly more effective than the PECS, with large effect sizes in facilitating turn taking and generalized initiation of joint attention; however, the latter finding was limited to children with at least some initiating joint attention at pretest. The PECS was more effective than RPMT in teaching generalized requests in children with little initiating joint attention prior to treatment. These findings are very intriguing because they offer evidence about the characteristics of children who responded differentially to two different communication interventions that required 1 hour of professional time per week for 6 months.

Collectively, the cumulative findings from these RCTs offer empirical evidence of the benefit of developmental interventions for children with ASD. Both the parent training and clinician-implemented programs were particularly impressive in that they entailed minimum professional time, and thus are feasible within the Part C service delivery system. Improvements in social communication outcomes were demonstrated in programs that were of low intensity and relatively short duration. Furthermore, group differences between treatment and control groups, with moderate to large effect sizes in social communication outcomes, were reported in four RCTs. Finally, these RCTs provide evidence that developmental interventions can lead to changes in the core deficits of joint attention and symbolic capacity in young children with ASD and suggest that they may be more effective than behavioral approaches for targeting these social communication goals. However, it is important to note that the children in all of these studies were also receiving community interventions, and therefore these intervention outcomes may reflect the combined effects of the targeted treatments and community interventions. It is not ethical to withhold treatment and therefore not possible to have a true no-treatment control group. To strengthen the causal conclusions that can be drawn from RCTs using interventions that are brief or of low intensity, future research should provide careful documentation of community interventions that families receive prior to and during treatment to document that groups are equivalent on this variable. Comparative treatment designs examining specific responses to treatment, as implemented by Kasari et al. (2006) and Yoder and Stone (2006), and that demonstrate group equivalence in community interventions, are well suited to document the effectiveness of developmental interventions.

CONCLUSIONS AND FUTURE DIRECTIONS

This chapter began by summarizing the core social communication deficits in infants and toddlers with ASD and underscoring the critical importance of early intervention to promote social communication skills and hence possibly prevent further abnormal brain development. A common key feature of developmental interventions is the use of naturalistic teaching strategies that follow the child's lead by means of responsive interaction. Teaching caregivers responsive interaction strategies may play a critical role in enhancing caregiver synchronization. Caregiver synchronization may, in turn, be a critical mediating variable impacting a child's social communication outcomes. There is now a body of research supporting the effectiveness of developmental interventions, and particularly noteworthy is that significant improvements have been documented in core social communication deficits, such as initiating and responding to joint attention. Joint attention appears to be a pivotal skill that, through a transactional process, has a cascading effect on later developmental outcomes (Wetherby et al., 2007). Further research is needed to systematically explore the mechanisms of change that occur with developmental interventions, particularly the impact of adult synchronization on child social communication outcomes.

Providing early intervention to infants and toddlers at risk for ASD and their families offers new challenges and promising opportunities for improving the children's outcomes. The challenges for professionals range from how to identify young children early and accurately, how to identify factors that determine amenability to treatment (to match strategy with the individual child), how to ensure that identified children receive intervention with sufficient intensity to maximize outcomes, to how to develop systems that ensure that services are coordinated with effective communication between professionals and families. Although the optimal intensity of intervention for infants and toddlers is yet undetermined, the family's unique role in the care and education of very young children must be recognized. There is little evidence to support the idea that once or twice weekly specialized therapy (e.g., speech–language therapy [SLP]; occupational therapy [OT]) will have an impact on child outcomes without responsive interactions by caregivers in the child's natural environment.

The research reviewed in this chapter highlights the effectiveness of parent-implemented developmental intervention for very young children with ASD. Working with family members in parent-implemented interventions will necessitate the "rethinking" of prevalent service delivery models and an increased emphasis on service provision in the child's and family's natural environment (Guralnick, 2001). The reality of designing and implementing embedded intervention within the child's routines and activities where they occur is not a common practice. It is not likely to be an easy shift for service providers to make without changes in program policies (e.g., reimbursement for parent training and travel) and practices (e.g., consultation with caregivers instead of direct "hands on" therapy). Personnel may need additional training in techniques for scaffolding with adults to make parent-implemented interventions maximally effective (Guralnick, 2000). Furthermore, there is much to learn about working collaboratively and effectively with families of low socioeconomic status, of diverse cultures, or with linguistic differences (Bernheimer & Keogh, 1995).

Agencies supporting service delivery, including Part C early intervention programs, will need to expand service options and opportunities for children and families. The determination of the intensity of services must not be based on the ability of the family to either access or afford them for a child. Early identification should be emphasized, with intervention available for all children according to their needs and the families' preferences. Again, although such services are costly, the outcomes indicated for children thus far are likely to result in savings in service delivery later and, more important, in increased potential for the children's success.

Developmental and contemporary behavioral intervention approaches have many common features, and developmental and behavioral features are often blended. Further intervention research is needed to study the relationship between child characteristics, specific treatment procedures, and specific outcomes. Future research should strive to document the relations between child characteristics, meaningful changes in core social communication deficits—skills that contribute to the capacity for joint attention and symbol use—and specific intervention strategies. Such research findings can help families and educators to prioritize intervention goals and select specific intervention strategies designed to best meet the goals targeted for children likely to be good responders. Interventions within the natural environment will need further delineation of "match" between strategies used by professionals and those that are comfortable and meaningful to the family members implementing them.

The list of future needs extends from increased public awareness of early red flags of ASD in young children to improved personnel training across the wide range of medical, educational, and social service personnel important to the child and family. It includes the need for the development of proactive approaches for identification of and intervention with young children and their families toward functional and meaningful outcomes and for careful evaluation of the services provided. Future needs will require a two-pronged approach—bridging the gap between existing knowledge and common practice for young children with ASD, and the pursuit of new knowledge to advance early identification and intervention efforts. As we are better able to identify children with ASD earlier and intervene earlier, early intervention may be viewed as a transactional process to prevent or minimize the unfolding of autism symptoms.

REFERENCES

Aldred, C., Green, J., & Adams, C. (2004). A new social communication intervention for children with autism: Pilot randomized controlled treatment study suggesting effectiveness. *Journal of Child Psychology and Psychiatry, 45,* 1420–1430.

Allen, R. I., & Petr, C. G. (1996). Toward developing standards and measurements for family-centered practice in family support programs. In G. H. S. Singer,

L. E. Powers, & A. I. Olson (Eds.), *Redefining family support: Innovations in public–private partnerships* (pp. 57–86). Baltimore: Brookes.

Baron-Cohen, S., Cox, A., Baird, G., Swettenham, J., Nightingale, N., Morgan, K., et al. (1996). Psychological markers in the detection of autism in infancy in a large population. *British Journal of Psychiatry, 168,* 158–163.

Bates, E. (1976). *Language and context: The acquisition of pragmatics.* New York: Academic Press.

Bates, E. (1979). *The emergence of symbols: Cognition and communication in infancy.* New York: Academic Press.

Bates, E., Camaioni, L., & Volterra, V. (1975). The acquisition of performatives prior to speech. *Merrill–Palmer Quarterly, 21,* 205–226.

Bates, E., O'Connell, B., & Shore, C. (1987). Language and communication in infancy. In J. Osofsky (Ed.), *Handbook of infant development* (pp. 149–203). New York: Wiley.

Bernheimer, L., & Keogh, B. (1995). Weaving interventions into the fabric of everyday life: An approach to family assessment. *Topics in Early Childhood Special Education, 15,* 415–433.

Bloom, L. (1993). *The transition from infancy to language.* New York: Cambridge University Press.

Bloom, L., & Lahey, M. (1978). *Language development and language disorders.* New York: Wiley.

Bondy, A., & Frost, L. (1994). *PECS: The Picture Exchange Communication System training manual.* Cherry Hill, NJ: Pyramid Educational Consultants.

Bono, M., Daley, T., & Sigman, M. (2004). Relations among joint attention, amount of intervention and language gain in autism. *Journal of Autism and Developmental Disorders, 34,* 495–505.

Boulware, G., Schwartz, I., Sandall, S., & McBride, B. (2006). Project DATA for toddlers: An inclusive approach to very young children with autism spectrum disorders. *Topics in Early Childhood Special Education, 26,* 94–105.

Bruner, J. (1978). From communication to language: A psychological perspective. In I. Markova (Ed.), *The social context of language* (pp. 17–48). Chichester, UK: Wiley.

Bruner, J. (1981). The social context of language acquisition. *Language and Communication, 1,* 155–178.

Buysse, V., & Wesley, P. (2005). *Consultation in early childhood settings.* Baltimore: Brookes.

Charlop, M. H., Schreibman, L., & Thibodeau, M. G. (1985). Increasing spontaneous verbal responding in autistic children using a time delay procedure. *Journal of Applied Behavior Analysis, 18,* 155–166.

Charlop, M. H., & Trasowech, J. E. (1991). Increasing children's daily spontaneous speech. *Journal of Applied Behavioral Analysis, 24,* 747–761.

Charman, T., Baron-Cohen, S., Swettenham, J., Baird, G., Drew, A., & Cox, A. (2003). Predicting language outcome in infants with autism and pervasive developmental disorder. *International Journal of Language and Communication Disorders, 38,* 265–285.

Charman, T., Swettenham, J., Baron-Cohen, S., Cox, A., Baird, G., & Drew, A. (1997). Infants with autism: An investigation of empathy, pretend play, joint attention, and imitation. *Developmental Psychology, 33,* 781–789.

Dawson, G., Toth, K., Abbott, R., Osterling, J., Munson, J., Estes, A., et al. (2004). Early social attention impairments in autism: Social orienting, joint attention, and attention to distress. *Developmental Psychology, 40,* 271–283.

Drew, A., Baird, G., Baron-Cohen, S., Cox, A., Slonims, V., Wheelwright, S., et al. (2002). A pilot randomized control trial of a parent training intervention for pre-school children with autism: Preliminary findings and methodological challenges. *European Child and Adolescent Psychiatry, 11,* 266–272.

Dunlap, G., & Fox, L. (1999). Supporting families of young children with autism. *Infants and Young Children, 12*(2), 48–54.

Dunst, C., Hamby, D., Trivette, C., Raab, M., & Bruder, M. B. (2000). Everyday family and community life and children's naturally occurring learning opportunities. *Journal of Early Intervention, 23*(3), 151–164.

Dunst, C., Lowe, L. W., & Bartholomew, P. C. (1990). Contingent social repsonsiveness, family ecology, and infant communicative competence. *National Student Speech Language Hearing Association Journal, 17,* 39–49.

Dunst, C., Trivette, C., & Deal, A. (Eds.). (1988). *Enabling and empowering families: Principles and guidelines for practice.* Cambridge, MA: Brookline Books.

Fenson, L., Dale, P., Reznick, S., Thal, D., Bates, E., Hartung, J., et al. (1993). *MacArthur–Bates Communicative Development Inventories: User's guide and technical manual.* Baltimore: Brookes.

Goldstein, H. (2002). Communication intervention for children with autism: A review of treatment efficacy. *Journal of Autism and Developmental Disorders, 32,* 373–396.

Greenspan, S. I. (1992). *Infancy and early childhood: The practice of clinical assessment and intervention with emotional and developmental challenges.* Madison, CT: International Universities Press.

Greenspan, S. I., & Wieder, S. (1997). Developmental patterns and outcomes in infants and children with disorders in relating and communicating: A chart review of 200 cases of children with autistic spectrum diagnoses. *Journal of Developmental and Learning Disorders. 1,* 87–141.

Greenspan, S. I., & Wieder, S. (1998). *The child with special needs: Intellectual and emotional growth.* Reading, MA: Addison Wesley Longman.

Greenspan, S. I., & Wieder, S. (2000). A developmental approach to difficulties in relating and communicating in autism spectrum disorders and related symptoms. In A. Wetherby & B. Prizant (Eds.), *Autism spectrum disorders: A transactional developmental perspective* (pp. 279–303). Baltimore: Brookes.

Guralnick, M. (2000). Early childhood intervention: Evolution of a system. *Focus on Autism and Other Developmental Disabilities, 15,* 68–79.

Guralnick, M. (Ed.). (2001). *Early childhood inclusion: Focus on change.* Baltimore: Brookes.

Gutstein, S., & Sheely, R. (2002). *Relationship development intervention with young children: Social and emotional development activities for Asperger syndrome, autism, PDD, and NLD.* Philadelphia: Kingsley.

Hancock, T. B., & Kaiser, A. P. (2002). The effects of trainer-implemented enhanced milieu teaching on the social communication of children with autism. *Topics in Early Childhood Special Education, 22,* 39–54.

Hart, B. (1985). Naturalistic language training strategies. In S. Warren & A.

Rogers-Warren (Eds.), *Teaching functional language* (pp. 63–88). Baltimore: University Park Press.

Hepting, N., & Goldstein, H. (1996). What's natural about naturalistic language intervention? *Journal of Early Intervention, 20,* 249–265.

Horner, R., O'Neill, R., & Flannery, K. (1993). Effective behavior support plans. In M. Snell (Ed.), *Instruction of students with severe disabilities* (pp. 184–214). New York: Merrill.

Howlin, P., & Moore, A. (1997). Diagnosis of autism: A survey of over 1200 patients in the UK. *Autism, 1,* 135–162.

Hwang, B., & Hughes, C. (2000). Increasing early social-communicative skills of preverbal preschool children with autism through social interactive training. *Journal of the Association for Persons with Severe Handicaps, 25,* 18–28.

Ingersoll, B., Dvortcsak, A., Whalen, C., & Sikora, D. (2005). The effects of a developmental, social-pragmatic language intervention on rate of expressive language production in young children with autistic spectrum disorders. *Focus on Autism and Other Developmental Disabilities, 20,* 213–222.

Kaiser, A. (1993). Functional language. In M. Snell (Ed.), *Instruction of students with severe disabilities* (pp. 347–379). New York: Macmillan.

Kaiser, A., Hancock, T., & Nietfeld, J. (2000). The effects of parent-implemented enhanced milieu teaching on the social communication of children who have autism. *Early Education and Development, 11,* 423–446.

Kaiser, A. P., Yoder, P. J., & Keetz, A. (1992). Evaluating milieu teaching. In S. F. Warren & J. Reichle (Eds.), *Causes and effects in communication and language intervention* (pp. 9–47). Baltimore: Brookes.

Kasari, C., Freeman, S., & Paparella, T. (2006). Joint attention and symbolic play in young children with autism: A randomized controlled intervention study. *Journal of Child Psychology and Psychiatry, 47,* 611–620.

Kashinath, S., Woods, J., & Goldstein, H. (2006). Enhancing generalized teaching strategy use in daily routines by caregivers of children with autism. *Journal of Speech, Language, and Hearing Research, 49,* 466–485.

Kazdin, A. (2003). *Research design in clinical psychology* (4th ed.). Boston: Allyn & Bacon.

Klinger, L., & Dawson, G. (1992). Facilitating early social and communicative development in children with autism. In S. Warren & J. Reichle (Eds.), *Causes and effects in communication and language intervention* (pp. 157–186). Baltimore: Brookes.

Koegel, L. (1995). Communication and language intervention. In R. Koegel & L. Koegel (Eds.), *Teaching children with autism* (pp. 17–32) Baltimore: Brookes.

Koegel, R., Bimbela, A., & Schreibman, L. (1996). Collateral effects of parent training on family interactions. *Journal of Autism and Developmental Disorders, 26,* 347–359.

Koegel, R., Camarata, S., Koegel, L., Ben-Tall, A., & Smith, A. (1998). Increasing speech intelligibility in children with autism. *Journal of Autism and Developmental Disorders, 28,* 241–251.

Koegel, R., Koegel, L., & Surratt, A. (1992). Language intervention and disruptive behavior in preschool children with autism. *Journal of Autism and Developmental Disorders: 22*, 141–153.

Koegel, R., O'Dell, M. C., & Koegel, L. K. (1987). A natural language paradigm for teaching nonverbal autistic children. *Journal of Autism and Developmental Disorders, 17*, 187–199.

Landa, R., & Garrett-Mayer, E. (2006). Development in infants with autism spectrum disorders: A prospective study. *Journal of Child Psychology and Psychiatry, 47*, 629–638.

Lord, C., Rutter, M., DiLavore, P., & Risi, S. (1999). *Autism Diagnostic Observation Schedule–Generic*. Los Angeles: Western Psychological Services.

Lovaas, O. I. (1977). *The autistic child: Language development through behavior modification*. New York: Irvington Press.

Lovaas, O. I. (1981). *Teaching developmentally disabled children. The "Me" book*. Baltimore: University Park Press.

Loveland, K., & Landry, S. (1986). Joint attention and language in autism and developmental language delay. *Journal of Autism and Developmental Disorders, 16*, 335–349.

MacDonald, J. (1989). *Becoming partners with children*. San Antonio, TX: Special Press.

MacDonald, J., & Carroll, J. (1992). A social partnership model for assessing early communication development: An intervention model for preconversational children. *Language, Speech, and Hearing Services in Schools, 23*, 113–124.

Mahoney, G., & Perales, F. (2005). Relationship-focused early intervention with children with pervasive developmental disorders and other disabilities: A comparative study. *Developmental and Behavioral Pediatrics, 26*, 77–85.

McClannahan, L. K., Krantz, P. J., & McGee, G. (1982). Parents as therapists for autistic children: A model for effective parent training. *Analysis and Intervention in Developmental Disabilities, 2*, 223–252.

McConachie, H., Randle, V., Hammal, D., & LeCouteur, A. (2005). A controlled trial of a training course for parents of children with suspected autism spectrum disorders. *Journal of Pediatrics, 147*, 335–340.

McEachin, J. J., Smith, T., & Lovaas, O. I. (1993). Long-term outcome for children with autism who received early intensive behavioral treatment. *American Journal on Mental Retardation, 97*(4), 359–372.

McGee, G., Krantz, P. J., & McClannahan, L. E. (1985). The facilitative effects of incidental teaching on preposition use by autistic children. *Journal of Applied Behavior Analysis, 18*, 17–31.

McGee, G., & Morrier, M. (2005). Preparation of autism specialists. In F. Volkmar, R. Paul, A. Klin, & D. Cohen (Eds.), *Handbook of autism and pervasive developmental disorders* (3rd ed., pp. 1123–1160). Hoboken, NJ: Wiley.

McGee, G., Morrier, M., & Daly, T. (1999). An incidental teaching approach to early intervention for toddlers with autism. *Journal of the Association for Persons with Severe Handicaps, 24*, 133–146.

McLean, J., & Snyder-McLean, L. (1978). *A transactional approach to early language training*. Columbus: Merrill.

McWilliam, R. A. (1992). *Family-centered intervention planning: A routines based approach*. Tuscon, AZ: Communication Skill Builders.

Mitchell, S., Brian, J., Zwaigenbaum, L., Roberts, W., Szatmari, P., Smith, I., et al. (2006). Early language and communication development of infants later diagnosed with autism spectrum disorders. *Developmental and Behavioral Pediatrics, 27,* S69–S78.

Mundy, P., & Burnette, C. (2005). Joint attention and neurodevelopmental models of autism. In F. Volkmar, R. Paul, A. Klin, & D. Cohen (Eds.), *Handbook of autism and pervasive developmental disorders* (3rd ed., pp. 650–681). Hoboken, NJ: Wiley.

Mundy, P., Sigman, M., & Kasari, C. (1990). A longitudinal study of joint attention and language development in autistic children. *Journal of Autism and Developmental Disorders, 20,* 115–128.

National Research Council. (2001). *Educating children with autism.* Washington, DC: National Academy Press.

Osterling, J., & Dawson, G. (1994). Early recognition of children with autism: A study of first birthday home videotapes. *Journal of Autism and Developmental Disorders, 24,* 247–257.

Osterling, J., Dawson, G., & Munson, J. (2002). Early recognition of one year old infants with autism spectrum disorder versus mental retardation: A study of first birthday party home videotapes. *Development and Psychopathology, 14,* 239–252.

Prizant, B., & Wetherby, A. (1993) Communication and language assessment for young children. *Infants and Young Children, 5,* 20–34.

Prizant, B. M., & Wetherby, A. M. (1998). Understanding the continuum of discrete-trial traditional behavioral to social-pragmatic developmental approaches in communication enhancement for young children with autism/ PDD. *Seminars in Speech and Language, 19,* 329–353.

Prizant, B., & Wetherby, A. (2005). Critical issues in enhancing communication abilities for persons with autism spectrum disorders. In F. Volkmar, R. Paul, A. Klin, & D. Cohen (Eds.), *Handbook of autism and pervasive developmental disorders* (3rd ed., pp. 925–945). Hoboken, NJ: Wiley.

Prizant, B., Wetherby, A., Rubin, E., Laurent, A., & Rydell, P. (2006). *The SCERTS model: A comprehensive educational approach for children with autism spectrum disorders.* Baltimore: Brookes.

Prizant, B., Wetherby, A., & Rydell, P. (2000). Issues in enhancing communication and related abilities for young children with autism spectrum disorders: A developmental transactional perspective. In A. Wetherby & B. Prizant (Eds.), *Autism spectrum disorders: A transactional developmental perspective* (pp. 193–234). Baltimore: Brookes.

Quill, K. A. (2000). *Do–Watch–Listen–Say: Social and communication intervention for children with autism.* Baltimore: Brookes.

Rogers, S. J., & DiLalla, D. (1991). A comparative study of a developmentally based preschool curriculum on young children with autism and young children with other disorders of behavior and development. *Topics in Early Childhood Special Education, 11,* 29–48.

Rogers, S. J., Hall, T., Osaki, D., Reaven, J., & Herbison, J. (2000). The Denver Model: A comprehensive, integrated educational approach to young children with autism and their families. In J. S. Handleman & S. L. Harris (Eds.), *Pre-*

school education programs for children with autism (2nd ed., pp. 95–133). Austin, TX: PRO-ED.

Rogers, S. J., Hayden, D., Hepburn, S., Charlifue-Smith, R., Hall, T., & Hayes, A. (2006). Teaching young nonverbal children with autism useful speech: A pilot study of the Denver Model and PROMPT interventions. *Journal of Autism and Developmental Disorders, 136,* 1007–1024.

Rogers, S. J., & Lewis, H. (1989). An effective day treatment model for young children with pervasive developmental disorders. *Journal of the American Academy of Child and Adolescent Psychiatry, 28,* 207–214.

Rowland, C., & Schweigert, P. (1993). Analyzing the communication environment to increase functional communication. *Journal of the Association for Persons with Severe Handicaps, 18,* 161–176.

Rutter, M., Bailey, A., Berument, S., Lord, C., & Pickles, A. (2001). *Social Communication Questionnaire–Research Edition.* Los Angeles: Western Psychological Services.

Sameroff, A. (1987). The social context of development. In N. Eisenburg (Ed.), *Contemporary topics in development* (pp. 273–291). New York: Wiley.

Sandall, S. R., McLean, M., & Smith, B. (2000). *DEC recommended practices in early intervention/early childhood special education.* Longmont, CO: Sopris West.

Schreibman, L., Kaneko, W., & Koegel, R. (1991). Positive affect of parents of autistic children: A comparison across two teaching techniques. *Behavior Therapy, 22,* 479–490.

Seifer, R., Clark, G. N., & Samaroff, A. (1991). Positive effects of interaction coaching on infants with developmental disabilities and their mothers. *American Journal of Mental Retardation, 96,* 1–11.

Short, A., & Schopler, E. (1988). Factors relating to age of onset in autism. *Journal of Autism and Developmental Disorders, 18,* 207–216.

Siegel, B., Pliner, C., Eschler, J., & Elliot, G. (1988). How children with autism are diagnosed: Difficulties in identification of children with multiple developmental delays. *Developmental and Behavioral Pediatrics, 9,* 199–204.

Sigman, M., Dijamco, A., Gratier, M., & Rozga, A. (2004). Early detection of core deficits in autism. *Mental Retardation and Developmental Disabilities Research Reviews, 10,* 221–233.

Sigman, M., Mundy, P., Sherman, T., & Ungerer, J. (1986). Social interactions of autistic, mentally retarded and normal children and their caregivers. *Journal of Child Psychology and Psychiatry and Allied Disciplines, 27*(5), 647–656.

Sigman, M., & Ruskin, E. (1999). Continuity and change in the social competence of children with autism, Down syndrome, and developmental delays. *Monographs of the Society for Research in Child Development, 64,* 1–113.

Siller, M., & Sigman, M. (2002). The behaviors of parents of children with autism predict subsequent development of children's communication. *Journal of Autism and Developmental Disorders, 32,* 77–89.

Smith, T., Scahill, L., Dawson, G., Guthrie, D., Lord, C., Odom, S., et al. (2007). Designing research studies on psychosocial interventions in autism. *Journal of Autism and Developmental Disorders, 37,* 354–366.

Sperry, L. A., Whaley, K. T., Shaw, E., & Brame, K. (1999). Services for young children with autism spectrum disorder: Voices of parents and providers. *Infants and Young Children, 11,* 17–33.

Stern, D. (1985). *The interpersonal world of the infant.* New York: Basic Books.

Stone, W., Ousley, O., Yoder, P., Hogan, K., & Hepburn, S. (1997). Nonverbal communication in 2- and 3-year old children with autism. *Journal of Autism and Developmental Disorders, 27,* 677–696.

Stone, W., & Yoder, P. (2001). Predicting spoken language level in children with autism spectrum disorders. *Autism, 5*(4), 341–361.

Strain, P., McGee, G., & Kohler, F. (2001). Inclusion of children with autism in early intervention environments. In M. J. Guralnick (Ed.), *Early childhood inclusion: Focus on change* (pp. 337–363). Baltimore: Brookes.

Sussman, F. (1999). *More than words: Helping parents promote communication and social skills in children with autism spectrum disorder.* Toronto, ON: Hanen Centre.

Swettenham, J., Baron-Cohen, S., Charman, T., Cox, A., Baird, G., Drew, A., et al. (1998). The frequency and distribution of spontaneous attention shifts between social and nonsocial stimuli in autistic, typically developing, and nonautistic developmentally delayed infants. *Journal of Child Psychology and Psychiatry, 39,* 747–753.

Tomasello, M., Kruger, A. C., & Ratner, H. H. (1993). Cultural learning. *Behavioral and Brain Sciences, 16,* 495–552.

Tronick, E. (1989). Emotions and emotional communication in infancy. *American Psychologist, 44,* 112–119.

Turnbull, A., & Ruef, M. (1997). Family perspectives on inclusive lifestyles for people with problem behavior. *Exceptional Children, 63,* 223–229.

U.S. Department of Education. (2004). The Individuals with Disabilities Education Improvement Act of 2004 (Public Law 108-446).

Vygotsky, L. (1986). *Thought and language* (A. Kozulin, Ed. and Trans.), Cambridge, MA: MIT Press. (Original work published 1934)

Wetherby, A., & Prizant, B. (2002). *Communication and Symbolic Behavior Scales Developmental Profile–First Normed Edition.* Baltimore: Brookes.

Wetherby, A. M., Prizant, B. M., & Hutchinson, T. (1998). Communicative, social-affective, and symbolic profiles of young children with autism and pervasive developmental disorder. *American Journal of Speech–Language Pathology, 7,* 79–91.

Wetherby, A., Schuler, A., & Prizant, B. (1997). Enhancing language and communication development: Theoretical foundations. In D. Cohen & F. Volkmar (Eds.), *Handbook of autism and pervasive developmental disorders* (2nd ed., pp. 513–538). New York: Wiley.

Wetherby, A., Watt, N., Morgan, L., & Shumway, S. (2007). Social communication profiles of children with autism spectrum disorders in the second year of life. *Journal of Autism and Developmental Disorders, 37,* 960–975.

Wetherby, A., & Woods, J. (2006). Effectiveness of early intervention for children with autism spectrum disorders beginning in the second year of life. *Topics in Early Childhood Special Education, 26,* 67–82.

Wetherby, A., Woods, J., Allen, L., Cleary, J., Dickinson, H., & Lord, C. (2004). Early indicators of autism spectrum disorders in the second year of life. *Journal of Autism and Developmental Disorders, 34,* 473–493.

Wimpory, D. C., Hobson, R. P., & Nash, S. (2007). What facilitates social engagement in preschool children with autism? *Journal of Autism and Developmental Disorders, 37,* 564–573.

Wimpory, D. C., Hobson, R. P., Williams, J. M. G., & Nash, S. (2000). Are infants with autism socially engaged? A study of recent retrospective parental reports. *Journal of Autism and Developmental Disorders, 30,* 525–536.

Woods, J., Kashinath, S., & Goldstein, H. (2004). Effects of embedding caregiver-implemented teaching strategies in daily routines on children's communication outcomes. *Journal of Early Intervention, 26,* 175–193.

Woods, J., & Wetherby, A. (2003). Early identification and intervention for infants and toddlers at-risk for autism spectrum disorders. *Language, Speech, and Hearing Services in Schools, 34,* 180–193.

Woods Cripe, J., & Venn, M. (1997). Family-guided routines for early intervention services. *Young Exceptional Children, 1*(1), 18–26.

Yirmiya, N., Gamliel, I., Pilowsky, T., Feldman, R., Baron-Cohen, S., & Sigman, M. (2006). The development of siblings of children with autism at 4 and 14 months: Social engagement, communication, and cognition. *Journal of Child Psychology and Psychiatry, 47,* 511–523.

Yoder, P., & Stone, W. (2006). Randomized comparison of two communication interventions for preschoolers with autism spectrum disorders. *Journal of Consulting and Clinical Psychology, 74,* 426–435.

Yoder, P., & Warren, S. (1999). Maternal responsivity mediates the relationship between prelinguistic intentional communication and later language. *Journal of Early Intervention, 22,* 126–136.

Yoder, P., & Warren, S. (2002). Effects of prelinguistic milieu teaching and parent responsivity education in dyads with children with intellectual disabilities. *Journal of Speech, Language, and Hearing Research, 45,* 1158–1174.

Yoder, P., Warren, S., McCathren, R., & Leew, S. (1998). Does adult responsivity to child behavior facilitate communication development? In A. M. Wetherby, S. F. Warren, & J. Reichle (Eds.), *Transitions in prelinguistic communication* (pp. 39–58). Baltimore: Brookes.

Zwaigenbaum, L., Bryson, S., Rogers, T., Roberts, W., Brian, J., & Szatmari, P. (2005). Behavioral manifestations of autism in the first year of life. *International Journal of Developmental Neuroscience, 23,* 143–152.

CHAPTER 8

Naturalistic Behavioral Approaches to Treatment

Lynn Kern Koegel
Robert L. Koegel
Rosy M. Fredeen
Grace W. Gengoux

Autism spectrum disorders (ASD) continue to be diagnosed at epidemic rates (Centers for Disease Control and Prevention, 2006). The literature suggests that the education of early health care providers coupled with the screening and diagnostic ability to identify children with ASD at very young ages (Baron-Cohen, Allen, & Gillberg, 1992; R. L. Koegel & Koegel, 2006; Lord & Risi, 2000) can lead to commencement of intervention at significantly younger ages. Consequently, this has created a new challenge for researchers and practitioners (Boulware, Schwartz, Sandall, & McBride, 2006). That is, how should infants and toddlers with ASD be supported in intervention, given their very young age and developmental needs? The need for evidence-based interventions for toddlers is critical, particularly in light of research showing that many childhood psychotherapies are no more effective than the passage of time (as discussed in Kazdin & Weisz, 2003). Furthermore, there is increasing empirical evidence suggesting that early intervention results in a much improved prognosis for children with ASD (Rogers, 1998).

Despite this ability to detect ASD at a young age (Baron-Cohen et al., 1992; Lord & Risi, 2000), and the fact that the majority of parents report that symptom onset occurs before the age of 2 (Baghadadli, Picot, Pascal, Pry, & Aussilloux, 2003), ASD is not often diagnosed until 2–3 years after parents begin to report symptoms (Filipek et al., 1999). There are several likely causes for the delays in the diagnosis of ASD and commencement of intervention. First, many parents first report their children's symptoms to their pediatricians. Developmental screenings are often not covered by insurance companies, and many pediatricians are not trained to diagnose the symptoms of ASD. Second, there appears to be some regression in about a third of the children diagnosed with ASD (Chawarska, Paul, et al., 2007). That is, the parents report that their children were developing typically, but then lost previously acquired skills (e.g., words, social skills, and so on). Third, because there is so much heterogeneity in children with ASD, children diagnosed with milder forms of the disorder may not be easily identified before the age of 3. Fourth, because some early milestones may be met on time, such as gross motor skills, parents may not realize the extent of delay in other areas. Fifth, a subset of children with ASD may not show symptoms in the first year of life (Chawarska, Paul, et al., 2007). For example, many parents report that delays in the onset of expressive verbal communication first alerted them to the possibility of a disability. Because first words usually do not appear until the second year of life, many prelinguistic symptoms of ASD may be missed. And finally, many families may not have access to specialists in the area of autism and, consequently, their child's disability may be un- or misdiagnosed.

In spite of the fact that most children are not diagnosed with ASD during the first few years of life, the literature suggests that there are a number of prelinguistic symptoms in children with ASD that are present during or close to the child's first year of life (Adrien et al., 1993; Chawarska, Paul, et al., 2007; Chawarska, Klin, Paul, & Volkmar, 2007; see also Volkmar, Chawarska, & Klin, Chapter 1; Bishop, Luyster, Richler, & Lord, Chapter 2; Chawarska & Bearss, Chapter 3; and Paul, Chapter 4, this volume). These prelinguistic symptoms, which suggest directions for treatment, include more neutral affect, less joint attention, fewer social interactions, limited response to the child's name being called, poor eye contact, lack of pointing, delays in play, and repetitive behaviors (cf. Adrien et al., 1993; Chawarska, Paul, et al., 2007). As a whole, this literature suggests that in the future the age of diagnosis of ASD may well be in the child's first year of life.

With a focus on, and efforts toward, early diagnosis (Osterling, Dawson, & Munson, 2002), there inherently is a pervasive need for empirical evaluation of effective interventions specifically designed for infants and toddlers (Boulware et al., 2006; Volkmar, Chawarska, & Klin, 2005; Wetherby & Woods, 2006). This gap in the literature continues for a number of reasons that are discussed later; however, a primary reason is that prior to this last decade "early intervention" in the treatment of ASD primarily consisted of intervention with children 3 years of age or older (Wetherby & Woods, 2006). Thus, the bulk of the published studies relating to intervention for young children with ASD include preschool and school-age participants (cf. Levy, Kim, & Olive, 2006).

Although few intervention studies have been published for toddlers, the variables that have produced the most positive outcomes for older children with ASD are most certainly relevant to toddlers with ASD and those at risk for this diagnosis. These include parent involvement, intensive behavioral intervention (i.e., applied behavior analysis), focus on language remediation, inclusion in the natural environment with typically developing children, long-term intervention, and multicomponent interventions (i.e., focus on language, social-emotional, cognition, and behavior; Levy et al., 2006). Within this general framework, there has been a search for interventions that can produce generalized improvements and target core or pivotal areas that may affect many broad areas of functioning. Hence, the goal is to hasten the habilitation process with more effective interventions beginning at an earlier age. This chapter attempts to synthesize the current knowledge of behavioral interventions for ASD and the application of these approaches to the growing number of toddlers being diagnosed. Furthermore, this chapter also presents considerations unique to this very young population of children and suggestions for treatment delivery. Finally, the chapter concludes with a conceptualization of the next steps for supporting these very young children.

CONSIDERATIONS IN THE TREATMENT OF TODDLERS WITH ASD

Throughout the last decade, there has been a growing call in the literature for developing standards and guidelines for the treatment of infants and toddlers with ASD (Volkmar et al., 2005; Wetherby & Woods, 2006). Although behavioral interventions have been widely effective in the treatment of symptoms in older children (Levy et al., 2006), research is currently needed to identify any necessary changes in these procedures for developmentally appropriate use with toddlers. For instance, researchers may need to consider developmental issues, such as teaching important prelinguistic skills (e.g., joint attention) and adapting behavioral protocols to take appropriate developmental processes and milestones into account (e.g., parent–toddler attachment), as well as other practical considerations (e.g., toilet training, sleep schedules).

Further reflection on typical toddler development may prove to be especially helpful. That is, the first couple years of life are marked by remarkable development, such as the emergence of intentional communication, which usually appears by 9 months of age in the form of joint attention skills and is completely in place by 18 months (Bates, 1976; Bates, Camaioni, & Volterra, 1975; Prizant & Wetherby, 1987). At this point in time, toddlers begin to comprehend that their behavior produces desired changes in their environment. However, the absence of these early social communication skills in toddlers with ASD (Osterling et al., 2002) may contribute to a failure to learn the response–reinforcer contingency. This, in turn, may lead to a state of learned helplessness, as suggested by cognitive-behavioral research (R. L. Koegel & Egel, 1979; R. L. Koegel, O'Dell, & Dunlap, 1988). This suggests that intervention for toddlers with ASD may require specific, frequent, and clear exposure to the response-reinforcer contingency in order to prevent the maladaptive behavior patterns associated with learned helplessness (Seligman, Maier, & Geer, 1968; R. L. Koegel, Opdenden, Fredeen, & Koegel, 2006). These and other issues related to the distinctive needs of toddlers with ASD are discussed throughout the rest of this chapter, particularly in the following section on behavioral approaches to early intervention in ASD.

BEHAVIORAL MODELS OF EARLY INTERVENTION

A variety of approaches have been attempted for the treatment of ASD, including physiological and nonphysiological (e.g., behavioral) approaches. Within nonphysiological approaches, the methods with the strongest empirical support are behavioral models based on operant conditioning theory, such as those used in applied behavior analysis (cf. Schreibman, 2000). Empirical validation is critical, as many ineffective interventions have caused great pain to families and either delayed the implementation of, or replaced altogether, important empirically based interventions. Prior to presenting and discussing the various models of applied behavior analysis (ABA) that have empirical evidence for supporting the development of children, including toddlers, with ASD, it can be helpful to briefly consider the historical aspects of early intervention that have enabled researchers and practitioners to advance the field to its current day status.

Historical Background

Prior to the 1960s most children with ASD were considered "uneducable," separated from their parents during treatment, and almost always institutionalized by adolescence or before (Rapin, 1991; Weiss, 1999). However, beginning in the early 1960s, scientific studies using behavioral interventions focusing on observable and quantifiable measurement began appearing in the literature (e.g., Ferster & DeMyer, 1961, 1962; Lovaas et al., 1966). These early studies primarily involved older children (e.g., age 5 and older) because it was rare to identify children with ASD much younger than school age. This initial research was necessary in order to prove to both the scientific and lay communities once and for all that children with ASD were indeed "educable," laying the foundation for future researchers to one day be able to reach toddlers (Wetherby & Woods, 2006).

In addition to primarily working with older children, these early studies focused on procedures for reducing problem behaviors, usually through punishment, and increasing positive behaviors by using rewards (Hewitt, 1965; Lovaas, 1977). Frequently, initial intervention steps focused on gross motor imitation and attempts to teach verbal communication to children with ASD through imitation of sounds and words, while rewarding closer approximations to the adult word through a strict operant shaping procedure. Correct responses were rewarded with extrinsic reinforcers, such as edibles paired with social praise. Overall, the underlying assumption and hope of these operant conditioning techniques was that once children were able to attend to and imitate others, they might be likely to demonstrate more global, generalized imitation (Lovaas, 1977). Though generalized imitation was achieved by some children, imitation taught in this way did not appear to reduce core symptom areas of ASD.

These early intervention procedures minimized distractions by using highly structured discrete trials in which an adult presented a series of learning tasks and rewarded successive correct responses (i.e., stimulus–response–consequence) in a one-on-one format. Although the approach was extremely effective, many children had difficulties such as cue dependency, lacked spontaneity and skill to initiate communicative bids and social approaches, engaged in rote responding, failed to generalize treatment gains to other settings, stimuli, and people, and had difficulty with long-term maintenance of their acquired skills (Schreibman, 2000; Horner, Dunlap, & Koegel, 1988).

To address these limitations, research focused on techniques for improving generalization and spontaneity began to emerge in the late 1970s and early 1980s. This next series of studies included procedures aimed at reducing the discriminability of the reinforcement schedules (R. L. Koegel & Rincover, 1974, 1977) by introducing the use of multiple exemplars (Gunter, Fox, Brady, Shores, & Cavanaugh, 1988; Matson, Sevin, Box, Francis, & Sevin, 1993), within-stimulus prompting (Schreibman, 1975), parent education (R. L. Koegel, Glahn, & Nieminen, 1978), and teaching responses that were likely to be rewarded outside the clinical setting (Schreibman & Carr, 1978), thereby improving the effectiveness of the intervention. Although these procedures often resulted in desirable behavioral change, they still focused on implementing the intervention in a highly structured context and were not easily incorporated into children's daily routines.

The ongoing issues of generalization, maintenance, spontaneity, and the desire to develop interventions that improved child affect, as well as decreased disruptive, escape, and avoidance behavior, led researchers in the 1980s, and particularly the 1990s, to focus on core areas for improving the motivation and responsivity of children with ASD (R. L. Koegel & Koegel, 2006). The line of research that emerged during this time not only demonstrated that previous limitations could be ameliorated but also documented collateral improvements in untargeted areas and produced generalized areas of responding (R. L. Koegel, O'Dell, & Koegel, 1987). These areas included improvements in child affect (R. L. Koegel et al., 1988), improvements in socialization (Gaylord-Ross, Haring, Breen, & Pitts-Conway, 1984; R. L. Koegel, Dyer, & Bell, 1987; R. L. Koegel & Frea, 1993), improvements in academic learning (Dunlap & Kern, 1993; Dunlap, Kern-Dunlap, Clarke, & Robbins, 1991), improvements in disruptive behaviors (R. L. Koegel, Koegel, & Surratt, 1992), and improvements in stereotypic and restrictive behaviors (Baker, Koegel, & Koegel, 1998).

The several decades of accumulating research in the area of ASD, as outlined above, suggested the efficacy of behavioral interventions, but some have argued that operant conditioning and discrete trial training may be so controlled that they result in a lack of generalization, are irrelevant outside the experimental setting, or may miss the child in behavioral reductionism (Schopler, 2001). Fortuitously, these and other concerns regarding the effectiveness of various interventions have been addressed by a Task Force on Promotion and Dissemination of Psychological Procedures of Division 12 of the American Psychological Association (APA; Task Force, 1995) that developed guidelines for empirically supported interventions. These guidelines emphasize interventions that have been demonstrated to be both efficacious (producing empirically documented change in target behavior) *and* effective (changes are demonstrated to be relevant to clinical populations in the natural environment; Chorpita, 2003). Simultaneously, behavioral researchers have stressed the importance of constructs such as social validation of intervention outcomes (so that changes are evidenced by the greater community; Geller, 1991; Hayes, Barlow, & Nelson-Gray, 1999; Kazdin, 1977; Schwartz & Baer, 1991; Wolf, 1978), goodness of fit with areas such as family and cultural values, individualization, and daily routines (Albin, Lucyshyn, Horner, & Flannery, 1996), stakeholder quality of life (Risley, 1996), and, in general, making meaningful differences in the lives of children and families (Carr et al., 2002; Strain & Schwartz, 2001). The following section discusses selected current evidence-based models and approaches.

Current Models

This section provides an overview of a number of empirically validated behavioral models and their applicability to toddlers with ASD, with a heavy emphasis on naturalistic behavioral approaches. The focus on naturalistic approaches is used in part to address the unique developmental needs of toddlers. That is, as reviewed in detail later, best practices for young children with ASD include such components as delivering interventions that can be incorporated into the daily family routine and resemble typical patterns of parent–child interactions (National Research Council, 2001; Wetherby & Woods, 2006). Given that naturalistic behavioral models inherently focus on embedding teaching opportunities throughout meaningful daily activities and routines, it seems appropriate to focus on this particular approach when addressing the needs of toddlers.

Nonetheless, before considering the specifics of each behavioral approach, it may be helpful to note the broader implications of interventions for young children with ASD. Specifically, in 2001, the National Research Council (NRC) performed a thorough review of the existing literature on ASD and concluded that there was significant evidence for educational interventions and that a considerable proportion of children with ASD respond to such interventions. Although the NRC reviewed a variety of teaching techniques for treating ASD, it identified a number of variables shared by these different approaches that seemed to constitute best practice. These include (1) entry into early intervention as soon as ASD is suspected; (2) intensive instruction for at least 5 hours per day, 5 days per week; (3) teaching opportunities that are delivered over brief periods of time and are repeated systematically; (4) ample individualized adult attention on a daily basis; (5) a family component, including parent education; (6) ongoing assessment and program evaluation, along with necessary programmatic adjustments; and (7) instructional priority in (a) functional and spontaneous communication, (b) social instruction delivered in a variety of settings, (c) play skills focused on peer interactions, (d) skill acquisition, maintenance, and generalization in natural settings, (e) functional assessment and positive behavioral support to address disruptive behaviors, and (f), if appropriate, functional academic skills (National Research Council, 2001; Wetherby & Woods, 2006). The current models discussed below are those identified by the NRC as empirically validated approaches and are all based on the principles of ABA. Given that these approaches have been used most often with preschool and school-age children, their relevance to toddlers is specifically discussed.

Early Intensive Behavior Intervention

Shea (2005) stated that the term *early intensive behavior intervention* (EIBI) has been used for a variety of techniques described in the literature, including the Lovaas method, discrete trial training, operant learning, and applied behavior analysis. However, the author quickly notes that the terms are not necessarily interchangeable and suggests that for further information about them that readers refer to Lovaas (2002),

McClannahan and Krantz (2001), and Smith (2001). Nonetheless, for the purpose of this chapter EIBI is discussed in the context of more traditional behavioral approaches versus the naturalistic behavioral approaches that are detailed below.

In spite of some specific definitional differences, the techniques of EIBI programming in general share a variety of common elements (Weiss, 1999; Shea, 2005). These include intensive one-on-one instruction for approximately 30–40 hours for at least 2 consecutive years (Green, 1996), initial interventions focusing on areas of severe deficits (e.g., imitation, matching, receptive language skills, expressive language skills, including early verbal imitation; see, e.g., Handleman & Harris, 2001), highly structured instructional settings (e.g., therapy room), and an overall use of discrete trial instruction with designated periods for incidental teaching (e.g., downtime; Anderson, Taras, & O'Malley Cannon, 1996). Research utilizing EIBI has documented compelling gains for children with ASD (Lovaas, 1987; Anderson, Avery, DiPierto, Edward, & Christian, 1987; Fenske, Zalenski, Krantz, & McClannahan, 1985); however, this approach and its reported results have not been without debate and controversy (Gresham & MacMillan, 1998; Mesibov, 1993; Shea, 2005). Boyd and Corley (2001) commented that most of the criticism of EIBI has been about methodological shortcomings, whereas Shea (2005) suggested that the most debated issue is related to the frequently cited expectation that 47% of children with ASD who receive services via this approach will become indistinguishable from typically developing peers.

Unfortunately, the scope of this chapter does not allow a comprehensive discussion of these issues (for more in-depth analyses, see Green, 1996, and Shea, 2005); however, we briefly discuss EIBI in relation to the treatment of toddlers with ASD. That is, original EIBI research was conducted with older preschool-age children (e.g., 4 years old and older; Lovaas, 1987; McEachin, Smith, & Lovaas, 1993). More recently, research on EIBI with toddlers has been emerging in the literature, with reports of gains in imitation skills and receptive and expressive language skills (Boyd & Corley, 2001; Weiss, 1999; Smith, 2001). Although each of these studies indicated benefits and included a few children of 24 months or younger as participants, the mean age of their participants was 4 years. Consequently, future research on the implementation of EIBI with toddlers is necessary in order to further clarify its applicability with this population.

Naturalistic Behavioral Interventions

The historical difficulties encountered by discrete trial approaches in achieving widespread and long-lasting gains in socially significant skills have led developers of many of the more recent behavioral approaches to develop methodologies that focus on generalization (R. L. Koegel &

Koegel, 2006). These more recent techniques have been highly effective in improving communication and emphasizing the reciprocal interactive nature of the communicative interaction and accentuating the child's role as an active participant. Because of the historical difficulties in early identification of ASD, much of the published empirical research has focused on older children (preschool- and elementary school-age). Current research is heavily emphasizing early intervention for toddlers, and emerging data are suggesting important variables for further study (R. L. Koegel & Schreibman, 2006). Although ongoing research is beginning to address the toddler population more specifically, there remains a need for empirical support of the types of changes needed when such interventions are applied to this population.

Several empirically validated methodologies have emerged that are similar in targeting core areas of ASD. Three researched methodology packages that are very similar are incidental teaching (Hart & Risley, 1968), milieu teaching (Halle, Baer, & Spradlin, 1981; Hancock & Kaiser, 2002; Hart & Risley, 1975; Warren, McQuarter, & Rogers-Warren, 1984), and pivotal response teaching, originally published as the Natural Language Paradigm (R. L. Koegel, O'Dell, et al., 1987). All have several common characteristics, which include child choice or following the child's lead, intervention in natural contexts, and the use of intrinsically related rewards. These areas are especially relevant to toddlers with ASD, as they are similar to parent–child interactions of typically developing children, hence these methods have been termed "naturalistic" approaches. That is, the less structured, more child-focused approaches in the child's natural settings not only result in faster learning, but also in less disruptive behavior (R. L. Koegel, O'Dell, et al., 1987; R. L. Koegel et al., 1992). It should also be noted that some of these components and similar strategies are also evident in other interventions, such as the Social Communication, Emotional Regulation, Transaction Supports (SCERTS) model (Prizant, Wetherby, Rubin, Laurent, & Rydell, 2006), and in-context teaching (Camarata & Nelson, 1992).

Some of these naturalistic interventions have been effective with toddlers with ASD. For example, Wetherby & Woods (2006) investigated the impact of their Early Social Interaction (ESI) project on the social-communication outcomes for a group of parent–toddler dyads (i.e., toddler ages were younger than 24 months). ESI consists of the following components: (1) routines-based intervention in natural environments, (2) individualized curriculum, and (3) parent-implemented intervention. Parent–toddler dyads participated in ESI for at least 12 months and agreed to a diagnostic evaluation again when the child was 36 months of age. Results indicated that the toddlers who participated in ESI showed dramatic improvements on 11 of 13 social-communication goals (e.g., gaze shifts, shared positive affect, rates of communicating), an overall far better outcome than for toddlers who had participated in a contrast group. Furthermore, at postintervention, 76.5% of the toddlers who participated in ESI were verbal (5.9% were verbal at preintervention), in comparison to only 55.6% of the toddlers who were in the contrast group. These findings are similar to data obtained by Boulware et al. (2006) in their analysis of Project DATA (Developmentally Appropriate Treatment for Autism) for toddlers. Project DATA consisted of parent–toddler dyads and the five following components: (1) services in inclusive environments, (2) family-centered services, (3) practices guided through transdisciplinary teaming, (4) empirical and value-driven interventions, and (5) programs that included developmentally appropriate practices. Children who participated in Project DATA received a minimum of 16 hours of intervention in a variety of arrangements (e.g., integrated play groups, individualized instruction, and in-home support). All eight toddlers studied received services for a minimum of 9 months. Results demonstrated that all eight children made gains on standardized measurements (e.g., Bayley Scales of Infant Development–Second Edition, BSID-II; Temperament and Atypical Behavior Scales; Communication and Symbolic Behavior Scales, CSBS) and/or on functional measures (e.g., gains in expressive language). These studies provide evidence for successful naturalistic behavioral interventions specifically designed for toddlers with ASD.

As discussed above, the empirical research conducted throughout the 1960s and 1970s not only demonstrated that children with ASD were indeed "educable" but also created the building blocks necessary for steering the intervention field into the direction of naturalistic methodologies aimed at addressing issues such as generalization, maintenance, and spontaneity (L. K. Koegel, 1995; Schreibman, 1988). Moreover, the naturalistic intervention approaches that developed from earlier methodologies focused research on factors that would lead to increased motivation, responsivity, parent education, and inclusion (L. K. Koegel, 1995). The following section discusses in detail three such naturalistic early intervention approaches: incidental teaching, milieu teaching, and pivotal response teaching.

INCIDENTAL TEACHING

Incidental teaching has a rich history of research in staff training, environmental arrangements, peer training, activity choices, and parent education (Doke & Risley, 1972; Hart & Risley, 1968; McClannahan, Krantz, & McGee, 1982; McGee, Almeida, Sulzer-Azaroff, & Feldman, 1992; McGee, Krantz, Mason, & McClannahan, 1983, 1986; Risley & Favell, 1979; Twardosz, Cataldo, & Risley, 1974). Incidental teaching consists of a systematic protocol of instruction that is delivered in the natural environment (i.e., everyday family and child activities, routines, and tasks). Moreover, incidental teaching requires that the environment be arranged so that it attracts the child's attention to desired toys, activities, and objects. The typical protocol of incidental teaching consists of child initiations, followed by instructor elaboration, and then natural reinforcement. In general, children initiate incidental teaching episodes by gesturing (e.g., reaching, pointing) or verbally requesting a desired object or activity. In response, the instructor (e.g., teacher, parent) prompts for an elaboration of the child's initiation and then follows the elaborated response with contingent access to the natural reinforcer (e.g., desired toy). As McGee, Morrier, and Daly (1999) discuss, incidental teaching offers the advantageous combination of applied behavior analysis with the benefit of delivering intervention in typical, everyday childhood routines and activities. For more specific details of incidental teaching, see McGee et al. (1999).

During the last couple of decades, much of the research in incidental teaching has been conducted at the Walden Early Childhood Programs, a division of the Emory Autism Resource Center at Emory University School of Medicine. One branch of the Walden Programs focused on very young children with ASD is the Walden Toddler Program. The Walden Toddler Model started in 1993 as a model demonstration grant from the U.S. Department of Education (Office of Special Education Programs) and consists of two components: a center-based program and a home-based program (McGee et al., 1999). The center-based component is an inclusive program that focuses on the developmental needs of children with ASD and typically developing peers. The home-based component focuses on parent education and the establishment of parent–professional collaboration. Between the center-based and home-based components, the Walden Toddler Program provides more than 30 hours per week of planned early intervention. McGee et al. (1999) highlight six hallmarks of the Walden Toddler Model: early is essential, more is better, family involvement is critical, social development requires early inclusion, early childhood should be fun, and incidental teaching should be planned. The results obtained by the Walden Toddler Program are nothing short of impressive. Specifically, 36% of toddlers (average age: 2.5 years) entered the Walden Toddler Program with elementary expressive language skills, although much of their language consisted of echolalia or perseverative speech. However, 82% of toddlers (average age: 3.5 years) exited the program with meaningful expressive verbalizations. In other words, the vast majority of the toddlers who participated in the Walden Toddler Program were subsequently able to start preschool with functional expressive language, a great contrast to reports that 50% of children with ASD never develop any form of spoken language (Lord & Paul, 1997). These results were so groundbreaking that the NRC highlighted them in its report on characteristics of effective interventions, noting that the extraordinary treatment outcomes were likely related to the children's young age at treatment entry (National Research Council, 2001).

More recently, Stahmer and Ingersoll (2004) reported similar results when they replicated the Walden Toddler Program. In particular, these authors used a quasi-experimental design to assess the effects of an inclusive program for toddlers with ASD (under 3 years of age). This replication of the Walden Toddler Program contributed to the present literature by reporting results for both standardized assessments and functional outcomes, which were consistent with those obtained by McGee et al. (1999). In particular, Stahmer and Ingersoll (2004) reported that 50% of the participating toddlers exhibited no functional expressive language at entry, but by the time they exited the Children's Toddler Program, 90% used a functional communication system (i.e., expressive language or augmentative language). Moreover, all of the toddlers demonstrated qualitative gains in their functional social and play behaviors after intervention. Specifically, none of the children engaged in social interaction with peers at entry, whereas at exit 60% engaged in social interaction, 25% could respond to peer initiations, and 35% could engage in reciprocal interactions. In terms of standardized assessments of cognitive skills (measured by scores on the BSID-II), 37% of the participating toddlers were functioning in the typical range at the time they exited the program, in comparison with only 11% at entry. Consistent with the results obtained by McGee and colleagues (1999), Stahmer and Ingersoll (2004) provided additional evidence that inclusion, paired with parent training and 2 hours per week of individualized instruction, may be an effective treatment model for toddlers, potentially providing new options for families with very young children with ASD.

MILIEU TEACHING

Milieu teaching is a naturalistic teaching approach targeting communication and social skills. Like incidental teaching, it emphasizes teaching in the context of ongoing, everyday activities both at home and in school, following the child's lead, and providing natural consequences for communication. The primary procedures of milieu teaching are modeling (i.e., demonstrating an action), mand modeling (i.e., demonstrating saying a word with the goal of having the child repeat that word to request something), time delay (i.e., presenting the desired item and allowing a period of time to pass for the child to respond spontaneously before providing any guidance), incidental opportunities, and environmental arrangements. Although incidental teaching also uses environmental arrangements, experts in milieu teaching emphasize this strategy as a defining and central feature of the milieu instructional approach (Kaiser, Ostrosky, & Alpert, 1993). In other words, environmental arrangements (i.e., arranging the environment to create opportunities for the child to engage in communication) are "a critical aspect of implementing milieu teaching" (Halle et al., 1981; Kaiser et al., 1993). Environmental arrangements are important for adults because they increase their awareness of opportunities for children to communicate (e.g., instead of having all the pieces to a puzzle on a table, placing some out of reach so the child needs to initiate a request of the adult). Likewise, environmental arrangements are important for children because they provide opportunities and nonverbal cues for initiating language (Kaiser et al., 1993). Examples of environmental arrangements include placing materials of interest within view but out of reach, assistance (i.e., giving the child materials that require assistance in order for them to be used), inadequate portions (e.g., giving small pieces of snacks so that the child is motivated to request more), sabotage (e.g., removing a necessary piece of a toy so the child is motivated to request it), protest (e.g., providing the wrong object so that the child is motivated to request a different one), and silly situations (e.g., providing an absurd object, such as a shovel, for a child to eat soup in order to motivate the child to request the correct object). For detailed definitions of the milieu teaching procedures, including the above mentioned environmental arrangements, see Kaiser et al. (1993).

Although many of the milieu teaching techniques have been implemented with preschool and elementary school children, many of the procedures are similar to those of incidental teaching, which has been effective with toddlers. Furthermore, milieu teaching has been shown to improve the social communication skills of children with ASD (Alpert & Kaiser, 1983; Kaiser, Yoder, & Keetz, 1992; Kaiser, Hancock, & Nietfeld, 2000) and to facilitate staff training (e.g., therapists, teachers; Kaiser et al., 1993), improve peer/sibling training (Hancock & Kaiser, 1996; Ostrosky & Kaiser, 1991), and incorporate parent education (Hemmeter & Kaiser, 1990; Kaiser et al., 1999). Studies have also found that children with ASD with some language (e.g., ability to produce 10 words) are likely to have especially positive gains when provided with milieu intervention (Yoder, Kaiser, Alpert, & Fischer, 1993).

A more recent application of milieu teaching is enhanced milieu teaching (EMT; Hancock & Kaiser, 2002; Hemmeter & Kaiser, 1994; Kaiser et al., 2000). Enhanced milieu teaching is a "hybrid approach to naturalistic, early language intervention" that includes components of behavioral and social interaction approaches (i.e., in which each partner's behavior affects the other's; Hancock & Kaiser, 2002). The EMT approach focuses on three specific areas: environmental arrangements, responsive interaction techniques, and teaching procedures used to promote new language use in their functional contexts (Hancock & Kaiser, 2002; Kaiser et al., 2000).

EMT is differentiated from incidental teaching and pivotal response teaching (which is discussed below) by having responsive interaction techniques (expansion, turn taking, etc.) as a foundation of the approach, whereby the responsiveness of both the therapist and the child are affected in a transactional manner. The specific components of EMT include expansions (e.g., child utterances that are expanded by an adult), balance of adult and child turns (mix of adult- and child-led situations), following the child's lead, pausing an appropriate amount of time (i.e., at least 3 seconds) for the child to respond, and responsive feedback (e.g., adult verbalizations that follow child's utterances). The standard milieu teaching procedures mentioned above (e.g., modeling, mand modeling, time delay) are maintained in EMT.

The focus on responsiveness in EMT changes the target from proactive instruction to responsive instruction (i.e., embedding prompting into ongoing conversation and play interactions). Hancock and Kaiser (2002) demonstrated that preschool children with ASD made gains in social communication skills by participating in EMT sessions with clinicians. Moreover, the participating children also generalized skills to new settings and to interactions with their parents, who had not received any specialized training. The authors discuss how, with a focus on responsive instruction, the flow of interaction between the child and adult is less prone or inclined to interruption as in discrete trials, therefore providing many more opportunities for teaching skills. In addition, the authors contend that the responsive engagement strategy utilized by EMT may be particularly helpful for children with ASD, who are frequently resistant to didactic interactions and/or direct instructions.

The application of EMT may be especially helpful when targeting toddlers with ASD because of its focus on "responsiveness" to the toddler's interests and behaviors as the means for directing instruction. As mentioned above, doing so may reduce the potential for avoidance responding, which is so characteristic of children with ASD, and may allow teaching episodes to be "gentler" for young children by motivating them to want to participate, thereby reducing the need for aversives. The next approach, pivotal response teaching (PRT), has been particularly strong in that area.

PIVOTAL RESPONSE TEACHING

Pivotal response teaching (PRT), also called the Natural Language Paradigm when it is focused specifically on language, is a highly efficient evidence-based approach that is founded on the scientific principles of applied behavior analysis (ABA). As noted earlier, its procedures were developed to address several concerns, including children's lack of generalization, slow rate of progress, poor affect during intervention, and high levels of disruptive behavior during intervention (R. L. Koegel, O'Dell, et al., 1987; R. L. Koegel et al., 1992). The studies focused on developing an intervention package that would address core "pivotal areas" that appear to be essential to vast areas of functioning instead of working on individual target behaviors one at a time (L. K. Koegel, Koegel, Shoshan, & McNerney, 1999; L. K. Koegel, Koegel, Harrower, & Carter, 1999). PRT targets key areas central to overall functioning and results in widespread, collateral gains in other untargeted domains (R. L. Koegel, O'Dell et al., 1987). Outcome data from the University of California at Santa Barbara related to specific PRT components, as well as to the overall approach, have led the National Research Council of the National Academy of Sciences (National Research Council, 2001) to describe PRT as an extremely effective comprehensive behavioral intervention. The intervention can be implemented in school, home, and community contexts throughout the child's daily routines and activities in order to foster ongoing opportunities for learning (L. K. Koegel, Koegel, Bruinsma, Brookman, & Fredeen, 2003). Moreover, PRT is intended to be implemented by family members so that children with ASD (like typical children) have learning opportunities throughout all their waking hours, as opposed to being instructed only during specific times of the day. PRT has been used extensively with toddlers with ASD, and long-term data suggest that approximately 90% of nonverbal children who begin PRT intervention for communication before the age of 3 are able to learn expressive verbal communication. If intervention begins between 3 and 5 years of age, approximately 80–85% of nonverbal children learn to use expressive verbal communication. If intervention begins after the age of 5, only about 20% of nonverbal children are able to use expressive verbal communication (L. K. Koegel, 2000). Again, these findings support the use of naturalistic procedures with toddlers.

Pivotal Area of Motivation. One of the primary pivotal areas that have been identified is the area of motivation for social communication and learning. Perhaps one of the greatest challenges facing researchers, practitioners, and families of toddlers with ASD is these children's apparent lack of motivation to learn and engage in social-communicative interactions with others (Churchill, 1971; R. L. Koegel & Egel, 1979; L. K. Koegel & Koegel, 1986; R. L. Koegel & Mentis, 1985). This characteristic lack of motivation is often exhibited by avoidance, inattention, noncompliance, and repeated temper tantrums, particularly in toddlers and preschoolers prior to intervention. There are a variety of theories in the literature as to why children with ASD exhibit lack of motivation to learn new tasks, the most common being that their frequent experience with failure leads to a state of learned helplessness (R. L. Koegel & Egel, 1979) in which it appears that the children are "giving up" (R. L. Koegel, Schreibman et al., 1989). The teaching methodology of PRT was designed specifically to address this characteristic lack of motivation by enhancing the response–reinforcer relationship within the context of communicative, social, and behavioral teaching goals. The specific motivational procedures of PRT include establishing attention and providing clear prompts, incorporating child choice of materials, interspersing maintenance and acquisition tasks, providing contingent and immediate reinforcement, reinforcing attempts, and employing natural reinforcers. A large body of empirical research supports the use of these individual motivational components with a variety of age groups and functioning levels (Dunlap & Koegel, 1980; R. L. Koegel, Dyer, et al., 1987; R. L. Koegel & Egel, 1979; R. L. Koegel et al., 1988; R. L. Koegel & Williams, 1980; Williams, Koegel, & Egel, 1981) and the pivotal role of this motivational package in producing widespread positive effects in the social-communicative behavior of children with ASD (R. L. Koegel, O'Dell, et al., 1987; R. L. Koegel et al., 1992). Logically, beginning to address motivation, particularly addressing the key problem areas in ASD, in the toddler years increases the likelihood of positive long-term prognoses (L. K. Koegel, Koegel, Shoshan, et al., 1999).

Pivotal Area of Attention to Multiple Cues. Research evidence indicates that children with ASD exhibit patterns of stimulus overselectivity, described as having difficulties in responding to multiple cues in their environments (R. L. Koegel & Wilhelm, 1973; Lovaas & Schreibman, 1971; Lovaas, Schreibman, Koegel, & Rehm, 1971; Reynolds, Newsom, & Lovaas, 1974). This pattern begins very early in life in all children, but seems to persist beyond normal developmental levels in children with ASD (R. L. Koegel & Koegel, 1995; Schover & Newsom, 1976). Given that multiple cues are typical of most learning environments, it has been suggested that stimulus overselectivity may be related to many of the deficits characteristic of ASD, including language deficits, prompt dependency, trouble with imitation and observational learning, and difficulty in generalizing newly learned behaviors (Lovaas, Koegel, & Schreibman, 1979; Schreibman & Koegel, 1982). However, studies have shown that children with ASD can be taught to respond to multiple cues (R. L. Koegel, Dunlap, Richman, & Dyer, 1981; R. L. Koegel & Schreibman, 1977; Schreibman, Koegel, & Craig, 1977) and that broadening their abilities in this area may allow children to benefit from more typical teaching environments (Burke & Cerniglia, 1990; R. L. Koegel, Koegel, & O'Neill, 1989; Schreibman, 1997; Schreibman, Charlop, & Koegel, 1982). In toddlers, targeting multiple cues in areas such as joint attention, appropriate toy play, socialization, and communication can affect the restricted interests evidenced in children with ASD (R. L. Koegel & Koegel, 2006). Consequently, responsivity to multiple cues has been identified as a pivotal area for intervention that, when targeted, can broadly improve outcomes for children with ASD by allowing them to learn more accurately and efficiently from their natural environments (L. K. Koegel, Koegel, Harrower, et al., 1999; Rosenblatt, Bloom, & Koegel, 1995).

Pivotal Area of Child Self-Initiations. Typically developing children begin initiating socially in the first months of life. During the toddler years, specific initiations, such as question asking (e.g., pointing to an item and saying "Dat?"—an early form of the question "What's that?"—as a request for information) generally emerges in a child's first group of words. Though children with ASD often show low rates or an absence of initiating social-communicative interactions relative to their typically developing peers, research has indicated that they can be taught to make initiations (L. K. Koegel, Camarata, Valdez-Menchaca, & Koegel, 1998; R. L. Koegel, Koegel, & Carter, 1999; Shukla, Surratt, Horner, & Albin, 1995; Taylor & Harris, 1995) and that learning to make initiations appears to be associated with dramatically more favorable long-term outcomes (L. K. Koegel, Koegel, Shoshan, et al., 1999). Given that the acquisition of this skill allows children to take advantage of widespread learning opportunities in natural environments, child self-initiations have been identified as a pivotal area (L. K. Koegel, Koegel, Harrower, et al., 1999; L. K. Koegel, Koegel, Shoshan, et al., 1999). When a child is motivated and has the skills necessary to initiate his or her own learning, that child can learn outside the adult-defined teaching context and thus can benefit from increased autonomy and opportunities for self-determination.

NATURALISTIC TEACHING PROCEDURES

The identification of the pivotal areas treated with naturalistic teaching procedures described above is consistent with the current focus in the behavioral literature on effective and efficient interventions that produce widespread gains in socially valid domains (Carr et al., 2002; Strain & Schwartz, 2001; Schwartz & Baer, 1991; Wolf, 1978). Each of these areas has been identified as pivotal because intervention has resulted in improvements in broad areas of functioning beyond those directly targeted (L. K. Koegel, Koegel, Harrower, et al., 1999). Furthermore, improvements in these areas result in children with ASD having increased access to reinforcement in the natural environment and increased opportunities for inclusion in their communities (R. L. Koegel, Openden, et al., 2006). Implementation of these procedures as early as possible in a child's life, before the gap between the child and his or her peers is too great, increases the likelihood of more positive long-term outcomes (R. L. Koegel, Bruinsma, & Koegel, 2006).

Like the results of both incidental teaching and milieu therapy, PRT results have been impressive in producing communication gains in young children. Again, group data for PRT reported at the Koegel Autism Center at the University of California at Santa Barbara are consistent with those of the other two approaches in that approximately 90% of children who began intervention before the age of 3 years acquired speech as their primary form of communication following intervention (L. K. Koegel, 1995). Further, some children were reported as having overcome many other, or even most, of their symptoms of ASD and participated in full-inclusion classrooms and extracurricular activities and had social circles including typically developing peers (R. L. Koegel & Koegel, 2006; L. K. Koegel, Koegel, Shoshan, et al., 1999). In addition, current research at the Koegel Autism Center funded by the National Institute of Mental Health is evaluating the use of PRT in teaching early communication skills to toddlers with ASD (R. L. Koegel & Schreibman, 2006), and results from this project will be available in the near future.

Overall, research studies relating to the naturalistic interventions tend to share a number of characteristics supporting the importance of these components. First, all of the naturalistic interventions discussed above emphasize teaching that occurs throughout ongoing, daily activities and routines that are meaningful to the child (e.g., at home, in school, and in other community settings). Second, each of these approaches suggests that the environment be arranged to enable both child communication and teaching opportunities. Third, following the child's lead and including child choice are extremely critical for improving child responsivity. That is, instruction should be in response to the child's interests, desires, and needs. In addition, in all of these newer approaches, natural reinforcers are described as being essential. In other words, communication attempts by the toddler should be reinforced with positive natural consequences (e.g., toddler says "uh" for "up": toddler should be picked up.). Incidental, milieu, and pivotal response teaching have been shown to be especially effective in teaching early expressive communication skills to children with ASD, and studies have documented success rates higher than those of previous, more structured discrete trial approaches (Kaiser et al., 1993; R. L. Koegel, O'Dell, et al., 1987; L. K. Koegel, 1995; McGee et al., 1992). As McGee and colleagues (1999) discuss, teaching throughout daily meaningful activities and routines in the child and family's natural environmental is a departure from traditional behavioral methods, which have usually emphasized drill instruction, distraction-free settings, teacher-directed learning trials, and artificial reinforcement (i.e., rewards and responses usually have no relationship). Although the reviewed naturalistic methodologies differ in a variety of ways from earlier, more traditional models of applied behavior analysis, it should be noted that the same principles of operant learning underscore both intervention orientations. That is, both naturalistic and more traditional "discrete trial" intervention approaches focus on the precision of reinforcement delivery, stimulus presentation that supports errorless learning, and many components of discrimination training (McGee et al., 1999). Furthermore, it is equally, if not more, important to note that naturalistic interventions did not arise as a rejection of more traditional discrete trial instruction, but as a response to the need to address issues of generalization, maintenance, and spontaneity. The research accomplished by the naturalistic approaches discussed above did exactly that; children with ASD are reported as being better able to generalize, maintain, and spontaneously use language when such naturalistic approaches are utilized (R. L. Koegel, O'Dell, et al., 1987; McGee et al., 1983).

CONTEXTUAL CONSIDERATIONS FOR TREATMENT DELIVERY

In considering treatment issues related to toddlers with ASD, it is also important to consider contextual factors affecting treatment delivery, such as when to begin treatment, where treatment should be conducted, how much treatment is needed, and who should deliver the treatment. For toddlers, issues such as the continuity between early detection and early intervention and issues of parent involvement, intensity, and individualization of intervention have become increasingly important.

Early Detection

There is no doubt that significant benefits result from beginning intervention at the earliest point possible. For instance, data from our large studies suggest that if PRT begins before the age of 3, more children will have positive outcomes in the area of communication than when intervention begins after 3 years of age (R. L. Koegel & Koegel, 1995; R. L. Koegel & Koegel, 2006). These data clearly support the advantage of beginning intervention in the toddler years; however, early intervention requires early detection.

There are a number of screening devices for early detection of ASD (e.g., Modified CHecklist for Autism in Toddlers, M-CHAT; Robins, Fein, Barton, & Green, 2001; Screening Tool for Autism in Two-Year-Olds, STAT; Stone, Coonrod, & Ousley, 2000). Clinical diagnosis made by an experienced clinician based on history information, direct multidomain assessment, and parent interview currently constitutes the gold standard in diagnosing young children with ASD (see Volkmar et al., Chapter 1, and Bishop et al., Chapter 2, this volume for discussion of early diagnosis). Current reports suggest that clinical diagnosis in the second and third years of life is relatively stable (e.g., Lord, 1995; Chawarska, Paul, et al., 2007). Again, studies suggest that symptoms appear before or about 12 months (Adrien et al., 1993; Chawarska, Klin, et al., 2007; Chawarska, Paul, et al., 2007; see the review in Goin & Myers, 2004; Osterling et al., 2002; see also Volkmar et al., Chapter 1, this volume) and that a vast majority of parents notice first symptoms by the age of 2 (De Giacomo & Fombonne, 1998; Shah, 2001; Siegel,

Pliner, Eschler, & Elliott, 1988). Concerns about the importance of early detection have resulted in the recent initiative of the Centers for Disease Control and Prevention, "Learn the Signs. Act Early," which calls for developmental screenings to include important behavioral, cognitive, and communication milestones (e.g., play skills, social communication skills) in order to identify developmental delays such as ASD at an earlier age (Centers for Disease Control and Prevention, 2006).

Overall, as the processes of screening and identification of toddlers with ASD become more efficient, intervention providers will be faced with increasing numbers of very young children in need of behavioral intervention services. Comprehensive developmental assessments of these children at the time of diagnosis will have important implications for treatment (Volkmar et al., 2005) and can play a crucial role in identifying strengths and important target areas for intervention.

Intensity of Intervention

There is no doubt that children with ASD benefit from intensive interventions. In a 1987 study, Lovaas suggested that 49% of the children who received more than 40 hours of one-to-one treatment per week achieved normal intellectual and educational functioning. Only 2% of the children in the control group, which received only 10 hours of intervention per week, achieved comparable intellectual and educational functioning. Although the total number of hours needed is economically and politically controversial, no one has doubted the fact that the children do need intensive intervention programs. One economical, practical, and developmentally desirable method of increasing the number of intervention hours a child receives is to incorporate parents as active participants in the intervention programs. Often this is accomplished with a "practice-with-feedback" model, wherein the parents select target goals and then are taught the intervention procedures while receiving feedback from a professional in the area of ASD (see, e.g., R. L. Koegel & Koegel, 2006). This has been both an effective and cost-efficient method of providing an intensive intervention program. Issues in parent education programs are discussed in the following section.

Parent Education

The literature is replete with studies documenting the effectiveness of parent education programs (Barlow & Stewart-Brown, 2000; Corcoran, 2000; Eyberg & Robinson, 1982; Forehand & Kotchick, 2002; MacKenzie, Fite, & Bates, 2004; Nixon, 2001; Sampers, Anderson, Hartung, & Scambler, 2001) and the lack of maintenance of behavioral gains when parents do not participate in their children's intervention programs (R. L. Koegel,

Schreibman, Britten, Burke, & O'Neill, 1982). In fact, the NRC highlighted the importance of family involvement and parent training by identifying this as one of the active ingredients in effective treatment programs for children with ASD (National Research Council, 2001). Because many parents desire to be involved in their children's development, and because this practice is economically advantageous and increases the number of hours of treatment, many programs now focus on parent education in treatment. In treatment of toddlers with ASD, some researchers have noted that parental involvement may be particularly important and developmentally appropriate, given the documented importance of intervention in the natural environment and the fact that parents play such an active role in the development of typical toddlers (Wetherby & Woods, 2006; Woods & Wetherby, 2003).

The basic assumption of behavioral parent training is that child behavior is learned and maintained through contingencies within the family context and that parents can be taught to change these contingencies in order to promote and reinforce appropriate behavior (Corcoran, 2000). In their meta-analysis of studies evaluating the effectiveness of behavioral parent training, Corcoran (2000) found improvements in child behavior based on behavioral observation and parent and teacher reports, and improvements in parent adjustment relative to no-treatment and control conditions. Behavioral parent education programs have resulted in promising outcomes in terms of child improvements (Barlow & Stewart-Brown, 2000; MacKenzie et al., 2004; Nixon, 2001), parent use of skills and adjustment (Eyberg & Robinson, 1982), and maintenance over time (Eyberg et al., 2001; Hood & Eyberg, 2003; Webster-Stratton & Reid, 2003). Another study examining the effects of parent management training (PMT) indicated changes in parenting practices, followed by decreases in child externalizing behaviors (DeGarmo, Patterson, & Forgatch, 2004). Additional follow-up data indicated that the decreases in externalizing behaviors mediated the relationship between PMT and the subsequent decreases in maternal depression. Additional research on parent education with families of children with ASD has demonstrated similar effects for parents, including generalized improvements in positive parent affect (Schreibman, Kaneko, & Koegel, 1991), positive family interactions (R. L. Koegel, Bimbela, & Schreibman, 1996), and decreases in maternal depression (Bristol, Gallagher, & Holt, 1993). Thus, actively including parents in the intervention process in the toddler years and beyond is not only helpful for the child, but also for maternal mental health as well.

However, the specific manner in which parents are incorporated into the intervention process is important, as well as individualizing the parent education program to consider different family needs and circumstances. That is, studies in the broader fields of psychology and education suggest that not all parents benefit from traditional behavioral parent education programs (Forehand & Kotchick, 2002) and that some parents may need supplemental assistance or support in order to parent more effectively (Corcoran, 2000; Singer, 1993). Parent education appears to work best with highly motivated and well-functioning adults who are not currently coping with additional psychological or life stressors (Blechman, 1998). Marital distress, parental depression, severe child problem behaviors (or behavioral problems), and lack of social support may prevent some families from benefiting from traditional parent training (Baker, Landen, & Kashima, 1991; Stern, 2000; Webster-Stratton & Reid, 2003). In the treatment of families with children with disabilities, Singer, Golberg-Hamblin, Peckham-Hardin, Barry, and Santarelli (2002) estimated that approximately 30% of families do not benefit from traditional behavioral parent training, possibly owing to social and psychological stress, which interferes with their acquisition and implementation of positive parenting strategies.

Research evidence indicates that individuals seeking parent education to help them provide treatment delivery for their child may be under particular stress and at risk for symptoms of depression. First, young adults between 25 and 44 years of age show the highest rates of depression (Clark, Beck, & Alford, 1999), and women may be about two times more likely to experience depression than men, especially in the presence of risk factors such as adverse life events, lack of social support, and poor or strained interpersonal relationships (Clark et al., 1999). In addition, having a child with a disability can put further stress on a family's functioning (Anastopoulos, 1998; Corcoran, 2000). Parents of children with severe disabilities, such as ASD, are prone to higher levels of stress (Moes, 1995). Evidence indicates that mothers show particularly high levels of stress and depression, possibly due to their differential daily responsibilities for care of the children (Bristol et al., 1993; Calzada, Eyberg, Rich, & Querido, 2004; Moes, Koegel, Schreibman, & Loos, 1992). In addition, marital conflict, social isolation, socioeconomic stressors, or family dysfunction may make effective parenting even more difficult without more comprehensive support (Briesmeister & Schaefer, 1998; Forehand & Kotchick, 2002; Singer et al., 2002), and this type of stress and poor family functioning has been identified as a predictor of low parent self-efficacy and empowerment (Scheel & Rieckmann, 1998). Therefore, parents of children referred for clinical treatment may be particularly at risk for feeling helpless and ineffective as parents, which in turn may further interfere with their ability to parent effectively.

Given this problem, there is a need for additional research to identify specific strategies (e.g., collaborative, strengths-based, directive vs. nondirective) to be incorporated into the process of parent education that may be more effective for families who have not benefited from traditional parent education approaches. That is, in order to better serve parents whose social and psychological distress may jeopardize their ability to fully benefit from traditional behavioral parent education programs, educational researchers have emphasized the importance of family support (Bass, 1996; Singer et al., 2002), empowerment (Fine & Gardner, 1991; Gerris, Van As, Wels, & Janssens, 1998; Jones, Garlow, Turnbull, & Barber, 1996), and family resilience (Schwartz, 2002). Future research focusing on how best to combine teaching actual behavioral procedures and focusing on empowerment, family support, and systems perspectives (Beutler, Alomohamed, Moleiro, & Romanelli, 2002; Cavell, 2000; Kaiser et al., 1999) should be especially fruitful for families of toddlers.

Cultural Considerations

Within the practice of parent education, another area that should receive research priority is the influence of cultural variables in parent education. This is particularly important, given the paucity of research on cultural considerations in providing services to children with ASD and their families (cf. Gorman & Balter, 1997). In fact, most research on parent education programs has been conducted with European American populations (Bennett & Grimley, 2001; Forehand & Kotchick, 1996). Given the negative influence of stress on parenting practices, and the consideration that families with minority status may experience particular stress as a result of discrimination or socioeconomic disadvantage, parent education and support may be especially important for these families (Forehand & Kotchick, 1996; McDermott, 2000).

Several researchers have begun to address cultural considerations in working with parents of children with ASD (Elder, Valcante, Won, & Zylis, 2003), but this continues to be an area in need of much continued empirical investigation. Santarelli, Koegel, Casas, and Koegel (2001) discussed the importance of considering the family ecology and "contextual fit" of parenting programs for parents of children with ASD, particularly when working with ethnically diverse populations. They emphasized the need for future research in identifying appropriate content for use with families from diverse backgrounds, as well as the need for additional research into instruction techniques that make up the process of parent education (Santarelli et al., 2001).

Though there is a lack of sufficient empirical evidence indicating exactly how parent education programs should be conducted in order to best benefit ethnically diverse families, some of the literature on differences in parenting practices among ethnic groups may have implications for parent education (Forehand & Kotchick, 1996). In fact, many popular parenting programs may differentially incorporate values from the dominant European American culture, such as the importance of individualism, competition, speed, action, explicit communication, and strong work ethic, and may require modifications for appropriate use with diverse families (McDermott, 2000). For example, Zegarra (1998) suggested that modifications to make popular parenting programs more effective with the Latino community should include not only translations of materials into Spanish, but also modifications, such as the inclusion of extended family members in treatment, and more complex changes to existing protocols to recognize the importance of family privacy and parental authority in these families.

These descriptions offer promising directions for parent education with diverse populations, but will require extensive research to clarify appropriate processes for designing effective, culturally relevant parenting programs. Future research must also attend to additional socioeconomic factors that may influence the acceptability and effectiveness of parenting techniques in diverse populations (Gorman & Balter, 1997; Kotchick & Forehand, 2002).

Individualization of the Treatment Program

The individualization of intervention services, as discussed earlier, is particularly important, given the heterogeneity in symptoms of children with ASD (Schreibman & Koegel, 2005). Targeted behaviors, the child's response to a given intervention, the child's age and cognitive and linguistic levels at intake and family factors, including any parent psychological or life stressors (discussed in detail above) need to be considered when developing an individualized, coordinated, and comprehensive program. Including the family in the development of treatment goals can increase the likelihood that intervention will be implemented and gains will be maintained. Addressing target behaviors that have the broadest and most socially significant impact for the child is essential. Finally, a thorough understanding of how the child's environment reinforces, maintains, and punishes behaviors allows interventionists to develop goals that result in maximum effectiveness.

CONCLUSION

Courts have held that, at minimum, a technically sound program must produce evaluation data to demonstrate an effective methodology that provides educational benefit for the child (Etscheidt, 2003). Program developers must have qualifications in the area of ASD and be able to develop appropriate treatment programs for toddlers with ASD that include procedural soundness, parent involvement, and documented outcomes (Etscheidt, 2003). Although naturalistic behavioral interventions have firm empirical support, future work focusing on the most effective and efficient components of these comprehensive interventions will be necessary in order to best address the individualized needs of toddlers with ASD.

REFERENCES

Adrien, J. L., Lenoir, P., Martineau, J., Perrot, A., Hameury, L., Larmande, C., et al. (1993). Blind rating of early symptoms of autism based upon family home movies. *Journal of the American Academy of Child and Adolescent Psychiatry, 32,* 617–626.

Albin, R. W., Lucyshyn, J. M., Horner, R. H., & Flannery, K. B. (1996). Contextual fit for behavioral support plan: A model for "goodness of fit." In L. K. Koegel, R. L. Koegel, & G. Dunlap (Eds.), *Positive behavioral support: Including people with difficult behavior in the community* (pp. 81–98). Baltimore: Brookes.

Alpert, C. L., & Kaiser, A. P. (1983). *Milieu teaching code.* Nashville, TN: Peabody College of Vanderbilt University.

Anastopoulos, A. D. (1998). A training program for parents of children with attention-deficit/hyperactivity disorder. In J. M. Briesmeister & C. E. Schaefer (Eds.), *Handbook of parent training: Parents as co-therapists for children's behavior problems* (pp. 27–60). New York: Wiley.

Anderson, S. R., Avery, D. L., DiPierto, E. K., Edward, G. L., & Christian, W. P. (1987). Intensive home-based early intervention with autistic children. *Education and Treatment of Children, 10,* 352–366.

Anderson, S. R., Taras, M., & O'Malley Cannon, B. (1996). Teaching new skills to young children with autism. In C. Maurice, G. Green, & S. C. Luce (Eds.), *Behavioral interventions for young children with autism: A manual for parents and professionals* (pp. 181–194) Austin, TX: PRO-ED.

Baghdadli, A., Picot, M. C., Pascal, C., Pry, R., & Aussilloux, C. (2003). Relationship between age of recognition of first disturbances and severity in young children with autism. *European Child and Adolescent Psychiatry, 12,* 122–127.

Baker, B. L., Landen, S. J., & Kashima, K. J. (1991). Effects of parent training on families of children with mental retardation: Increased burden or generalized benefit? *American Journal on Mental Retardation, 96,* 127–136.

Baker, M. J., Koegel, R. L., & Koegel, L. K. (1998). Increasing the social behavior of young children with autism using their obsessive behaviors. *Journal of the Association for Persons with Severe Handicaps, 23,* 300–308.

Barlow, J., & Stewart-Brown, S. (2000). Behavior problems and group-based parent education programs. *Journal of Developmental and Behavioral Pediatrics, 21,* 356–370.

Baron-Cohen, S., Allen, J., & Gillberg, C. (1992). Can autism be detected at 18 months?: The needle, the haystack, and the CHAT. *British Journal of Psychiatry, 161,* 839–843.

Bass, D. (1996). Family support across programs and populations. In G. H. S. Singer, L. E. Powers, & A. L. Olson (Eds.), *Redefining family support: Innovations in public–private partnerships* (pp. 39–55). Baltimore: Brookes.

Bates, E. (1976). *Language and context: The acquisition of pragmatics.* San Diego: Academic Press.

Bates, E., Camaioni, L., & Volterra, V. (1975). The acquisition of performatives prior to speech. *Merrill–Palmer Quarterly, 21,* 205–226.

Bennett, J., & Grimley, L. K. (2001). Parenting in the global community: A cross-cultural/international perspective. In M. J. Fine & S. W. Lee (Eds.), *Handbook of diversity in parent education* (pp. 97–132). San Diego: Academic Press.

Beutler, L. E., Alomohamed, S., Moleiro, C., & Romanelli, R. (2002). Systematic treatment selection and prescriptive therapy. In F. W. Kaslow (Ed.), *Comprehensive handbook of psychotherapy: Integrative/eclectic* (Vol. 4, pp. 255–271). New York: Wiley.

Blechman, E. A. (1998). Parent training in moral context: Prosocial family therapy. In J. M. Briesmeister & C. E. Schaefer (Eds.), *Handbook of parent training: Parents as co-therapists for children's behavior problems* (pp. 509–548). New York: Wiley.

Boulware, G., Schwartz, I. S., Sandall, S. R., & McBride, B. J. (2006). Project DATA for toddlers: An inclusive approach to very young children with autism spectrum disorder. *Topics in Early Childhood Special Education, 26,* 94–105.

Boyd, R. D., & Corley, M. J. (2001). Outcome survey of early intensive behavioral intervention for young children with autism in a community setting. *Autism, 5,* 430–441.

Briesmeister, J. M., & Schaefer, C. E. (1998). *Handbook of parent training: Parents as co-therapists for children's behavior problems.* New York: Wiley.

Bristol, M. M., Gallagher, J. J., & Holt, K. D. (1993). Maternal depressive symptoms in autism: Response to psychoeducational intervention. *Rehabilitation Psychology, 38,* 3–10.

Burke, J. C., & Cerniglia, L. (1990). Stimulus complexity and autistic children's responsivity: Assessing and training a pivotal behavior. *Journal of Autism and Developmental Disorders, 20,* 233–253.

Calzada, E. J., Eyberg, S. M., Rich, B., & Querido, J. G. (2004). Parenting disruptive preschoolers: Experiences of mothers and fathers. *Journal of Abnormal Child Psychology, 32,* 203–213.

Camarata, S. M., & Nelson, K. E. (1992). Treatment efficiency as a function of target selection in the remediation of child language disorders. *Clinical Linguistics and Phonetics, 6,* 167–178.

Carr, E. G., Dunlap, G., Horner, R. H., Koegel, R. L., Turnbull, A. P., Sailor, W., et al. (2002). Positive behavior support: Evolution of an applied science. *Journal of Positive Behavior Interventions, 4,* 4–16.

Cavell, T. A. (2000). *Working with parents of aggressive children: A practitioner's guide.* Washington, DC: American Psychological Association.

Centers for Disease Control and Prevention: National Center on Birth Defects and Developmental Disabilities. (2006). *Learn the signs. Act early.* Retrieved December 12, 2006, from *www.cdc.gov/ncbddd/autism/ActEarly/*.

Chawarska, K., Klin, A., Paul, R., & Volkmar, F. (2007). Autism spectrum disorder in the second year: Stability and change in syndrome expression. *Journal of Child Psychology and Psychiatry, 48*(2), 128–138.

Chawarska, K., Paul, R., Klin, A., Hannigen, A., Dichtel, L. E., & Volkmar, F. (2007). Parental recognition of developmental problems in toddlers with autism spectrum disorders. *Journal of Autism and Developmental Disorders, 37*(1), 62–72.

Chorpita, B. F. (2003). The frontier of evidence-based practice. In A. E. Kazdin, & J. R. Weisz (Eds.), *Evidence-based psychotherapies for children and adolescents* (pp. 42–59). New York: Guilford Press.

Churchill, D. W. (1971). Effects of success and failure in psychotic children. *Archives of General Psychiatry, 25,* 208–214.

Clark, D. A., Beck, A. T., & Alford, B. A. (1999). *Scientific foundations of cognitive theory and therapy of depression.* New York: Wiley.

Corcoran, J. (2000). Family treatment of preschool behavior problems. *Research on Social Work Practice, 10,* 547–588.

DeGarmo, D. S., Patterson, G. R., & Forgatch, M. S. (2004). How do outcomes in a specified parent training intervention maintain or wane over time? *Prevention Science, 5,* 73–89.

De Giacomo, A., & Fombonne, E. (1998). Parental recognition of developmental abnormalities in autism. *European Child and Adolescent Psychiatry, 7*(3), 131–136.

Doke, L. A., & Risley, T. R. (1972). The organization of daycare environments: Required versus optional activities. *Journal of Applied Behavior Analysis, 5,* 405–420.

Dunlap, G., & Kern, L. (1993). Assessment and intervention for children within the instructional curriculum. In J. Reichle & D. P. Wacker (Eds.), *Communication and language intervention series: Vol. 3. Communicative alternatives to challenging behavior: Integrating functional assessment and intervention strategies* (pp. 177–203). Baltimore: Brookes.

Dunlap, G., Kern-Dunlap, L., Clarke, S., & Robbins, F. R. (1991). Functional assessment, curricular revision, and severe behavior problems: Social validity: Multiple perspectives [Special issue]. *Journal of Applied Behavior Analysis, 24*(2), 387–397.

Dunlap, G., & Koegel, R. L., (1980). Motivating autistic children through stimulus variation. *Journal of Applied Behavior Analysis, 13,* 619–627.

Elder, J. H., Valcante, G., Won, D., & Zylis, R. (2003). Effects of in-home training for culturally diverse fathers of children with autism. *Issues in Mental Health Nursing, 24,* 273–295.

Etscheidt, S., (2003). An analysis of legal hearings and cases related to individualized education programs for children with autism. *Research and Practice for Persons with Severe Disabilities, 28*(2), 51–69.

Eyberg, S. M., Funderburk, B. W., Hembree-Kigin, T. L., McNeil, C. B., Querido, J. G., & Hood, K. K. (2001). Parent–child interaction therapy with behavior problem children: One and two year maintenance of treatment effects in the family. *Child and Family Behavior Therapy, 23,* 1–20.

Eyberg, S. M., & Robinson, E. A. (1982). Parent–child interaction training: Effects on family functioning. *Journal of Clinical Child Psychology, 11,* 130–137.

Fenske, E. C., Zalenski, S., Krantz, P. J., & McClannahan, L. E. (1985). Age at intervention and treatment outcomes for autistic children in a comprehensive intervention program. *Analysis and Intervention in Developmental Disabilities, 5,* 49–58.

Ferster, C. B., & DeMyer, M. K. (1961). The development of performances in autistic children in an automatically controlled environment. *Journal of Chronic Diseases, 13,* 312–345.

Ferster, C. B., & DeMyer, M. K. (1962). A method for the experimental analysis of the behavior of autistic children. *American Journal of Orthopsychiatry, 32,* 89–98.

Filipek P. A., Accardo, P. J., Baranek, G. T., Cook, E. H., Dawson, G., Gordon, B., et al. (1999). The screening and diagnosis of autistic spectrum disorders. *Journal of Autism and Developmental Disorders, 29,* 439–484.

Fine, M. J., & Gardner, P. A. (1991). Counseling and education services for families: An empowerment perspective: School counseling services for pre-kindergarten children [Special issue]. *Elementary School Guidance and Counseling, 26,* 33–44.

Forehand, R., & Kotchick, B. A. (1996). Cultural diversity: A wake-up call for parent training. *Behavior Therapy, 27,* 187–206.

Forehand, R., & Kotchick, B. A. (2002). Behavioral parent training: Current challenges and potential solutions. *Journal of Child and Family Studies, 11,* 377–384.

Gaylord-Ross, R. J., Haring, T. G., Breen, C., & Pitts-Conway, V. (1984). The training and generalization of social interaction skills with autistic youth. *Journal of Applied Behavior Analysis, 17,* 229–247.

Geller, E. S. (1991). Where is the validity in social validity? Social validity: Multiple perspectives [Special issue]. *Journal of Applied Behavior Analysis, 24,* 179–184.

Gerris, J. R. M., Van As, N. M. C., Wels, P. M. A., & Janssens, J. M. A. M. (1998). From parent education to family empowerment programs. In L. L'Abate (Ed.), *Family psychopathology: The relational roots of dysfunctional behavior* (pp. 401–426). New York: Guilford Press.

Goin, R. P., & Myers, B. J. (2004). Characteristics of infantile autism: Moving toward earlier detection. *Focus on Autism and Other Developmental Disabilities, 19,* 5–12.

Gorman, J. C., & Balter, L. (1997). Culturally sensitive parent education: A critical review of quantitative research. *Review of Educational Research, 67,* 339–369.

Green, G. (1996). Early behavioral intervention for young children with autism: What does research tell us? In C. Maurice, G. Green, & S. C. Luce (Eds.), *Behavioral interventions for young children with autism: A manual for parents and professionals* (pp. 29–44). Austin, TX: PRO-ED.

Gresham, F. M., & MacMillan, D. L. (1998). Early intervention project: Can its claims be substantiated and its effects replicated? *Journal of Autism and Developmental Disorders, 28,* 5–13.

Gunter, P., Fox, J. J., Brady, M. P., Shores, R. E., & Cavanaugh, K. (1988). Nonhandicapped peers as multiple exemplars: A generalization tactic for promoting autistic students' social skills. *Behavioral Disorders, 13,* 116–126.

Halle, J. W., Baer, D. M., & Spradlin, J. E. (1981). Teachers' generalized use of delay as a stimulus control procedure to increase language use in handicapped children. *Journal of Applied Behavior Analysis, 14,* 389–409.

Hancock, T. B., & Kaiser, A. P. (1996). Siblings' use of milieu teaching at home. *Topics in Early Childhood Special Education, 16,* 168–190.

Hancock, T. B., & Kaiser, A. P. (2002). The effects of trainer-implemented enhanced milieu teaching on the social communication of children with autism. *Topics in Early Childhood Special Education, 22,* 39–54.

Handleman, J. S., & Harris, S. L. (Eds.). (2001). *Preschool education programs for children with autism.* Austin, TX: PRO-ED.

Hart, B. M., & Risley, T. R. (1968). Establishing use of descriptive adjectives in the spontaneous speech of disadvantaged preschool children. *Journal of Applied Behavior Analysis, 1,* 109–120.

Hart, B. M., & Risley, T. R. (1975). Incidental teaching of language in the preschool. *Journal of Applied Behavior Analysis, 8,* 411–420.

Hayes, S. C., Barlow, D. H., & Nelson-Gray, R. O. (1999). *The scientist practitioner: Research and accountability in the age of managed care* (2nd ed.). Needham Heights, MA: Allyn & Bacon.

Hemmeter, M. L., & Kaiser, A. P. (1990). Environmental influences on children's language: A model and case study. *Education and Treatment of Children, 13,* 331–346.

Hemmeter, M. L., & Kaiser, A. P. (1994). Enhanced milieu teaching: An analysis of parent-implemented language intervention. *Journal of Early Intervention, 18,* 269–289.

Hewitt, F. M. (1965). Teaching speech to autistic children through operant conditioning. *American Journal of Orthopsychiatry, 34,* 927–936.

Hood, K. K., & Eyberg, S. M. (2003). Outcomes of parent–child interaction therapy: Mothers' reports of maintenance three to six years after treatment. *Journal of Clinical Child and Adolescent Psychology, 32,* 419–429.

Horner, R. H., Dunlap, G., & Koegel, R. L. (Eds.). (1988). *Generalization and maintenance: Life-style changes in applied settings.* Baltimore: Brookes.

Jones, T. M., Garlow, J. A., Turnbull, H. R., & Barber, P. A. (1996). Family empowerment in a family support program. In G. H. S. Singer, L. E. Powers, & A. L. Olson (Eds.), *Redefining family support: Innovations in public–private partnerships* (pp. 87–112). Baltimore: Brookes.

Kaiser, A. P., Hancock, T. B., & Nietfeld, J. P. (2000). The effects of parent-implemented enhanced milieu teaching on the social communication of children who have autism. *Early Education and Development, 11,* 423–446.

Kaiser, A. P., Mahoney, G., Girolametto, L., MacDonald, J., Robinson, C., Safford, P., et al. (1999). Rejoinder: Toward a contemporary vision of parent education. *Topics in Early Childhood Special Education, 19,* 173–176.

Kaiser, A. P., Ostrosky, M. M., & Alpert, C. L. (1993). Training teachers to use environmental arrangement and milieu teaching with nonvocal preschool children. *Journal of the Association for Persons with Severe Handicaps, 18,* 188–199.

Kaiser, A. P., Yoder, P. J., & Keetz, A. (1992). Evaluating milieu teaching. In S. F. Warren & J. Reichle (Eds.), *Causes and effects in communication and language intervention* (Vol. 1, pp. 9–47). Baltimore: Brookes.

Kazdin, A. E. (1977). Assessing the clinical or applied importance of behavior change through social validation. *Behavior Modification, 1,* 427–452.

Kazdin, A. E., & Weisz, J. R. (Eds.). (2003). *Evidence-based psychotherapies for children and adolescents.* New York: Guilford Press.

Koegel, L. K. (1995). Communication and language intervention. In R. L. Koegel, & L. K. Koegel (Eds.), *Teaching children with autism: Strategies for initiating positive interactions and improving learning opportunities* (pp. 17–32). Baltimore: Brookes.

Koegel, L. K. (2000). Interventions to facilitate communication in autism: Treatments for people with autism and other pervasive developmental disorders: Research perspectives [Special issue]. *Journal of Autism and Developmental Disorders, 35,* 383–391.

Koegel, L. K., Camarata, S. M., Valdez-Menchaca, M., & Koegel, R. L. (1998). Setting generalization of question-asking by children with autism. *American Journal on Mental Retardation, 102,* 346–357.

Koegel, L. K., & Koegel, R. L. (1986). The effects of interspersed maintenance tasks on academic performance in a severe childhood stroke victim. *Journal of Applied Behavior Analysis, 19,* 425–430.

Koegel, L. K., Koegel, R. L., Bruinsma, Y., Brookman, L., & Fredeen, R. (2003). *Teaching first words.* Santa Barbara: University of California.

Koegel, L. K., Koegel, R. L., Harrower, J. K., & Carter, C. M. (1999). Pivotal response intervention: I. Overview of approach. *Journal of the Association for Persons with Severe Handicaps, 24,* 174–185.

Koegel, L. K., Koegel, R. L., Shoshan, Y., & McNerney, E. (1999). Pivotal response intervention: II. Preliminary long-term outcome data. *Journal of the Association for Persons with Severe Handicaps, 24,* 186–198.

Koegel, R. L., Bimbela, A., & Schreibman, L. (1996). Collateral effects of parent training on family interactions. *Journal of Autism and Developmental Disorders, 26,* 347–359.

Koegel, R. L., Bruinsma, Y. E. M., & Koegel, L. K. (2006). Developmental trajectories with early intervention. In R. L. Koegel & L. K. Koegel (Eds.), *Pivotal response treatments for autism: Communication, social, and academic development* (pp. 131–140). Baltimore: Brookes.

Koegel, R. L., Dunlap, G., Richman, G., & Dyer, K. (1981). The use of specific orienting cues for teaching discrimination tasks. *Analysis and Intervention in Developmental Disabilities, 1,* 187–198.

Koegel, R. L., Dyer, K., & Bell, L. K. (1987). The influence of child preferred activities on autistic children's social behavior. *Journal of Applied Behavior Analysis, 20,* 243–252.

Koegel, R. L., & Egel, E. L. (1979). Motivating autistic children. *Journal of Abnormal Psychology, 88,* 418–426.

Koegel, R. L., & Frea, W. D. (1993). Treatment of social behavior in autism through the modification of pivotal social skills. *Journal of Applied Behavior Analysis, 26,* 369–377.

Koegel, R. L., Glahn, T. J., & Nieminen, G. S. (1978). Generalization of parent training results. *Journal of Applied Behavior Analysis, 11,* 95–109.

Koegel, R. L., & Koegel, L. K. (Eds.). (1995). *Teaching children with autism: Strategies for initiating positive interactions and improving learning opportunities.* Baltimore: Brookes.

Koegel, R. L., & Koegel, L. K. (Eds.). (2006). *Pivotal response treatments for autism: Communication, social, and academic development.* Baltimore: Brookes.

Koegel, R. L., Koegel, L. K., & Carter, C. M. (1999). Pivotal teaching interactions for children with autism. *School Psychology Review, 28,* 576–594.

Koegel, R. L., Koegel, L. K., & O'Neill, R. E. (1989). Generalization in the treatment of autism. In L. V. McReynolds & J. E. Spradlin (Eds.), *Generalization strategies in the treatment of communication disorders* (pp. 116–131). Toronto: B.C. Decker.

Koegel, R. L., Koegel, L. K., & Surratt, A. (1992). Language intervention and disruptive behavior in preschool children with autism. *Journal of Autism and Developmental Disorders, 22,* 141–153.

Koegel, R. L., & Mentis, M. (1985). Motivation in childhood autism: Can they or won't they? *Journal of Child Psychology and Psychiatry, 26,* 185–191.

Koegel, R. L., O'Dell, M. C., & Dunlap, G. (1988). Producing speech use in nonverbal autistic children by reinforcing attempts. *Journal of Autism and Developmental Disorders, 18,* 525–538.

Koegel, R. L., O'Dell, M. C., & Koegel, L. K. (1987). A natural language paradigm for teaching non-verbal autistic children. *Journal of Autism and Developmental Disorders, 17,* 187–199.

Koegel, R. L., Openden, D., Fredeen, R., & Koegel, L. K. (2006). The basics of pivotal response treatment. In R. L. Koegel & L. K. Koegel (Eds.), *Pivotal response treatments for autism: Communication, social, and academic development* (pp. 3–30). Baltimore: Brookes.

Koegel, R. L., & Rincover, A. (1974). Treatment of psychotic children in a classroom environment: I. Learning in a large group. *Journal of Applied Behavior Analysis, 7,* 45–59.

Koegel, R. L., & Rincover, A. (1977). Research on the difference between generalization and maintenance in extra-therapy responding. *Journal of Applied Behavior Analysis, 10,* 1–12.

Koegel, R. L., & Schreibman, L. (1977). Teaching autistic children to respond to simultaneous multiple cues. *Journal of Experimental Child Psychology, 24,* 299–311.

Koegel, R. L., & Schreibman, L. (2006). *Research in autism: Parent intervention.* Washington, DC: National Institute of Mental Health.

Koegel, R. L., Schreibman, L., Britten, K. R., Burke, J. C., & O'Neill, R. E. (1982). A comparison of parent training to direct child treatment. In R. L. Koegel, A. Rincover, & A. L. Egel (Eds.), *Educating and understanding autistic children* (pp. 260–279). San Diego: College-Hill Press.

Koegel, R. L., Schreibman, L., Good, A., Cerniglia, L., Murphy, C., & Koegel, L. K. (1989). *How to teach pivotal behaviors to children with autism: A training manual.* Santa Barbara: University of California.

Koegel, R. L., & Wilhelm, H. (1973). Selective responding to the components of multiple visual cues by autistic children. *Journal of Experimental Child Psychology, 15,* 442–453.

Koegel, R. L., & Williams, J. A. (1980). Direct vs. indirect response–reinforcer relationships in teaching autistic children. *Journal of Abnormal Child Psychology, 8,* 537–547.

Kotchick, B. A., & Forehand, R. (2002). Putting parenting in perspective: A discussion of the contextual factors that shape parenting practices. *Journal of Child and Family Studies, 11,* 255–269.

Levy, S., Kim, A., & Olive, M. L. (2006). Interventions for young children with autism: A synthesis of the literature. *Focus on Autism and Other Developmental Disabilities, 21,* 55–62.

Lord, C. (1995). Follow-up of two-year-olds referred for possible autism. *Journal of Child Psychology and Psychiatry, 36*(8), 1365–1382.

Lord, C., & Paul, R. (1997). Language and communication in autism. In D. J.

Cohen & F. R. Volkmar (Eds.), *Handbook of autism and pervasive developmental disorders* (2nd ed., pp. 195–225). New York: Wiley.

Lord, C., & Risi, S. (2000). Diagnosis of autism spectrum disorders in young children. In A. M. Wetherby & B. M. Prizant (Eds.), *Communication and language intervention: Vol. 9. Autism spectrum disorders: A transactional developmental perspective* (pp. 11–30). Baltimore: Brookes.

Lovaas, O. I. (1977). *The autistic child: Language development through behavior modification.* Oxford, UK: Irvington.

Lovaas, O. I. (1987). Behavioral treatment and normal education and intellectual functioning in young autistic children. *Journal of Consulting and Clinical Psychology, 55,* 3–9.

Lovaas, O. I. (2002). *Teaching individuals with developmental delays: Basic intervention techniques.* Austin, TX: PRO-ED.

Lovaas, O. I., Freitag, G., Kinder, M. I., Rubenstein, B. D., Schaeffer, B., & Simmons, J. Q. (1966). Establishment of social reinforcers in two schizophrenic children on the basis of food. *Journal of Experimental Child Psychology, 4,* 109–125.

Lovaas, O. I., Koegel, R. L., & Schreibman, L. (1979). Stimulus overselectivity in autism: A review of research. *Psychological Bulletin, 86,* 1236–1254.

Lovaas, O. I., & Schreibman, L. (1971). Stimulus overselectivity of autistic children in a two stimulus situation. *Behaviour Research and Therapy, 9,* 305–310.

Lovaas, O. I., Schreibman, L., Koegel, R. L., & Rehm, R. (1971). Selective responding by autistic children to multiple sensory input. *Journal of Abnormal Psychology, 77,* 211–222.

MacKenzie, E. P., Fite, P. J., & Bates, J. E. (2004). Predicting outcome in behavioral parent training: Expected and unexpected results. *Child and Family Behavior Therapy, 26,* 37–53.

Matson, J. L., Sevin, J. A., Box, M. L., Francis, K. L., & Sevin, B. M. (1993). An evaluation of two methods for increasing self-initiated verbalizations in autistic children. *Journal of Applied Behavior Analysis, 26,* 389–398.

McClannahan, L. E., & Krantz, P. J. (2001). Behavior analysis and intervention for preschoolers at the Princeton Child Development Institute. In J. S. Handleman & S. L. Harris (Eds.), *Preschool education programs for children with autism* (pp. 191–213). Austin, TX: PRO-ED.

McClannahan, L. E., Krantz, P. J., & McGee, G. G. (1982). Parents as therapists for autistic children: A model for effective training. *Analysis and Intervention in Developmental Disabilities, 2,* 223–252.

McDermott, D. (2000). Parenting and ethnicity. In M. J. Fine & S. W. Lee (Eds.), *Handbook of diversity in parent education* (pp. 73–96). San Diego: Academic Press.

McEachin, J. J., Smith, T., & Lovaas, O. I. (1993). Long-term outcomes for children with autism who received early intensive behavioral treatment. *American Journal on Mental Retardation, 4,* 359–372.

McGee, G. G., Almeida, M. C., Sulzer-Azaroff, B., & Feldman, R. S. (1992). Promoting reciprocal interactions via peer incidental teaching. *Journal of Applied Behavior Analysis, 25,* 117–126.

McGee, G. G., Krantz, P. J., Mason, D., & McClannahan, L. E. (1983). A modified incidental-teaching procedure for autistic youth: Acquisition and generalization of receptive object labels. *Journal of Applied Behavior Analysis, 16*, 329–338.

McGee, G. G., Krantz, P. J., Mason, D., & McClannahan, L. E. (1986). An extension of incidental teaching procedures to reading instruction for autistic children. *Journal of Applied Behavior Analysis, 19*, 147–157.

McGee, G. G., Morrier, M. J., & Daly, T. (1999). An incidental teaching approach to early intervention for toddlers with autism. *Journal of the Association for Persons with Severe Handicaps, 24*, 133–146.

Mesibov, G. B. (1993). Treatment outcome is encouraging. *American Journal on Mental Retardation, 97*, 379–380.

Moes, D. (1995). Parent education and parenting stress. In R. L. Koegel & L. K. Koegel (Eds.), *Teaching children with autism: Strategies for initiating positive interactions and improving learning opportunities* (pp. 79–93). Baltimore: Brookes.

Moes, D., Koegel, R. L., Schreibman, L., & Loos, L. M. (1992). Stress profiles for mothers and fathers of children with autism. *Psychological Reports, 71*, 1272–1274.

National Research Council. (2001). *Educating children with autism*. Washington, DC: National Academy Press.

Nixon, R. D. V. (2001). Changes in hyperactivity and temperament in behaviorally disturbed preschoolers after parent–child interaction therapy (PCIT). *Behaviour Change, 18*, 168–176.

Osterling, J. A., Dawson, G., & Munson, J. A. (2002). Early recognition of 1-year-old infants with autism spectrum disorder versus mental retardation. *Development and Psychopathology. 14*, 239–251.

Ostrosky, M. M., & Kaiser, A. P. (1991). Preschool classroom environments that promote communication. *Teaching Exceptional Children, 23*(4), 6–10.

Prizant, B. M., & Wetherby, A. M. (1987). Communicative intent: A framework for understanding social-communicative behavior in autism. *Journal of the American Academy of Child and Adolescent Psychiatry, 26*, 472–479.

Prizant, B. M., Wetherby, A. M., Rubin, E., Laurent, A. C., & Rydell, P. J. (2006). *The SCERTS Model: A comprehensive educational approach for children with autism spectrum disorders: Vol. II. Program planning and intervention*. Baltimore: Brookes.

Rapin, I. (1991). Autistic children: Diagnosis and clinical features. *Pediatrics, 87*, 751–760.

Reynolds, B. S., Newsom, C. D., & Lovaas, O. I. (1974). Auditory overselectivity in autistic children. *Journal of Abnormal Child Psychology, 2*, 253–263.

Risley, T. (1996). Get a life!: Positive behavioral intervention for challenging behavior through life arrangement and life coaching. In L. K. Koegel, R. L. Koegel, & G. Dunlap (Eds.), *Positive behavioral support: Including people with difficult behavior in the community* (pp. 425–437). Baltimore: Brookes.

Risley, T. R., & Favell, J. E. (1979). Constructing a living environment in an institution. In L. A. Hamerlynch (Ed.), *Behavioral systems for the developmentally disabled* (Vol. 2, pp. 3–24). New York: Brunner/Mazel.

Robins, D. L., Fein, D., Barton, M. L., & Green, J. A. (2001). The Modified Checklist for Autism in Toddlers: An initial study investigating the early detection of autism and pervasive developmental disorders. *Journal of Autism and Developmental Disorders, 31*, 131–144.

Rogers, S. (1998). Empirically supported comprehensive treatments for young children with autism. *Journal of Clinical Child Psychology, 27*, 168–179.

Rosenblatt, J., Bloom, P., & Koegel, R. L. (1995). Overselective responding: Description, implications, and intervention. In R. L. Koegel & L. K. Koegel (Eds.), *Teaching children with autism: Strategies for initiating positive interactions and improving learning opportunities* (pp. 33–42). Baltimore: Brookes.

Sampers, J., Anderson, K. G., Hartung, C. M., & Scambler, D. J. (2001). Parent training programs for young children with behavior problems. *Infant–Toddler Intervention, 11,* 91–110.

Santarelli, G., Koegel, R. L., Casas, J. M., & Koegel, L. K. (2001). Culturally diverse families participating in behavior therapy parent education programs for children with developmental disabilities. *Journal of Positive Behavior Interventions, 3,* 120–123.

Scheel, M. J., & Rieckmann, T. (1998). An empirically derived description of self-efficacy and empowerment for parents of children identified as psychologically disordered. *American Journal of Family Therapy, 26,* 15–27.

Schopler, E. (2001). Treatment for autism: From science to pseudo-science or anti-science. In E. Schopler, N. Yirmiya, C. Shulman, & L. M. Marcus (Eds.), *The research basis for autism intervention* (pp. 9–24). New York: Kluwer Academic/Plenum Press.

Schover, L. R., & Newsom, C. D. (1976). Overselectivity, developmental level, and overtraining in autistic and normal children. *Journal of Abnormal Child Psychology, 4,* 289–298.

Schreibman, L. (1975). Effects of within-stimulus and extra-stimulus prompting on discrimination learning in autistic children. *Journal of Applied Behavior Analysis, 8,* 91–112.

Schreibman, L. (1988). *Autism.* Newbury Park, CA: Sage.

Schreibman, L. (1997). The study of stimulus control in autism. In D. M. Baer & E. M. Pinkston (Eds.), *Environment and behavior* (pp. 203–209). Boulder, CO: Westview Press.

Schreibman, L. (2000). Intensive behavioral/psychoeducational treatments for autism: Research needs and future directions. Treatments for people with autism and other pervasive developmental disorders: Research perspective [Special issue]. *Journal of Autism and Developmental Disorders, 30,* 373–378.

Schreibman, L., & Carr, E. G. (1978). Elimination of echolalic responding to questions through the training of a generalized verbal response. *Journal of Applied Behavior Analysis, 11,* 453–463.

Schreibman, L., Charlop, M. H., & Koegel, R. L. (1982). Teaching autistic children to use extra-stimulus prompts. *Journal of Experimental Child Psychology, 33,* 475–491.

Schreibman, L., Kaneko, W. M., & Koegel, R. L. (1991). Positive affect of parents of autistic children: A comparison across two teaching techniques. *Behavior Therapy, 22,* 479–490.

Schreibman, L., & Koegel, R. L. (1982). Multiple-cue responding in autistic children. In J. J. Steffen & P. Karoly (Eds.), *Autism and severe psychopathology* (pp. 81–99). Lexington, MA: Heath.

Schreibman, L., & Koegel, R. L. (2005). Training for parents of children with autism: Pivotal responses, generalization, and individualization of interventions. In E. D. Hibbs & P. S. Jensen (Eds.), *Psychosocial treatments for child and adolescent disorders: Empirically based strategies for clinical practice* (2nd ed., pp. 605–631). Washington, DC: American Psychological Association.

Schreibman, L., Koegel., R. L., & Craig, M. S. (1977). Reducing stimulus over-selectivity in autistic children. *Journal of Abnormal Child Psychology, 5,* 425–435.

Schwartz, I. S., & Baer, D. M. (1991). Social validity assessments: Is current practice state of the art?: Social validity: Multiple perspectives [Special issue]. *Journal of Applied Behavior Analysis, 24,* 189–204.

Schwartz, J. P. (2002). Family resilience and pragmatic parent education. *Journal of Individual Psychology, 58,* 250–262.

Seligman, M. E. P., Maier, S. F., & Greer, J. (1968). The alleviation of learned help-lessness in the dog. *Journal of Abnormal and Social Psychology, 73,* 256–262.

Shah, K. (2001). What do medical students know about autism? *Autism, 5,* 127–133.

Shea, V. (2005). A perspective on the research literature related to early intensive behavioral interventions (Lovaas) for young children with autism. *Communication Disorders Quarterly, 26,* 102–111.

Shukla, S., Surratt, A. V., Horner, R. H., & Albin, R. W. (1995). Examining the relationship between self-initiations of an individual with disabilities and directive behavior of staff persons in a residential setting. *Behavioral Interventions, 10,* 101–110.

Siegel, B., Pliner, C., Eschler, J., & Elliott, G. R. (1988). How children with autism are diagnosed: Difficulties in identification of children with multiple developmental delays. *Journal of Developmental and Behavioral Pediatrics, 9,* 199–204.

Singer, G. H. S. (1993). When it's not so easy to change your mind: Some reflections on cognitive interventions for parents of children with disabilities. In A. P. Turnbull, J. M. Patterson, S. K. Behr, D. L. Murphy, J. G. Marquis, et al. (Eds.), *Cognitive coping, families, and disability* (pp. 207–220). Baltimore: Brookes.

Singer, G. H. S., Golberg-Hamblin, S. E., Peckham-Hardin, K. D., Barry, L., & Santarelli, G. E. (2002). Toward a synthesis of family support practices and positive behavior support. In J. M. Lucyshyn, G. Dunlap, & R. W. Albin (Eds.), *Families and positive behavior support: Addressing problem behavior in family contexts* (pp. 155–183). Baltimore: Brookes.

Smith, T. (2001). Discrete trial training in the treatment of autism. *Focus on Autism and Other Developmental Disabilities, 16,* 86–92.

Stahmer, A. C., & Ingersoll, B. (2004). Inclusive programming for toddlers with autism spectrum disorder: Outcomes from the children's toddler school. *Journal of Positive Behavioral Interventions, 6,* 67–83.

Stern, J. (2000). Parent training. In J. R. White & A. S. Arthur (Eds.), *Cognitive-behavioral group therapy: For specific problems and populations* (pp. 331–360). Washington, DC: American Psychological Association.

Stone, W. L., Coonrod, E. E., & Ousley, O. Y. (2000). Screening Tool for Autism Two-Year-Olds (STAT): Development and preliminary data. *Journal of Autism and Developmental Disorders, 30,* 607–612.

Strain, P. S., & Schwartz, I. (2001). ABA and the development of meaningful social relations for young children with autism. *Focus on Autism and Other Developmental Disabilities, 16,* 120–128.

Task Force on Promotion and Dissemination of Psychological Procedures. (1995). Training in and dissemination of empirically-validated psychological treatments. *Clinical Psychologist, 48*(1), 3–23.

Taylor, B. A., & Harris, S. L. (1995). Teaching children with autism to seek information: Acquisition of novel information and generalization of responding. *Journal of Applied Behavior Analysis, 28,* 3–14.

Twardosz, S., Cataldo, M. F., & Risley, T. R. (1974). Open environment design for infant and toddler day care. *Journal of Applied Behavior Analysis, 7,* 529–549.

Volkmar, F., Chawarska, K., & Klin, A. (2005). Autism in infancy and early childhood. *Annual Review of Psychology, 56,* 315–336.

Warren, S. F., McQuarter, R. J., & Rogers-Warren, A. K. (1984). The effects of teacher mands and models on the speech of unresponsive language-delayed children. *Journal of Speech and Hearing Research, 49,* 43–52.

Webster-Stratton, C., & Reid, M. J. (2003). The incredible years parents, teachers and children training series: A multifaceted treatment approach for young children with conduct problems. In A. E. Kazdin, Yale University School of Medicine, Child Study Center, et al. (Eds.), *Evidence-based psychotherapies for children and adolescents* (pp. 224–240). New York: Guilford Press.

Weiss, M. J. (1999). Differential rates of skill acquisition and outcomes of early intensive behavioral intervention for autism. *Behavioral Interventions, 14,* 3–22.

Wetherby, A. M., & Woods, J. J. (2006). Early social interaction project for children with autism spectrum disorders beginning in the second year of life: A preliminary study. *Topics in Early Childhood Special Education, 26,* 67–82.

Williams, J. A., Koegel, R. L., & Egel, A. L. (1981). Response–reinforcer relationships and improved learning in autistic children. *Journal of Applied Behavior Analysis, 14,* 53–60.

Wolf, M. M. (1978). Social validity: The case for subjective measurement or how applied behavior analysis is finding its heart. *Journal of Applied Behavior Analysis, 11,* 203–214.

Woods, J. J., & Wetherby, A. M. (2003). Early identification of and intervention for infants and toddlers who are at risk for autism spectrum disorder. *Language, Speech, and Hearing Services in Schools, 34,* 180–193.

Yoder, P. J., Kaiser, A. P., Alpert, C., & Fischer, R. (1993). Following the child's lead when teaching nouns to preschoolers with mental retardation. *Journal of Speech and Hearing Research, 36,* 158–167.

Zegarra, G. (1998). Educando a la familia Latina: Ideas for making parent education programs accessible to the Latino community. *Family and Conciliation Courts Review, 36,* 281–293.

CHAPTER 9

————•◦•————

Controversial Treatments

TRISTRAM SMITH
JENNIFER WICK

Children with autism spectrum disorder (ASD) often receive controversial treatments—interventions that are popular despite an absence of scientific or theoretical support. As many as one-third of all newly diagnosed children with ASD participate in such treatments (Levy, Mandell, Merhar, Ittenbach, & Pinto-Martin, 2003). Many others start soon after they begin conventional therapies such as behavioral or educational services, and some undergo multiple ones (Smith & Antolovich, 2000), which may continue into adolescence (Witwer & Lecavelier, 2005). The use of controversial treatments for children with ASD is a long-standing issue (Rimland, 1964), and the number of different treatments and their rate of use have grown over time (Levy & Hyman, 2003).

The most common controversial treatments for children with ASD are sensory–motor therapies such as auditory integration training, bonding therapies such as Options (also called Son-Rise; Kaufman, 1976), and several forms of complementary and alternative medicine (CAM) interventions such as vitamin therapies and special diets. The proliferation of controversial treatments for children with ASD is probably due to many factors. Among them is that the precise etiology or etiologies of ASD remain unknown, fueling speculation and debate about possible causes and remedies (Levy & Hyman, 2005). Another is that ASD is a complex behavioral syndrome with many areas of need, each of which is potentially a focus of intervention (Lovaas & Smith, 2003). Moreover, caregivers may be eager to try a variety of treatments in search of a favorable outcome for their children. Their hopes may be high because, in some cases, the onset of ASD occurs after a period of apparently typical development (Luyster et al., 2005), and children may be free of obvious physical abnormalities and retain isolated areas of age-appropriate skills. Reports of children who improve markedly may add to caregivers' hopes (e.g., Seroussi, 2000). In addition, caregivers often feel a sense of urgency, which may be fueled by the significant behavioral difficulties associated with ASD and the stress on caregiver–child relationships arising from a disorder characterized above all by impaired reciprocal social interaction (Bouma & Schweitzer, 1990; Hoppes & Harris, 1990).

Caregivers may hear more about controversial treatments than about treatments with rigorous, scientific evidence for safety and efficacy. Controversial treatments attract far more media publicity than evidence-based treatments, which include behavioral and educational interventions (Lord et al., 2002) and psychopharmacological therapies (McCracken et al., 2002; Research Units on Pediatric Psychopharmacology Autism Network, 2005). Moreover, controversial treatments are frequently touted as cures, whereas evidence-based treatments yield only limited improvement, as they increase adaptive functioning for most children with ASD but do not eliminate the disorder. Some controversial treatments are relatively straightforward to implement; in contrast, evidence-based treatments are hard to obtain in many communities because they require supervision from highly trained professionals and may be expensive.

Because all of these factors are likely to persist into the foreseeable future, practitioners and families can expect controversial treatments for children with ASD to remain popular. Therefore, to make informed decisions, it is essential to be able to distinguish controversial from established treatments and to be aware of the most common controversial treatments. To resolve controversies and advance the field, the scientific community must identify constructive ways to respond to advocates of controversial treatments, and practitioners and families must find ways to work together when controversial treatments are being considered for a child with ASD.

DISTINGUISHING CONTROVERSIAL FROM ESTABLISHED TREATMENTS

Standards of Evidence

The only evidence for many controversial treatments consists of subjective information such as case reports, anecdotes, testimonials from parents or practitioners, and surveys. Reports that a child improved or that families gave high marks for a treatment in a survey are encouraging and may indicate that a treatment deserves further study. Unfortunately, this is not proof that the treatment is effective. Many other explanations are plausible. For example, additional interventions that the children were concurrently receiving, such as behavioral and educational services, may account for favorable outcomes. Furthermore, as children grow up, they may develop new abilities regardless of treatment. It is even possible that reported improvements can reflect parents' or practitioners' desires to see gains, rather than real progress.

Scientific studies incorporate methodologies that make it possible to test whether a treatment is truly associated with improved outcomes. For instance, participants may be randomly assigned to two groups. One group receives the treatment, and the other is untreated; then the outcomes of the two groups are statistically compared. This design, called a randomized clinical trial (RCT), can offer the strongest test of whether a treatment is effective. The randomization maximizes the probability that children in the treatment group are similar to those in the no-treatment group prior to intervention. If the groups are similar prior to treatment but differ afterward, the posttreatment difference is likely to be attributable to the intervention. Optimally, an RCT includes a large number of children in each group (at least 20, often considerably more) so that the statistical analyses have adequate power to detect differences in outcome between groups. It may also include multiple treatment sites and practitioners to assess the consistency of results at different sites, with different personnel.

Another appropriate research strategy is the use of single-case designs. These designs involve comparing a baseline phase, in which an individual receives no treatment, with one or more intervention phases in which treatment is provided to the individual. Data are collected continuously on the outcome measure. If scores on the outcome measure consistently improve during intervention relative to baseline, one may conclude that the treatment was effective for that individual. However, because the design involves only one individual, multiple studies by independent investigators are required to confirm the findings. A series of single-case studies may need to be followed by an RCT in order to test the treatment with a sufficiently large number of individuals (Smith et al., 2007).

In both RCTs and single-case studies, standardized measures such as the Autism Diagnostic Interview–Revised (ADI-R; Rutter, LeCouteur, & Lord, 2003) and the Autism Diagnostic Observation Schedule–Generic (ADOS-G; Lord, Rutter, DiLavore, & Risi, 2001) should be used to confirm the diagnosis. In addition, investigators should show that the outcome measures are valid indicators of improvement, and the measures should reflect readily observable gains in functioning such as increased communication or reduced aggression, rather than vague constructs such as "greater focus" or "improved sense of self." Moreover, to ensure unbiased data collection, individuals who are unaware of the purpose of the study or the children's treatment histories should administer and score the measures. Assessments should also be conducted to ascertain whether treatment was delivered as intended, in keeping with a standard protocol or set of procedures.

When possible, intervention should be administered in a double-blind, placebo-control design. In this approach, children and practitioners are unaware of whether the children are receiving treatment or a placebo. For example, in a study of a medication or vitamin therapy, the pills that contain the active ingredient can be made identical to placebo pills. Investigators can postpone telling the children and practitioners which pill the children received until the completion of the study. Although this strategy is not viable for most behavioral or educational studies because the interventions cannot be disguised, it is feasible for most CAM treatments.

Table 9.1 presents a standard system for rating the evidence from scientific studies and shows that anecdotal reports are considered the weakest form of evidence, and favorable results from multiple studies that incorporate strong designs constitute the strongest evidence. When only anecdotal evidence is available, a treatment is considered to be essentially unproven; if studies were conducted, they could find that the treatment was helpful, harmful, or neither. Families and practitioners should consider such treatment experimental and should be very cautious about implementing it (or decide not to try it). However, when multiple, well-designed studies indicate that a treatment is effective, one can be confident that the treatment really is effective. Table 9.2 summarizes the criteria for a strong scientific study.

TABLE 9.1. Levels of Evidence for the Effectiveness of a Treatment

Grade	Criteria
I	Evidence from studies of strong design, with minor flaws at most and free from serious doubts about bias. Results are both clinically important and consistent. Results are free from concerns about generalizability. Studies with negative results have sufficiently large samples to have adequate statistical power.
II	Evidence from studies of strong design, but there is some uncertainty owing to inconsistencies in findings, or concern about generalizability, bias, research design flaws, or sample size (for negative findings, again). OR, consistent evidence, but from studies of weaker design.
III	Evidence from a limited number of studies of weaker design. Studies with strong design have not been done or are inconclusive.
IV	Support solely from informed professional commentators based on clinical experience without substantiation from the published literature.

Note. Adapted from Joint Commission Resources. (2000). Copyright 2000 by Joint Commission Resources. Adapted by permission.

TABLE 9.2. Characteristics of Scientifically Sound Studies on Treatment

1. Participants are assigned randomly to groups (or use of single-subject experimental designs, with multiple replications by independent investigators).

2. The study includes a large enough number of participants to support meaningful statistical analyses.

3. Diagnosis is based on standardized measures.

4. Validated outcome measures relating to improvements in functioning are collected.

5. Measures are collected in an unbiased manner.

6. Assessments are conducted to determine whether treatment adheres to a standard, predetermined set of procedures.

7. When possible, the study is performed double-blind (participants and practitioners are unaware of whether the treatment or a placebo is being provided).

Plausibility

Although scientific evidence is the primary criterion for evaluating a treatment, the theoretical basis of the treatment is another important consideration. To be plausible, a treatment must address a problem known to be associated with ASD, and its mechanism for producing change must be consistent with principles of behavior or biology. For example, Floortime is an intervention that involves playfully obstructing children's activities (Greenspan & Wieder, 1999). Although it has not been evaluated in studies with strong scientific designs (Greenspan & Wieder, 1997), it is viewed as a possibly effective intervention (National Research Council [NRC], 2001). Its purpose is to improve reciprocal social interactions, which are a major area of difficulty for children with ASD, via sustained back-and-forth communication during unstructured games. Playful obstruction is similar to a scientifically validated instructional method called incidental teaching (Hart & Risley, 1980), which is often a useful component of intervention programs for children with ASD. In contrast, "gentle teaching" is a therapy that is said to provide "unconditional and authentic valuing" of individuals with ASD in order to facilitate bonding or attachment to caregivers (McGee & Gonzales, 1990). However, most individuals with ASD already display attachment to caregivers (Sigman & Mundy, 1989), and it is unclear as to what unconditional and authentic valuing is or how it would be beneficial. Because it does not address a known problem in ASD and does not include interventions known to change behavior, gentle teaching is not usually regarded as a plausible treatment.

These criteria are also applicable to biomedical interventions. For example, mood swings are a problem for some children with ASD. Psychotropic medication may be a reasonable intervention even if the medication has not been studied in children with ASD. Because of government regulations, all medications undergo extensive testing for safety and efficacy before becoming available in clinical practice. Psychotropic medications alter the function of neurotransmitters in the brain, and some have been shown to be effective in reducing mood swings associated with disorders other than ASD. For these reasons, such medications are potentially effective for children with ASD, though close monitoring by the prescribing physician is necessary. In contrast, although ASD is known to be a neurological disorder that affects brain development, many CAM interventions focus on entirely different parts of the body, such as the gastrointestinal system. It is unclear whether individuals with ASD are at any greater risk than other individuals for such problems. It is also unknown whether interventions such as hormone injections or dietary changes are safe or effective in addressing these problems if they do exist, and whether improvement in gastrointestinal functioning is relevant to the underlying neurological difficulties in ASD. Thus, the theoretical basis for many CAM interventions is often questionable.

Potential "Red Flags"

Unfortunately, families and professionals often view particular treatments as having support from scientific studies and theories even when the consensus of the scientific community advises otherwise (Smith & Antolovich, 2000). Treatments may be pseudoscientific (described as proven and well-grounded in established theory yet lacking any such basis), and it may be difficult to distinguish between scientific and pseudoscientific approaches. However, one study identified a set of 10 "red flags" that may increase nonspecialists' ability to spot pseudoscientific treatments (Finn, Bothe, & Bramlett, 2005; see Table 9.3):

1. *Does the evidence in support of the treatment rely on personal experience and anecdotal accounts?* As discussed, anecdotes may suggest that scientific testing of a treatment would be worthwhile but in themselves are weak evidence that the treatment is effective.

2. *Is the treatment approach disconnected from well-established scientific models or paradigms?* As noted, a treatment should address problems known to be associated with ASD and should be consistent with principles of behavior and biology.

3. *Is the treatment unable to be tested or disproved?* To qualify as scientific, assertions about treatment effects must be stated in such a way that direct observation and experiments can either confirm or falsify them.

TABLE 9.3. Red Flags for Identifying a Treatment as Pseudoscientific

1. Does the evidence in support of the treatment rely on personal experience and anecdotal accounts?
2. Is the treatment approach disconnected from well-established scientific models or paradigms?
3. Is the treatment unable to be tested or disproved?
4. Does the treatment remain unchanged even in the face of contradictory evidence?
5. Is the rationale for the treatment based only on confirming evidence, with disconfirmatory evidence ignored or minimized?
6. Are the treatment claims incommensurate with the supporting evidence for those claims?
7. Are the treatment claims unsupported by evidence that has undergone critical scrutiny?
8. Is the treatment described by terms that appear to be scientific but upon further examination are determined not to be?
9. Is the treatment based on grandiose claims or poorly described outcomes?
10. Is the treatment claimed to make sense only within a vaguely described holistic framework?

Note. Adapted from Finn, Bothe, and Bramlett (2005). Copyright 2005 by the American Speech–Language–Hearing Association. Adapted by permission.

Otherwise, the credibility of the treatment depends solely on the authority of its developer. However, assertions about controversial treatments are often untestable and therefore pseudoscientific. For example, the developer of one controversial treatment contended that any intervention for children with ASD would be impossible to study because treatment "cannot observe the rigors of a 'scientific' experiment since it must, in its course, pursue the vagaries of life which are nothing if not unpredictable" (Bettelheim, 1967, p. 6). Proponents of another controversial treatment maintained that negative research findings could never be used as evidence against the intervention because the presence of an objective observer (as required for research) disrupted the therapeutic relationship so severely that treatment gains were lost (Biklen & Cardinal, 1997).

4. *Does the treatment remain unchanged even in the face of contradictory evidence?* Established treatments such as behavioral interventions continually evolve as a result of new research findings. However, many controversial treatments originated many years ago and are still implemented in essentially their original form, without revisions based on scientific advances (see, e.g., Kaufman, 1976).

5. *Is the rationale for the treatment based only on confirming evidence, with disconfirmatory evidence ignored or minimized?* Scientific evaluation of a

treatment requires consideration of all evidence from relevant well-designed studies, including both positive and negative results. However, advocates of controversial treatments sometimes focus only on supporting evidence. For example, proponents of vitamin therapies sometimes cite a large number of uncontrolled studies that appear to support these therapies but do not cite relevant RCTs, all of which so far indicate that the therapies are not effective (see, e.g., Rimland, 2000).

6. *Are the treatment claims incommensurate with the supporting evidence for those claims?* Advocates of a controversial treatment may recommend the treatment for children with ASD solely on the basis of anecdotal information. They also may divert attention away from this weak evidence by criticizing other treatments, arguing that skepticism about their treatment reflects opposition from a narrow-minded establishment (Rimland, 1992) or insisting that scientific tests of the treatment are superfluous (Biklen & Cardinal, 1997).

7. *Are treatment claims unsupported by evidence that has undergone critical scrutiny?* Before publication in a scholarly journal, reports of scientific studies undergo careful peer review. The report is read by several experts, whose identities are usually withheld from the authors of the report so that they can give honest feedback. The experts critique the adequacy of the research methodology, soundness of the conclusions, and contribution to scientific knowledge. Based on the experts' critique, an editor makes a recommendation for or against publishing the report. Although not a perfect process, peer review increases the likelihood that published reports are reliable and useful sources of information. Many controversial treatments, however, do not receive this kind of scrutiny and are instead publicized through press releases to the popular media, websites, advertisements, workshops, and the like.

8. *Is the treatment described by terms that appear to be scientific but upon further examination are found not to be scientific at all?* Controversial treatments often use scientific-sounding jargon to describe ideas that lack a scientific foundation. For example, the developer of sensory integration therapy (SIT) asserted, "Sensations [from activities such as riding a scooter board] and the resulting movements leave memories stored in his brain, and so the child gradually makes his body percept more accurate" (Ayres, 1979, p. 143). However, no direct evidence of changes in the brain or behavior is provided. Thus, despite the technical terms, the reported benefits are merely the subjective impressions of one practitioner, rather than the results of scientific study.

9. *Is the treatment based on grandiose claims or poorly described outcomes?* Many controversial treatments are said to produce a "cure," "miracle," "breakthrough," "transformation," or "revolution." Such unabashed self-promotion should be a warning that marketing rather than science is the main impetus for the treatment. Outcomes for other treatments are

described in fuzzy terms. For example, in addition to improving "body percept," SIT is said to help children pull their lives together, develop sensory maps, and improve postural and equilibrium responses (Ayres, 1979, pp. 143–147). Because these outcomes are so nebulous, it is impossible to test whether the intervention achieves them.

10. *Is the treatment claimed to make sense only within a vaguely described holistic framework?* Controversial treatments are often portrayed as "natural," "organic," "purifying," or "cleansing." They may also be depicted as designed to help the "whole person" through processes such as "unconditional and authentic valuing" (as in gentle teaching). The use of such feel-good words cannot substitute for a clear, concrete explanation of how the treatment works.

COMMON CONTROVERSIAL TREATMENTS FOR ASD

Sensory–Motor Therapies

Children with ASD often react incongruously to sensory input. They may be so unresponsive when their names are called that caregivers wonder whether they are deaf, yet they may cover their ears and appear pained in response to other sounds such as noises made by household appliances (Kanner, 1943). Many practitioners infer that these reactions are a sign of a sensory dysfunction that causes children with ASD to be either under-aroused or overaroused by everyday sounds, sights, and other environmental events. Many also suggest that children with ASD have a motor apraxia—difficulty in producing an adaptive response to sensory input despite having the desire and physical ability to do so. It remains unknown whether these hypotheses are correct, as research has yielded conflicting findings regarding the presence or absence of sensory dysfunction and apraxia in children with ASD (Rogers & Ozonoff, 2005). It is therefore unclear whether or how to intervene for these proposed areas of difficulty. Nevertheless, many children with ASD receive sensory–motor treatments.

Sensory Integration Therapy

Sensory integration therapy (SIT) is designed to address sensory dysfunction through activities that provide vestibular, proprioceptive, or tactile senations (Ayres, 1972, 1979). Vestibular activities focus on the movement of the body through space and include swinging, rolling, jumping on a trampoline, and riding on scooter boards. Proprioceptive activities emphasize stimulating the muscles and joints and may consist of "smooshing" the child between gymnasium pads or pillows to provide "deep pressure" or providing "joint compression" by repeatedly tightening the individual's joints at the wrist or elbow. Tactile activities pertain to the child's responses to being touched; examples include brushing the child's body and providing textured toys for the child to use during play.

The application of a "sensory diet" is a related clinical practice in which practitioners develop individualized plans to meet the presumed sensory needs of the child with ASD. Such a plan may include a schedule for having children play gross motor games, wear weighted vests or wrist bands, put on a body sock, brush their gums and massage their faces, and modify their environment (e.g., adjusting the lighting) in order to improve or alter arousal states and affect (Alhage-Kientz, 1996).

SIT practitioners are usually occupational therapists (OTs). These practitioners typically conduct 30- to 60-minute sessions one to three times per week and often direct parents and paraprofessionals such as classroom aides to carry out the intervention at other times throughout the day (Bundy & Murray, 2002). Most OTs view SIT as a standard part of treatment for children with ASD (Watling, Dietz, Kanny, & McLaughlin, 1999), and SIT takes place in a variety of settings, including many public schools, residential placements, and independent agencies (Smith, Mruzek, & Mozingo, 2005).

Four published reports contained objective data on SIT for children with autism: one case study (Ray, King, & Grandin, 1988), two uncontrolled studies with small samples and no comparison groups (Case-Smith & Bryan, 1999; Linderman & Stewart, 1998), and one study with a larger sample that failed to demonstrate gains in speech following participation in sensory activities (Reilly, Nelson, & Bundy, 1984). Dawson and Watling (2000) commented, "There exist so few studies that conclusions cannot be drawn" (p. 419).

Auditory Integration Training

Auditory integration training (AIT; Berard, 1993) is based on the view that the hypersensitive hearing displayed by some children with ASD causes them to avoid social interactions and tune out what others say. AIT practitioners are human service professionals who complete a training workshop and obtain certification. The Tomatis and Berard methods are the most influential forms of AIT. Both begin with an audiogram (observations by an AIT practitioner) to determine the frequencies at which a child's hearing appears to be too sensitive. Children then listen to music played through a device that filters out the threshold frequencies identified by the audiogram. In the Tomatis method, children may also speak into a microphone as their own filtered speech is played back. This method typically involves 60–90 hours of intervention in sessions lasting 1–3 hours. The Berard method involves a total of 10 hours of intervention over a 2-week period. Several small RCTs of AIT have obtained mixed results, with some studies showing benefits and others failing to do so

(Sinha, Silove, Wheeler, & Williams, 2005). Additional studies are needed to evaluate AIT more conclusively.

Facilitated Communication

Facilitated communication (FC; Biklen, 1993) derives from the hypothesis that individuals with ASD have a motor apraxia that prevents them from expressing themselves despite a sophisticated understanding of spoken and written language. To overcome this conjectured problem, trained facilitators (professionals or nonprofessionals who complete a workshop on the treatment) hold a person's hands, wrists, or arms to spell messages on a keyboard or a board with printed letters. FC practitioners assert that this intervention suddenly and dramatically increases appropriate language displayed by individuals with ASD. Investigators have evaluated this assertion in numerous studies by testing whether the facilitator or the individual with ASD produced the communications made during FC. For example, in some evaluations, the facilitators and children were simultaneously but separately asked questions. Sometimes the questions were the same for both the facilitators and the children; other times, they differed. When the questions were the same, the child's answers were often correct; but when the questions were different, most answers were in response to the facilitator's questions, not the child's. This evidence, replicated across several hundred children with ASD, shows that the facilitators rather than the individuals with ASD control the communication and that FC does not improve language skills (Mostert, 2001). Therefore, FC is an inappropriate intervention for individuals with ASD.

Rapid Prompting Method

In the rapid prompting method (RPM), practitioners attempt to compensate for the hypothesized sensory overload and apraxia in children with ASD by continually speaking and requesting responses so that the children stay attentive (Mukhopadhyay, 2003). To encourage successful responding, they initially focus on having children observe correct responses. As the children progress, practitioners begin to ask children to point to correct responses. Subsequently, they teach children to spell answers on a keyboard or write them down, often attaching a rubber band to the children's hands to help them hold the pen or pencil. No scientific studies have evaluated RPM.

Vision Therapy

Many children with ASD have poor eye contact. Some also flap their hands or fingers in front of their eyes repeatedly, look at objects out of the corners of their eyes, and display unusually intense interest in visual stimuli such as spinning objects. Vision therapy is intended to address these problems through the use of tinted eyeglasses, prisms, or eye exercises (Kaplan, Edelson, & Seip, 1998). Tinted eyeglasses, such as Irlen lenses, are thought to reduce "perceptual stress" by filtering out certain colors, decreasing glare, or dimming the light. Prisms are used to displace children's field of vision to the left, right, up, or down. Eye exercises emphasize relaxing the eyes or activities such as following a series of blinking lights, gazing at a string of objects, or working on hand–eye coordination. There are no studies on vision therapy for children with ASD. Studies of other populations such as children with learning disabilities indicate that it is likely to be ineffective (Rawstron, Burley, & Elder, 2005).

Bonding Therapies

Although impaired reciprocal social interaction is a central feature of ASD, most children with ASD form attachments to their caregivers. Like typically developing children, children with ASD may become distressed upon separation, are eager to see caregivers when reunited, and stay nearer to caregivers than to unfamiliar adults (Sigman & Mundy, 1989). Nevertheless, a number of interventions are intended to facilitate attachment or bonding between individuals with ASD and their caregivers. In holding therapy (Tinbergen & Tinbergen, 1983; Welch, 1987), the mother forcibly holds the child close to her so as to cause "the autistic defense . . . to crumble" (Welch, 1987, p. 48). Options (also called Son-Rise) offers individualized, loving attention to a child in a residential setting for most of the child's waking hours (Kaufman, 1976). As described earlier, "gentle teaching" focuses on providing unconditional support and encouragement to individuals with ASD (McGee & Gonzales, 1990). None of these therapies have been evaluated in scientific studies on children with ASD, although one study suggests that gentle teaching may be nonbeneficial for children with other developmental disabilities (Mudford, 1995). Given that attachment difficulties are not characteristic of most children with ASD, the theoretical rationale for bonding therapies is suspect.

CAM Interventions

Diets

Many children with ASD have idiosyncratic eating habits: Some are very picky about what they eat, and others crave large amounts of certain foods. A few professionals suggest that these behaviors reflect a serious underlying problem, namely, a difficulty in tolerating certain substances found in various foods. They argue that eliminating these substances from children's diets may alleviate physical discomfort, which may lead to an improvement in their behavior (Reiten, 1987).

The most common special diet for children with ASD is the gluten-free–casein-free (GfCf) diet. Gluten is an elastic protein in wheat that gives cohesiveness to dough. Casein is a protein in milk, cheese, and other dairy products. Numerous parents and professionals aver that the GfCf diet cures a few people with ASD and helps many others. The diet reportedly improves communication, social interaction, and sleep patterns while reducing autistic behaviors and digestive problems such as diarrhea. These benefits are said to occur rapidly, often within a few days of starting the diet (Seroussi, 2000).

Supporters of the GfCf diet propose that people with autism have a metabolic disorder that causes them to break down gluten and casein into opioids, which are peptides produced by the body and found in drugs such as morphine (Shattock, Kennedy, Rowell, & Berney, 1990). They also suggest that people with autism have leaky guts, which allow some of the opioids to escape from the digestive system and circulate to other parts of the body, including the brain (Horvath, Papadimitriou, Rabsztyn, Drachenberg, & Tildon, 1999). According to the theory, these problems create an addiction to foods that contain gluten and casein, as evidenced by the strong cravings that people with autism often have for such foods. The cravings are thought to be symptomatic of pervasive toxic effects in the brain, thus resulting in autism. The intended purpose of the GfCf diet is to reverse the damage by detoxifying the brain.

Although some investigators have presented evidence that people with autism overproduce opioids and have leaky guts (Reichelt, Knivsberg, Nodland, & Lind, 1994), other investigators have failed to replicate these findings (Williams & Marshall, 1992). Only two small RCTs have evaluated the GfCf diet. Knivsberg, Reichelt, Hoien, and Nodland (2002) found that although the diet did not significantly improve cognitive, language, or motor skills, it may have reduced autistic behaviors such as repetitive statements. Elder et al. (2006) reported that the diet did not produce significant changes for children with autism in their study. Additional study of the theoretical basis and efficacy of the GfCf diet is an important area for research (Millward, Ferriter, Calver, & Connell-Jones, 2004). Because the removal of gluten and casein may compromise a child's nutritional intake, dietary counseling is recommended for families who place their children on the diet (Levy & Hyman, 2003).

Vitamin Therapies

A few investigators assert that some children with autism require much higher doses of certain nutrients than can be obtained from any traditional diet (Rimland, 1987). According to these investigators, children with autism have a genetic or acquired medical disorder (as yet unspeci-fied) that increases their need for specific nutrients. Research based on this hypothesis has centered on the use of a combination of vitamin B_6 (pyridoxine) and magnesium. B_6 is a chemical whose primary function is to aid in protein digestion; magnesium is a mineral that helps build bones, maintain nerve and muscle cells, and enhance the function of vari-ous enzymes in the body. Three small-scale RCTs indicated that B_6 with magnesium is ineffective in changing behavior (Findling et al., 1997; Kuriyama et al., 2002; Tolbert, Haigler, Waits, & Dennis, 1993), but fur-ther study may be warranted (Nye & Brice, 2005).

Other common vitamin therapies include (1) dimethylglycine (DMG), which assists in the metabolism of amino acids and other sub-stances, (2) vitamin A (often in tablets of fish oil or omega-3 fatty acids), (3) vitamin B_{12} (folic acid or folate), and (4) vitamin C. The theoretical basis for these vitamin therapies is unclear, and none have been evaluated in well-designed studies of children with ASD.

Treatment of Infections

Some researchers contend that children with ASD may have impaired immune systems (see Lawler, Croen, Grether, & van de Water, 2004, for a review), though evidence for such an impairment remains inconclusive. One small study indicated that an antibiotic, vancolycin, may increase the amount of communication initiated by children with ASD (Sandler et al., 2000), but until this finding is replicated, it is premature to recommend antibiotic treatment. Antifungal or antiyeast medications such as mycos-tatin (Nystatin) or fluconazole (Diflucan) are sometimes also prescribed. However, well-designed studies have not been conducted to examine the effectiveness of these medications in changing the behavior of children with ASD (Levy & Hyman, 2005). Moreover, the diagnostic tests used to identify fungal or yeast infections have not been empirically validated and must be viewed with skepticism. Intravenous injections of immunoglobu-lin treatments (IV-Ig) have been proposed as a way to improve immune functioning but have also not been evaluated in well-designed studies (Levy & Hyman, 2005).

Immunizations and Nonvaccination

Much concern has arisen among the general public that vaccines cause autism (Kennedy, 2005), and this concern has significant public health implications, as it has apparently contributed to a reduction in vaccination rates in many countries (Fleck, 2003). Initially, it was suggested that some vaccines, particularly diphtheria–tetanus–pertusis (DTaP) and measles-mumps–rubella (MMR), may trigger out-of-control infections or immune responses, leading to brain damage and the onset of autism (Coulter, 1990). This view was largely set aside and replaced with a new hypothesis, that the MMR vaccine may cause bowel inflammation, hindering the absorption of essential vitamins and nutrients (Wakefield et al., 1998). The Wakefield et al. hypothesis generated enormous publicity and led to numerous studies evaluating the putative links among the MMR vaccine, bowel inflammation, and ASD. A review of 31 well-designed studies found no evidence for the proposed links (Demicheli, Jefferson, Rivetti, & Price, 2005). For instance, a Japanese city stopped administering the MMR vaccine in 1993, but the prevalence of ASD did not decrease after the vaccine's removal (Honda, Shimzu, & Rutter, 2005). Further weakening the MMR hypothesis, 10 of the 13 authors of the Wakefield et al. (1998) report retracted their initial conclusion that findings in the report showed a possible connection between MMR and ASD (Murch et al., 2004). Thus, many studies have failed to find an association between the MMR vaccine and ASD (Demicheli et al., 2005).

As evidence began to accumulate against a link between the MMR vaccine and ASD, another hypothesized connection between vaccines and ASD was advanced: Bernard, Enayati, Redwood, Roger, and Binstock (2000) and subsequent writers proposed that vaccines containing thimerosal, which is a mercury compound used as a preservative, may cause autism. In 1999, the U.S. Food and Drug Administration (FDA) mandated the removal of this substance from all childhood vaccines, including DTaP, haemophilus influenza type b (Hib), and hepatitis B. (The MMR vaccine never contained thimerosal; some influenza vaccines continue to include trace amounts.) This action is sometimes cited as an indication that the FDA had evidence of a link between thimerosal and ASD or other conditions (Kennedy, 2005). However, studies indicate that thimerosal is *not* associated with ASD (Institute of Medicine, 2004). Doses of thimerosal in vaccines are excreted quickly and appear to pose little risk (Pichichero, Cernichiari, Lopreiato, & Treanor, 2002). More generally, these studies confirm that vaccines are safe and that withholding them poses much greater risk than administering them to children with or without ASD.

Secretin

Secretin is a hormone that is secreted by the lining of the duodenum (part of the small intestine) and assists with food digestion. In 1998, news stories publicized a report that intravenous injections of secretin led to symptom improvement in three children with ASD (Horvath et al., 1998). Some news stories also described a child whose ASD was said to be cured by secretin. Subsequently, secretin attracted a great deal of interest from families and practitioners, and many researchers began to study it. Investigators discovered that secretin receptors resided in both the gut and the brain and that secretin can cross the blood–brain barrier, indicating that it could potentially influence brain function (Levy & Hyman, 2005). However, an authoritative review identified 14 RCTs of secretin, all of which found secretin to be ineffective, and concluded, "There is no evidence that single or multiple dose intravenous secretin is effective and as such it should not currently be recommended or administered as a treatment for autism" (Williams, Wray, & Wheeler, 2005).

Chelation

Chelation therapy involves administering a substance that binds to metal ions so that the metal can be excreted from the body. The substance, called the chelating agent, can be administered intravenously, intramuscularly, orally, or rectally. With the increased interest in the (unproven) hypothesis that ASD is caused by exposure to mercury, chelation has become a common intervention for children with ASD. Chelating agents that are used for children with ASD include disodium versante (Na_2-EDTA), calcium disodium versante ($CaNa_2$-EDTA), dimercaptosuccinic acid (DMSA), sodium dimercaptopropanesulfonate (DMPS), and thiamine tetrahydrofurfyl disulfide (TTFD). However, none of these agents cross the blood–brain barrier in significant amounts; thus, their theoretical basis is dubious, as there is no mechanism by which any chelating agent could reverse the brain damage associated with ASD (Levy & Hyman, 2005). Only Na_2-EDTA and DMSA have been approved by the FDA to treat acute poisoning from heavy metals, and Na_2-EDTA is not effective in removing mercury from the body. These and other chelating agents have significant risks of side effects. For example, in August 2005, a 5-year-old boy died as a result of chelation therapy with intravenous Na_2-EDTA (Kane, 2006). Thus, although no RCTs have evaluated any form of chelation therapy for children with ASD, and although other chelating agents may not be as dangerous as Na_2-EDTA, this therapeutic approach appears implausible and unacceptably risky. It should not be used as a treatment for ASD.

Discussion

Table 9.4 summarizes common controversial therapies and their intended outcomes. The preceding sections reveal that several of these therapies have undergone extensive evaluation in well-controlled studies (providing Grade I evidence, according to the criteria in Table 9.1) and have clearly been refuted: facilitated communication, secretin, and nonvaccination. Therefore, a strong recommendation can be made *against* implementing these treatments. Chelation, although not evaluated in well-controlled

TABLE 9.4. Common Controversial Treatments for ASD

Intervention	Example of method	Intended outcome
Sensory–motor therapies		
Sensory integration therapy	Repeated exposure to vestibular, proprioceptive, and tactile activities	Organize sensory input and reduce anxiety associated with hypersensitivity to sensations
Auditory integration therapy	Headphones to listen to filtered sound frequencies	Reduce sensitivity to sounds, thereby increasing social interaction and attentiveness
Facilitated communication	Physical support given by placing a practitioner's hand on the child's arm or hand; with support, child expresses ideas via picture board, typewriter, or computer	Overcome motor apraxia to enable communication
Rapid prompting method	Continuous verbal requesting in order to maintain attending behavior; children initially observe correct responses to requests, then are required to emit progressively more active responses	Compensate for sensory overload and apraxia to improve communication
Vision therapy	Use of tinted eyeglasses, prism lenses, or eye exercises	Improve eye contact and diminish repetitive behaviors that involve visual stimuli such as spinning objects
Bonding therapies		
Options or Son-Rise, holding therapy, gentle teaching	Giving unconditional loving attention to the child	Increase attachment to familiar adults
CAM interventions		
Diets	Removal of gluten and casein from the diet	Heal leaky gut and detoxify the brain of opiods
Vitamin therapies	Vitamin or nutritional supplements: vitamin B_6 + magnesium; DMG; vitamin A; vitamin B_{12} (folate); vitamin C	Alter neurotransmitter levels to produce global improvements in behavior
Treatment of infections	Antibiotic or antifungal treatments; IV-Ig	Eliminate infectious disease, improve immune functioning

(continued)

TABLE 9.4. *(continued)*

Intervention	Example of method	Intended outcome
CAM interventions *(cont.)*		
Nonvaccination	Withholding vaccines such as MMR	Avoid bowel inflammation or metal toxicity to prevent ASD
Secretin	Intravenous injection	Alter activity of secretin receptors in gut and brain
Chelation	Oral or intravenous administration of a chelating agent such as DMSA or EDTA	Remove heavy metals such as mercury from the body to restore brain functioning

studies, has a faulty theoretical basis and an intolerable level of risk; as such, it is also an intervention to avoid. The remaining controversial therapies have received little or no scientific testing, leaving only Grade III or Grade IV evidence, as outlined in Table 9.1. These treatments have unknown effects, and families and practitioners should be cautious about them (either deciding not to implement them or monitoring them carefully). Some treatments, such as bonding therapies, are based on obsolete theories about ASD, and interventions such as some sensory–motor therapies, diets, and vitamins are based on unproven theories that may merit further research.

IMPLICATIONS FOR THE SCIENTIFIC COMMUNITY

Ideally, the scientific community could settle controversies about treatments by providing evidence on their effectiveness or lack thereof. The reality, however, is somewhat more complicated. As detailed in the preceding section, controversial treatments are many and varied, and new ones continually emerge. Therefore, it is not feasible to evaluate all controversial treatments adequately. Even when a treatment has been studied extensively and found to be ineffective, some families and practitioners remain steadfast in their belief that the treatment is beneficial. For example, FC, secretin, and nonvaccination still have many ardent supporters in spite of devastating evidence against them. One study revealed that, despite being informed of the negative results from a secretin study in which they participated, 69% of families remained interested in receiving secretin as a treatment for their children with ASD (Sandler et al., 1999). This enduring support shows that the hope for effective interventions and the appeal of pseudoscientific claims may be so strong that they override any amount of scientific data that researchers may produce.

Nevertheless, the scientific community can play a constructive role in responding to controversial treatments. Research that pertains to the theoretical basis of the treatments may be especially useful. For example, until the 1980s, many bonding therapies were proposed for children with ASD (discussed by Smith, 1993). However, with the increase in research during the 1980s regarding social deficits displayed by children with ASD, interest in bonding therapies may have waned as it became apparent that bonding was not a primary concern for most of these children. In contrast, unusual sensory–motor behaviors, which are also a central feature of ASD, have generated much less research, and no generally accepted scientific theory accounts for these behaviors (Rogers & Ozonoff, 2005). Perhaps as a result, sensory–motor and dietary interventions continue to proliferate. Other controversial treatments, particularly CAM interventions, are based in part on the belief that there is an epidemic of ASD and that recent changes in children's environments, such as the introduction of new vaccines or exposure to toxic substances, must be responsible. Although estimates of the prevalence of ASD have certainly increased since the 1980s (Fombonne, 2003), it remains unclear whether this increase reflects an actual rise in the prevalence in ASD or merely improved detection and broadened diagnostic criteria for the disorder. Extensive research is now under way to resolve this issue, and such investigations may influence the extent to which the belief in an autism epidemic continues to drive the development of new CAM interventions.

Scientific evaluations of treatments, as well as position statements by professional organizations based on these evaluations, can also have an effect on controversial treatments, albeit a limited one. For example, a search of the database Lexis/Nexis was conducted for reports on several controversial treatments in the popular media (newspapers and magazines, television, and radio); these reports were rated as having a positive, neutral, or negative stance toward a particular treatment. Figure 9.1 shows reports on FC. This intervention was virtually unknown prior to 1990 but suddenly became a topic of many favorable media reports in the early 1990s. Reports often described miraculous improvements in the communications made by children with ASD. From the start, scientists expressed skepticism about the validity of FC and responded quickly by conducting single-case studies of FC involving many children with autism. By 1994, studies had unequivocally shown FC to be ineffective (Green & Shane, 1994), and professional organizations presented position statements advising against its use (American Psychological Association, 1994). As shown in Figure 9.1, positive media references to FC sharply decreased at that time, suggesting that the studies and position statements may have created doubts about the intervention. However, the reports remained mostly favorable and rose in frequency again in 2004, perhaps because a film on FC was nominated for an Academy Award that year. Thus, evidence from scientific evaluations did not put an end to public interest in FC, but did appear to have an impact on media coverage (perhaps only temporarily).

Figure 9.2 displays media reports on secretin, which attracted a flurry of publicity in 1998 when an article described favorable outcomes in three children with ASD. Within weeks, the National Institutes of Health (1998) issued a call for the scientific evaluation of secretin, and scientists responded with three RCTs published in 1999, all finding secretin to be ineffective. At that time, as revealed in Figure 9.2, skeptical media reports on secretin began to surface, but positive reports also continued to flourish. As with FC, negative research findings appear to have dampened enthusiasm about this treatment, though they did not eliminate it.

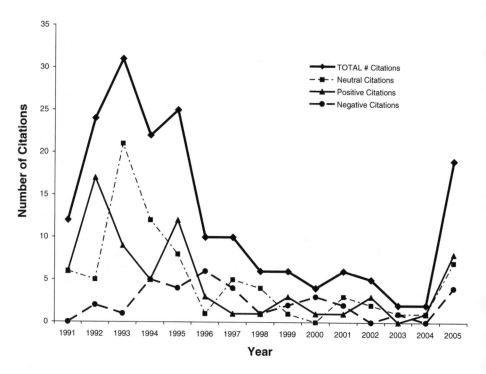

FIGURE 9.1. References to facilitated communication in the popular media (1991–2005).

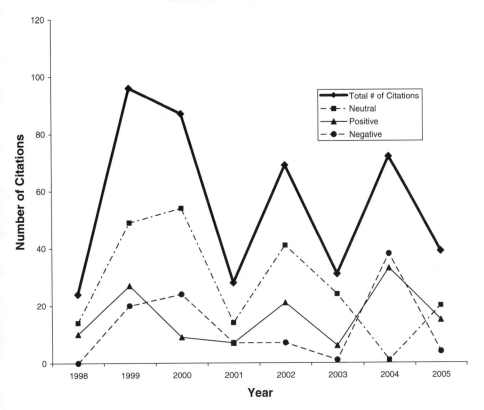

FIGURE 9.2. References to secretin in the popular media (1997–2005).

The influence of research findings on public opinion may be enhanced by illustrating them with case examples. For example, media reports on FC supplemented discussions of research findings with demonstrations on television that the facilitators rather than the children with ASD were controlling the communication (Palfreman, 1993). As another example, the media report of a death resulting from chelation in 2005 was followed by a number of other media reports cautioning against this intervention, as shown in Figure 9.3. Many of these reports cited scientific evidence for the risks and limitations of chelation, in addition to commenting on the tragic death.

In sum, although not a perfect solution, research on characteristics of ASD, scientific evaluation of controversial treatments, and position statements by professional organizations can influence public interest in a treatment, particularly if presented in an accessible format (e.g., with case reports).

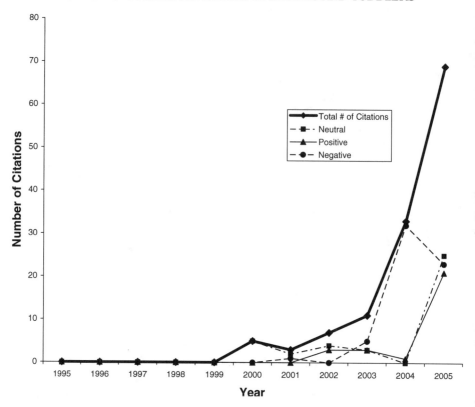

FIGURE 9.3. References to chelation therapy in the popular media (1995–2005).

IMPLICATIONS FOR CLINICAL PRACTICE

Given the prevalence and durability of controversial treatments for ASD, practitioners who assess and treat children with ASD can neither ignore nor dismiss such treatments. Instead, they must anticipate that the treatments will be appealing to many families. To be in a position to help families make informed decisions, practitioners can encourage families to discuss controversial treatments by asking direct, nonjudgmental questions about treatments that families have tried or considered. Practitioners can also show an awareness of and compassion for the many understandable motives that families may have for trying unproven or even disproven approaches (Committee on Children with Disabilities, 2001).

Open discussion on controversial treatments creates an opportunity for practitioners to present information on how to distinguish between scientific and pseudoscientific treatments, and to review what is known and unknown from relevant research. Research supports clear recommendations against some treatments, notably FC, secretin, and nonvaccination. It also provides reasons to be skeptical about other treatments such as AIT. However, because of the large number of controversial treatments available, practitioners may not always be familiar with a particular treatment or have up-to-date knowledge of the research on that treatment. Under this circumstance, practitioners can express a willingness to learn about the treatment, review information that families bring, and describe criteria they would use to gauge whether the treatment appears promising.

Finally, practitioners can advocate for and, if resources are available, assist with an objective evaluation of a controversial treatment so that families can assess the treatment efficacy themselves. Guidelines for conducting this evaluation include the following (Hyman & Levy, 2000): First, make only one treatment change at a time and hold other treatments constant. Second, identify specific target behaviors to be addressed by the treatment, and use objective measures to obtain a baseline of this behavior prior to treatment. Finally, monitor ongoing changes in the target behavior with objective measures obtained by raters who are blind to the treatment (e.g., a teacher who is unaware of changes in vitamin consumption rate).

In some settings, such as schools, it is often possible to go a step further and conduct single-case experiments in which a child with ASD serves as his or her own control (Smith et al., 2005). The multielement design (also called alternating treatment design) may be especially useful because it yields quick results. The design involves implementing a treatment on alternate days or in alternate sessions. During the other days or sessions, a baseline is in effect (i.e., no intervention is provided) or another treatment is provided. Kay and Vyse (2005) used this approach to evaluate the effects of prism glasses on appropriate walking by an 8-year-old boy with ASD. Data are shown in Figure 9.4 and reveal that prism glasses interfered with appropriate walking, rather than helping. As a result, the intervention was discontinued.

A limitation of the alternating treatment design is that it is appropriate only when treatment effects are observable within a single day or session. Thus, if an intervention is said to require multiple days or weeks to change the target behavior, other designs must be considered. A useful example is the reversal design, in which a baseline phase is followed by a treatment phase, followed by a return to the baseline phase, and so on. Each phase lasts several sessions, days, or weeks. Figure 9.5 illustrates the use of a reversal design to evaluate the effects of an SIT intervention (brushing) for a 4-year-old boy with ASD who engaged in tantrums (screaming, crying, throwing objects, falling to the floor). During the baseline phases, Robert played with favorite toys or briefly watched vid-

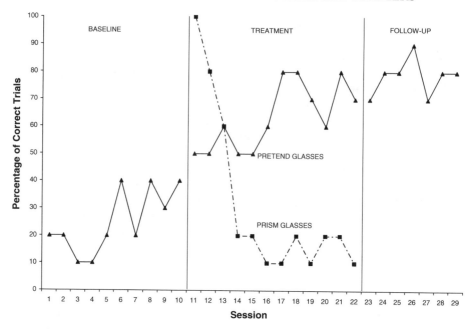

FIGURE 9.4. Alternating treatment design to evaluate the effect of prism lenses on appropriate walking by an 8-year-old boy with ASD. From Kay and Vyse (2005). Copyright 2005. Reprinted by permission of Lawrence Erlbaum Associates, Inc., a division of Taylor & Francis Group.

eos when he had breaks in learning activities. During treatment phases, Robert's mother performed the brushing at break times. Instructors, who were unaware of whether Robert was in the baseline or treatment condition, collected frequency data on tantrums during teaching sessions. Figure 9.5 shows that SIT failed to reduce this behavior (and possibly increased it). After the findings were discussed with the family, a decision was made to discontinue SIT.

CONCLUDING COMMENTS

Beyond acknowledging the many reasons for the ubiquity of controversial treatments in ASD and considering how to confront them, an important next step is to increase support for developing treatments that scientists view as promising. Until the late 1990s, little funding was available for research on ASD. The funds that did become available were devoted

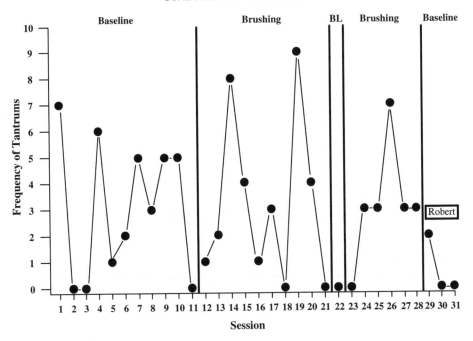

FIGURE 9.5. Reversal design to evaluate the effect of brushing on a 4-year-old boy with ASD. From Smith, Mruzek, and Mozingo (2005). Copyright 2005. Reprinted by permission of Lawrence Erlbaum Associates, Inc., a division of Taylor & Francis Group.

mainly to studies of the characteristics and causes of ASD, rather than to treatment. More recently, however, private foundations have begun to sponsor pilot studies on innovative treatments, and federal agencies have formed multisite networks to carry out large-scale clinical trials evaluating treatments that have shown promise in preliminary investigations (Vitiello & Wagner, 2004). These initiatives are encouraging. Although treatment studies often take years to complete, and although they are not infallible, they ultimately provide the firmest foundation for enabling families and practitioners to choose from an array of appropriate treatment options and for improving outcomes achieved by children with ASD.

ACKNOWLEDGMENTS

Preparation of this chapter was supported by Grant No. U54 MH066397 (Genotype and Phenotype of Autism).

REFERENCES

Alhage-Kientz, M. (1996). Sensory-based need in children with autism: Motivation for behavior and suggestions for intervention. *AOTA Developmental Disabilities Special Interest Section Newsletter, 19*(3), 1–3.

American Psychological Association (1994). *Council policy manual: M. Scientific affairs.* Retrieved January 20, 2006, from *www.apa.org/about/division/cpmscientific. html#6.*

Ayres, A. J. (1972). *Sensory integration and learning disorders.* Los Angeles: Western Psychological Services.

Ayres, A. J. (1979). *Sensory integration and the child.* Los Angeles: Western Psychological Services.

Berard, G. (1993). *Hearing equals behavior.* New Canaan, CT: Keats.

Bernard, S., Enayati, A., Redwood, L., Roger, H., & Binstock, T. (2000). Autism: a novel form of mercury poisoning. *Medical Hypotheses, 56,* 452–471.

Bettelheim, B. (1967). *The empty fortress.* New York: Free Press.

Biklen, D. (1993). *Communication unbound: How facilitated communication is challenging traditional views of ability/disability.* New York: Teachers College Press.

Biklen, D., & Cardinal, D. N. (Eds.). (1997). *Contested words, contested science: Unraveling the facilitated communication controversy.* New York: Teachers College Press.

Bouma, R., & Schweitzer, R. (1990). The impact of chronic childhood illness on family stress: A comparison between autism and cystic fibrosis. *Journal of Clinical Psychology, 46,* 722–730.

Bundy, A. C., & Murray, E. A. (2002). Sensory integration: A. Jean Ayres' theory revisited. In A. C. Bundy, S. J. Lane, & E. A. Murray (Eds.), *Sensory integration: theory and practice* (2nd ed., pp. 3–34). Philadelphia: Davis.

Case-Smith, J., & Bryan, T. (1999). The effects of occupational therapy with sensory integration emphasis on preschool-age children with autism. *American Journal of Occupational Therapy, 53,* 489–497.

Committee on Children with Disabilities, American Academy of Pediatrics. (2001). The pediatrician's role in the diagnosis and management of autism spectrum disorder in children. *Pediatrics, 107,* 1221–1226.

Coulter, H. L. (1990). *Vaccination, social violence, and criminality: The medical assault on the American brain.* Berkeley, CA: North Atlantic Books.

Dawson, G., & Watling, R. (2000). Interventions to facilitate auditory, visual, and motor integration in autism: A review of the evidence. *Journal of Autism and Developmental Disorders, 30,* 415–421.

Demicheli, V., Jefferson, T., Rivetti, A., & Price, D. (2005). Vaccines for measles, mumps and rubella in children. *Cochrane Database of Systematic Reviews, 4,* 1–36.

Elder, J. H., Shankar, M., Shuster, J., Theriaque, D., Burns, S., & Sherrill, L. (2006). The gluten-free, casein-free diet in autism: Results of a preliminary double blind clinical trial. *Journal of Autism and Developmental Disorders, 36,* 413–420.

Findling, R. L., Maxwell, K., Scotese-Wojtila, L., Huang, J., Yamashita, T., & Wiznitzer, M. (1997). High-dose pyridoxine and magnesium administration in children with autistic disorder: An absence of salutary effects in a double-blind, placebo-controlled study. *Journal of Autism and Developmental Disorders, 27*, 467–478.

Finn, P., Bothe, A. K., & Bramlett, R. E. (2005). Science and pseudoscience in communication disorders: Criteria and applications. *American Journal of Speech–Language Pathology, 14*, 172–186.

Fleck, F. (2003). UK and Italy have low MMR uptake. *British Medical Journal, 327*, 1124.

Fombonne, E. (2003). Epidemiological surveys of autism and other pervasive developmental disorders: An update. *Journal of Autism and Developmental Disorders, 34*, 365–382.

Green, C., & Shane, H. C. (1994). Science, reason, and facilitated communication. *Journal of the Association for Persons with Severe Handicaps, 19*, 151–172.

Greenspan, S., & Wieder, S. (1997). Developmental patterns and outcomes in infants and children with disorders in relating and communicating: A chart review of 200 cases of children with autistic spectrum diagnoses. *Journal of Developmental and Learning Disorders, 1*, 87–141.

Greenspan, S., & Wieder, S. (1999). A functional developmental approach to autism spectrum disorders. *Journal of the Association for Persons with Severe Handicaps, 24*, 147–161.

Hart, B., & Risley, T. R. (1980). In vivo language intervention: Unanticipated general effects. *Journal of Applied Behavior Analysis, 13*, 407–432.

Honda, H., Shimizu, Y., & Rutter, M. (2005). No effect of MMR withdrawal on the incidence of autism: A total population study. *Journal of Child Psychology and Psychiatry, 46*, 572–579.

Hoppes, K., & Harris, S. L. (1990). Perceptions of child attachment and maternal gratification in mothers of children with autism and Down syndrome. *Journal of Clinical Child Psychology, 19*, 365–370.

Horvath, K., Papadimitriou, J. C., Rabsztyn, A., Drachenberg, C., & Tildon, J. T. (1999). Gastrointestinal abnormalities in children with autistic disorder. *Journal of Pediatrics, 135*, 559–563.

Horvath, K., Stefanatos, G., Sokolski, K. N., Wachtel, R., Nabors, L., & Tildon, J. T. (1998). Improved social and language skills after secretin administration in patients with autistic spectrum disorders. *Journal of the Association for Academic Minority Physicians, 9*, 9–15.

Hyman, S. L., & Levy, S. E. (2000). Autism spectrum disorders: When traditional medicine is not enough. *Contemporary Pediatrics, 17*(10), 101–116.

Institute of Medicine. (2004). *Immunization safety review: Vaccines and autism.* Washington, DC: National Academies Press.

Joint Commission Resources. (2000). A practical system for evidence grading. *Joint Commission Journal on Quality Improvement, 26*, 700–712.

Kane, K. (2006, January 6). Death of 5-year-old boy linked to controversial chelation therapy. *Pittsburgh Post Gazette.* Retrieved January 30, 2006, from *www.post-gazette.com/pg/06006/633541.stm.*

Kanner, L. (1943). Autistic disturbances of affective contact. *Nervous Child, 2*, 217–250.

Kaplan, M., Edelson, S. M., & Seip, J. A. (1998). Behavioral changes in autistic individuals as a result of wearing ambient transitional prism lenses. *Child Psychiatry and Human Development, 29*, 65–76.

Kaufman, B. N. (1976). *Son-Rise*. New York: Harper & Row.

Kay, S., & Vyse, S. (2005). Helping parents separate the wheat from the chaff: Putting autism treatments to the test. In J. W. Jacobson & R. M. Foxx (Eds.), *Fads, dubious and improbable treatments for developmental disabilities* (pp. 265–277). Mahwah, NJ: Erlbaum.

Kennedy, R. F. (2005, June 16). Deadly immunity. *Salon.com*. Retrieved December 15, 2005, from *www.salon.com/news/feature/2005/06/16/thimerosal/index_np.html*.

Knivsberg, A-M., Reichelt, K. L., Hoien, T., & Nodland, M. (2002). A randomised, controlled study of dietary intervention in autistic syndromes. *Nutritional Neuroscience, 5,* 251–261.

Kuriyama, S., Kamiyama, M., Watanabe, M., Tamahashi, S., Muraguchi, I., Watanabe, T., et al. (2002). Pyridoxine treatment in a subgroup of children with pervasive developmental disorders. *Developmental Medicine and Child Neurology, 44,* 284–246.

Lawler, C. P., Croen, L. A., Grether, J. K., & Van de Water, J. (2004). Identifying environmental contributions to autism: Provocative clues and false leads. *Mental Retardation and Developmental Disabilities Research Reviews, 10,* 292–302.

Levy, S. E., & Hyman, S. L. (2003). Use of complementary and alternative treatments for children with autism spectrum disorders is increasing. *Pediatric Annals, 32,* 685–691.

Levy, S. E., & Hyman, S. L. (2005). Novel treatments for autistic spectrum disorders. *Mental Retardation and Developmental Disabilities Research Reviews, 11,* 131–142.

Levy, S. E., Mandell, D. S., Merhar, S., Ittenbach, R. F., & Pinto-Martin, J. A. (2003). Use of complementary and alternative medicine among children recently diagnosed with autistic spectrum disorder. *Journal of Developmental and Behavioral Pediatrics, 24,* 418–423.

Linderman, T. M., & Stewart, K. B. (1998). Sensory-integrative based occupational therapy and functional outcomes in young children with pervasive developmental disorders: A single-subject design. *American Journal of Occupational Therapy, 53,* 207–213.

Lord, C., Bristol-Power, M., Cafiero, J. M., Filipek, P. A., Gallagher, J. J., Harris, S. L., et al. (Eds.). (2002). *JADD* special issue: NAS workshop papers. *Journal of Autism and Developmental Disorders, 32,* 349–508.

Lord, C., Rutter, M., DiLavore, P., & Risi, S. (2001). ADOS: Autism Diagnostic Observation Schedule. Los Angeles: Western Psychological Services.

Lovaas, O. I., & Smith, T. (2003). Early and intensive behavioral intervention in autism. In A. E. Kazdin & J. Weisz (Eds.), *Evidence-based psychotherapies for children and youth* (pp. 325–340). New York: Guilford Press.

Luyster, R., Richler, J., Risi, S., Hsu, W. L., Dawson, G., Bernier, R., et al. (2005). Early regression in social communication in autism spectrum disorders: A CPEA Study. *Developmental Neuropsychology. 27,* 311–336.

McCracken, J. T., McGough, J., Shah, B., Cronin, P., Hong, D., Aman, M. G., et al. (2002). Risperidone in children with autism and serious behavior problems. *New England Journal of Medicine, 347,* 314–321.

McGee, J. J., & Gonzales, L. (1990). Gentle teaching and the practice of human interdependence: A preliminary group study of 15 persons with severe behavior disorders and their caregivers. In A. C. Repp & N. N. Singh (Eds.), *Perspectives on the use of nonaversive and aversive interventions for people with developmental disabilities* (pp. 215–230). Sycamore, IL: Sycamore.

Millward, C., Ferriter, M., Calver, S., & Connell-Jones, G. (2004). Gluten- and casein-free diets for autistic spectrum disorder. *Cochrane Database of Systematic Reviews, 3,* 1–14.

Mostert, M. P. (2001). Facilitated communication since 1995: A review of published studies. *Journal of Autism and Developmental Disorders, 31,* 287–313.

Mudford, O. C. (1995). Review of the gentle teaching data. *American Journal on Mental Retardation, 99,* 345–355.

Mukhopadhyay, T. R. (2003). *The Mind Tree: A miraculous boy breaks the silence of autism.* New York: Arcade.

Murch, S. H., Anthony, A., Casson, D. H., Malik, M., Berelowitz, M., Dhillon, A. P., et al. (2004). Retraction of an interpretation. *Lancet, 363,* 750.

National Institutes of Health. (1998, October 16). *The use of secretin to treat autism.* Retrieved January 27, 2006, from *www.nichd.nih.gov/new/releases/secretin.cfm.*

National Research Council. (2001). *Educating children with autism.* Washington, DC: National Academy Press.

Newsom, C., & Hovanitz, C. A. (2005). The nature and value of empirically validated interventions. In J. W. Jacobson & R. M. Foxx (Eds.), *Fads, dubious and improbable treatments for developmental disabilities* (pp. 31–44). Mahwah, NJ: Erlbaum.

Nye, C., & Brice, A. (2005). Combined vitamin B_6-magnesium treatment in autism spectrum disorder. *Cochrane Database of Systematic Reviews, 3,* 1–17.

Palfreman, J. (Director). (1993, October 19). Prisoners of silence. In J. Palfreman (Producer), *Frontline.* Washington, DC: Public Broadcasting Service.

Pichichero, M. E., Cernichiari, E., Lopreiato, J., & Treanor, J. (2002). Mercury concentrations and metabolism in infants receiving vaccines containing thimerosal: A descriptive study. *Lancet, 360,* 1737–1741.

Rawstron, J. A., Burley, C. D., & Eldeer, M. J. (2005). A systematic review of the applicability and efficacy of eye exercises. *Journal of Pediatric Ophthalmology and Strabismus, 42,* 82–88.

Ray, T. C., King, L. K., & Grandin, T. (1988). The effectiveness of self-initiated vestibular stimulation in producing speech sounds in an autistic child. *Occupational Therapy Journal of Research, 8,* 186–190.

Reichelt, K. L., Knivsberg, A. M., Nodland, M., & Lind, G. (1994). Nature and consequences of hyperpeptiduria and bovine casomorphins found in autistic syndromes. *Developmental Brain Dysfunction, 7,* 71–85.

Reilly, C., Nelson, D. L., & Bundy, A. C. (1984). Sensorimotor versus fine motor activities in eliciting vocalization in autistic children. *Occupational Therapy Journal of Research, 3,* 199–212.

Reiten, D. J. (1987). Nutrition and developmental disabilities: Issues in chronic care. In E. Schopler & G. B. Mesibov (Eds.), *Neurobiological issues in autism* (pp. 373–388). New York: Plenum Press.

Research Units on Pediatric Psychopharmacology Autism Network. (2005). Randomized, controlled, crossover trial of methylphenidate in pervasive developmental disorders with hyperactivity. *Archives of General Psychiatry, 62,* 1266–1274.

Rimland, B. (1964). *Infantile autism: The syndrome and its implication for a neural theory of behavior.* New York: Appleton-Century-Crofts.

Rimland, B. (1987). Megavitamin B₆ and magnesium in the treatment of autistic children and adults. In E. Schopler & G. B. Mesibov (Eds.), *Neurobiological issues in autism* (pp. 390–405). New York: Plenum Press.

Rimland, B. (1992). The FDA's war against health. *Autism Research Review International, 6*(2), 4.

Rimland, B. (2000). The most air-tight study in psychiatry?: Vitamin B₆ in autism. *Autism Research Review International, 14*(3), 3.

Rogers, S. J., & Ozonoff, S. (2005). What do we know about sensory dysfunction in autism?: A critical review of the empirical evidence. *Journal of Child Psychology and Psychiatry, 46,* 1255–1268.

Rutter, M., LeCouteur, A., & Lord, C. (2003). *ADI-R: The Autism Diagnostic Interview–Revised.* Los Angeles: Western Psychological Services.

Sandler, A. D., Sutton, K. A., DeWeese, J., Girardi, M. A., Sheppard, V., & Bodfish, J. W. (1999). Lack of benefit of a single dose of synthetic human secretin in the treatment of autism and pervasive developmental disorder. *New England Journal of Medicine, 341,* 1801–1806.

Sandler, R. H., Finegold, S. M., Bolte, E. R., Buchanan, C. P., Maxwell, A. P., Vaisanen, M. L., et al. (2000). Short-term benefit from oral vancomycin treatment of regressive-onset autism. *Journal of Child Neurology, 15,* 429–435.

Seroussi, K. (2000). *Unraveling the mystery of autism and pervasive developmental disorder: A mother's story of research and recovery.* New York: Simon & Schuster.

Shattock, P., Kennedy, A., Rowell, F., & Berney, T. (1990). Role of neuropeptides in autism and their relationships with classical neurotransmitters. *Brain Dysfunction, 3,* 328–345.

Sigman, M., & Mundy, P. (1989). Social attachments in autistic children. *Journal of the American Academy of Child and Adolescent Psychiatry, 28,* 74–81.

Sinha, Y., Silove, N., Wheeler, D., & Williams, K. (2005). Auditory integration training and other sound therapies for autism spectrum disorders. *Cochrane Database of Systematic Reviews, 3,* 1–22.

Smith, T. (1993). Autism. In T. Giles (Ed.), *Effective psychotherapies* (pp. 107–133). New York: Plenum Press.

Smith, T., & Antolovich, M. (2000). Parental perceptions of supplemental interventions received by young children with autism in intensive behavior analytic treatment. *Behavioral Interventions, 15,* 83–97.

Smith, T., Mruzek, D., & Mozingo, D. (2005). Sensory integrative therapy. In J. W. Jacobson & R. M. Foxx (Eds.), *Fads, dubious and improbable treatments for developmental disabilities* (pp. 331–350). Mahwah, NJ: Erlbaum.

Smith, T., Scahill, L., Dawson, G., Guthrie, D., Lord, C., Odom, S., et al. (2007). Designing research studies on psychosocial interventions in autism. *Journal of Autism and Developmental Disorders, 37,* 354–366.

Tinbergen, W., & Tinbergen, E. A. (1983). *Autistic children: New hope for a cure.* London: Allen and Unwin.

Tolbert, L., Haigler, T., Waits, M. M., & Dennis, T. (1993). Brief report: Lack of response in an autistic population to a low dose clinical trial of pyridoxine plus magnesium. *Journal of Autism and Developmental Disabilities, 23,* 193–199.

Vitiello, B., & Wagner, A. (2004). Government initiatives in autism clinical trials. *CNS Spectrums, 9,* 66–70.

Wakefield, A. J., Murch, S. H., Anthony, A., Linnell, J., Casson, D. M., Malik, M., et al. (1998). Ileal-lymphoid-nodular hyperplasia, non-specific colitis, and pervasive developmental disorder in children. *Lancet, 351,* 637–641.

Watling, R., Deitz, J., Kanny, E. M., & McLaughlin, J. F. (1999). Current practice of occupational therapy for children with autism. *American Journal of Occupational Therapy, 53,* 489–497.

Welch, M. G. (1987). Toward prevention of developmental disorders. *Pennsylvania Medicine, 90,* 47–52.

Williams, K. M., & Marshall, T. (1992). Urinary protein patterns in autism as revealed by high resolution two-dimensional electrophoresis. *Biochemical Society Transactions, 20,* 189S.

Williams, K. W., Wray, J. J., & Wheeler, D. M. (2005). Intravenous secretin for autism spectrum disorder. *Cochrane Database of Systematic Reviews, 4,* 1–35.

Witwer, A., & Lecavelier, L. (2005). Treatment incidence and patterns in children and adolescents with autism spectrum disorders. *Journal of Child and Adolescent Psychopharmacology, 15,* 671–681.

CHAPTER 10

Medical Issues

FRED R. VOLKMAR
ALEXANDER WESTPHAL
ABHA R. GUPTA
LISA WIESNER

Autism is an early-onset condition characterized by impaired social skills, impaired communication skills, and associated unusual restricted interests and behavior (*Diagnostic and Statistical Manual of Mental Disorders*, fourth edition [DSM-IV]; American Psychiatric Association, 1994). Autistic Disorder remains the prototypic condition within the autism spectrum disorders (ASD), although more recently other conditions in the group have been recognized. This chapter focuses on selected aspects of autism and related conditions relevant to medical care. These issues include early diagnosis and screening, etiology of autism, medical evaluations of infants with possible autism, and challenges for provision of health care in this population.

DIAGNOSTIC AND SCREENING ISSUES

Leo Kanner's (1943) initial impression was that children were born with autism, that is, that it was congenital, and although some cases of probable later onset are now recognized (see Volkmar, Chawarska, & Klin, Chapter 1, this volume) it is clear that autism is a disorder of very early onset. In addition, it is increasingly clear that outcome, in many but not all cases, can be substantially improved with early intervention (National Research Council, 2001). However, the diagnosis can be more difficult to make in infants and toddlers, reflecting both the rapid pace of developmental change and issues relative to clinical presentation before age 3 (see Volkmar et al., Chapter 1, Bishop, Luyster, Richler, & Lord, Chapter 2, this volume). Until relatively recently various factors delayed recognition of the condition and service delivery (Siegel, Pliner, Eschler, & Elliott, 1988); these included lack of awareness of the condition and the importance of early intervention, combined with the tendency to adopt a "wait and see" approach. Given these factors, delays in diagnosis were common. Fortunately, with greater awareness on the part of professionals and the public, the age of first diagnosis is now clearly decreasing, with diagnoses often made about 2 years of age or even earlier (Chawarska & Volkmar, 2005; Klin et al., 2004). At the same time, difficulties remain with early diagnosis, and at present a diagnosis is made with greatest certainty after age 3 (Lord, 1995, 2007). It is clear that despite some difficulties in the application of DSM-type diagnostic criteria (Stone et al., 1999) and the problems posed by the rapid pace of developmental change, the diagnosis can be made in infancy. Some children, however, do not exhibit all features of autism spectrum disorder (ASD) until about 3 years of age (Lord, 1995) and, much less commonly, a child who appears to have autism can dramatically and substantially improve before age 3 (Chawarska & Volkmar, 2005; Lord, 1995). As discussed by Volkmar et al., Bishop et al., and Chawarska and Bearss (Chapters 1, 2, and 3, this volume), a growing body of work has focused on early signs and symptoms of autism using a number of complementary methods—for example, prospective studies of infants at risk and retrospective methods. The features identified have been incorporated in various screening instruments, and a wide range of screening approaches are now available (Coonrod & Stone, 2005; Filipek et al., 2000).

Screening approaches vary in a number of respects—for example, specificity to autism or focused on more general developmental problems, the age of the child at screening, organization and format of the screener, and level of informant (for an exhaustive review, see Coonrod & Stone, 2005). These instruments are discussed by Bishop et al. (Chapter 2, this volume). They augment but do not replace clinical judgment. New approaches to screening are actively being developed to rely on more physiologically based approaches (Klin, Jones, Schultz, & Volkmar, 2003). The Centers for Disease Control and Prevention (*www.cdc.gov/ncbddd/dd/ ddautism.htm*) also provide useful information, including materials (in English and Spanish) for distribution to parents.

CAUSES OF AUTISM

Although Kanner's original report suggested that autism was congenital, several decades passed before the neurobiological basis of autism was clearly established (Volkmar & Klin, 2005). Kanner's observation of high levels of parental educational and occupational success in his original sample suggested an unusual high-socioeconomic-status predominance and this, along with strong interest at the time in experiential factors in pathogenesis, led to speculation that autism was caused by experience— for example, by a "refrigerator" mother unresponsive to the child's emotional needs. The early belief that autism was a form of schizophrenia complicated research studies. Typically, intensive psychotherapy for mother and child was recommended with little benefit, and an entire generation of parents felt blamed for their children's difficulties.

Beginning in the 1970s various factors helped to focus researchers on the neurobiological basis of autism. The work of Kolvin (1971) and Rutter (1972) suggested that autism was a distinctive condition and not a form of schizophrenia. As children with autism were then followed, various lines of evidence strongly suggested an important role for neurobiology in pathogenesis, such as the high rate of seizure disorders and the recognition that various medical and/or genetic conditions are sometimes associated with autism. Figure 10.1 presents data on rates of epilepsy (recurrent seizure disorder) in two samples of children with autism/ASD and a normative British sample; as is clear, infants with autism are at a much higher than expected risk for developing seizures of all types. This risk continues throughout the developmental period. Additional studies have suggested

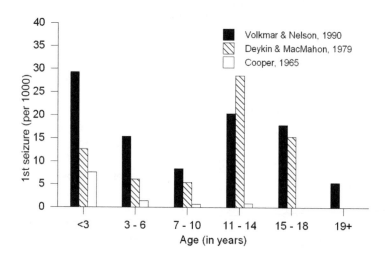

FIGURE 10.1. Rates of epilepsy (recurrent seizures) in two samples of individuals with autism/PDD (Volkmar & Nelson, 1990, and Deykin & MacMahon, 1979) and a normative British sample (Cooper, 1965). From Volkmar et al. (2007). Copyright 2007 by Lippincott Williams & Wilkins. Reprinted by permission.

changes in brain cytoarchitechure (Casanova et al., 2006), in other aspects of brain functioning (Minshew, Sweeney, Bauman, & Webb, 2005) and even in the way that the brain processes social information like human faces (Schultz et al., 2000). The present consensus is that autism is a behavioral syndrome caused by one or more factors acting on the central nervous system. Beginning with the first twin study of autism (Folstein & Rutter, 1977) there appeared to be a strong genetic basis for these problems as well.

Evidence for a Genetic Basis

Several lines of evidence support a genetic basis for ASD. Epidemiological studies reveal that ASD are the most strongly genetic of psychiatric disorders, with a heritability factor greater than 90% (Bailey, LeCouteur, Gottesman, & Bolton, 1995). Heritability, which is the proportion of phenotypic variance attributable to genetic causes, is calculated from the results of twin and family studies. Twin studies compare the rate at which a diagnosis is shared by monozygotic (MZ) twins versus dizygotic (DZ) twins. Because MZ twins are genetically identical and DZ twins share on average 50% of their genetic material, a higher rate of concordance in MZ twins suggests a genetic component to the disorder. Bailey et al. (1995) found that, for autism, the concordance rates are 60% (MZ) versus 0% (DZ), which would likely approach the sibling recurrence rate in a larger sample size. For broader spectrum diagnoses, the concordance rates are 92% versus 10%. These figures are highly divergent and indicate a strong genetic contribution to the etiology of ASD. Of note, however, is that the concordance rates for MZ twins are not 100%, which would be expected if the etiology was entirely genetic. This suggests that environmental factors also play a role. Family studies determine if the relatives of individuals with ASD more commonly have the disorder than the general population. Chakrabarti and Fombonne (2001) calculated the sibling recurrence risk for ASD to be approximately 4%, which is higher than the general prevalence rate.

Another line of evidence is the observation that there is a higher rate of chromosomal abnormalities in ASD (Veenstra-Vanderweele, Christian, & Cook, 2004). Furthermore, a proportion of cases have been associated with disorders that have well-defined genetic etiologies, such as fragile-X and tuberous sclerosis (Rutter, 2005b). However, the proportion is small; the vast majority of cases do not follow simple Mendelian patterns of inheritance, such as dominant, recessive, or X-linked. It is widely accepted that multiple genes interact to produce the disorder, with more than 15 genes likely involved (Risch et al., 1999). Along with the wide phenotypic variability, these factors make ASD very complex disorders genetically.

The intense efforts of numerous groups over the past decade are finally beginning to yield insights into the genetic basis of ASD. Researchers use a variety of techniques, such as linkage analysis, cytogenetic analysis, and candidate gene studies, to identify disease genes.

Linkage Analysis

The goal of linkage analysis is to identify chromosomal regions (loci) that are inherited by affected individuals more frequently than expected by chance. Loci are marked by DNA polymorphisms, short variable sequences that are distributed throughout the genome. The closer a marker is to a disease gene, the less chance there is for meiotic recombination between the two sites, causing them to cosegregate in families and appear to be linked. This is reflected in the logarithm of the odds (LOD) score, the likelihood that a given chromosomal locus is linked to the phenotype of interest. A LOD score of 3.0, for example, would indicate 1,000:1 odds that the locus is linked to a disease gene. A score of 3.6 is generally accepted as significant evidence for linkage in complex genetic traits (Lander & Kruglyak, 1995).

Several linkage studies have been published for ASD. The results are generally difficult to compare because of differences in the sizes of the study populations, the diagnostic instruments, inclusion and exclusion criteria, polymorphic markers, and the statistical methods used for assessing linkage. Evidence for linkage has been reported for the majority of chromosomes, although most of the LOD scores do not approach the threshold for significance. In addition, there has been little direct agreement between studies (Gupta & State, 2006). This likely reflects the differences in study design listed above and the phenotypic and genetic heterogeneity of ASD.

Still, some patterns do emerge. Among the chromosomes that are cited by multiple studies and/or have yielded the highest LOD scores are 7 and 17. Chromosome 7 contains two genes, *EN2* (engrailed 2) and *MET* (*MET* receptor tyrosine kinase), which have been associated with ASD (Benayed et al., 2005; Gharani, Benayed, Mancuso, Brzustowicz, & Millonig, 2004, Campbell et al., 2006). Chromosome 17 became an area of interest after some groups stratified their study populations by sex. Researchers have attempted to address the problem of heterogeneity in ASD by analyzing subsets of their samples that are more phenotypically homogeneous and, therefore, perhaps more genetically homogeneous, to increase the chances that common loci will be detected. Given the male predominance in ASD, it has been hypothesized that stratifying samples by sex may uncover loci that predispose boys to the disorder. This approach yielded significant LOD scores on chromosome 17 (Cantor et al., 2005, Stone et al., 2004), near the serotonin transporter gene.

Cytogenetic Analysis

Individuals with ASD carry chromosomal abnormalities at a greater frequency than the typically developing population. A recent review calculated that 4.3% of karyotypes were abnormal (Veenstra-Vanderweele et al., 2004). Abnormalities have been found on every chromosome, so that no single rearrangement is likely to account for a major fraction of cases. The advantage of cytogenetic analysis is that it can rapidly pinpoint candidate genes that may be disrupted by the chromosomal rearrangement.

The most frequent site of chromosomal abnormalities in ASD is 15q11-13, the locus for Angelman and Prader–Willi syndromes, which have some phenotypic overlap with autism. Several candidate genes are located in this region. However, none have been clearly associated with ASD. Moreover, multiple genes have been found to be physically disrupted by chromosomal rearrangements in patients with ASD (Gupta & State, 2006). None of these genes are clearly associated with the disorder either.

The promise of cytogenetic analysis was realized by the identification of the first gene reported to have clearly functional mutations in ASD. A deletion of the chromosomal region Xp22.3 in three girls with autism (Thomas et al., 1999) identified *NLGN4X* (neuroligin 4 on the X chromosome) as a candidate gene. DNA sequencing revealed deleterious mutations in this gene and *NLGN3*, another member of the neuroligin family, in individuals with ASD (Jamain et al., 2003).

Candidate Gene Studies

Studies of candidate genes are generally of two types. Association studies aim to identify common DNA variations (defined as present in 1% of the general population), and mutation screening aims to identify rare functional mutations in disease genes. Both common and rare alleles likely underlie the genetic architecture of ASD. Common variants would be expected to contribute to this relatively common group of disorders, especially to milder phenotypes and if multiple genes, each contributing a small increment of risk, are involved. Such variants would not be predicted to be subject to strong negative selection pressure. Rare mutations would be expected in genes of major effect, those that contribute to most of the phenotypic expression, and in severe phenotypes that lead to reduced social capability for reproduction. The frequency of these gene variants would be suppressed owing to natural selection.

More than one hundred genes have been tested for involvement in ASD (Wassink, Brzustowicz, Bartlett, & Szmatmari, 2004). Only recently has promising evidence for a few genes been produced. Common variants of the genes *EN2* (Benayed et al., 2005; Gharani et al., 2004) and *MET*

(Campbell et al., 2006) have been associated with ASD. *EN2* encodes a homeobox protein involved in development of the cerebellum. Mice that have been engineered to express *EN2* abnormally develop cerebellar defects (Kuemerle, Zanjani, Joyner, & Herrup, 1997; Millen, Wurst, Herrup, & Joyner, 1994; Millen, Hui, & Joyner, 1995) that are reminiscent of histopathological findings in ASD (Palmen, van Engeland, Hof, & Schmitz, 2004). *MET* is involved in cerebral (Powell, Muhlfriedel, Bolz, & Levitt, 2003) and cerebellar (Ieraci, Forni, & Ponzetto, 2002) cortex development, which have shown disruptions in ASD (Courchesne, Redcay, & Kennedy, 2004, Palmen et al., 2004). Furthermore, *MET* is involved in immune (Okunishi et al., 2005) and gastrointestinal (Ido et al., 2005) functions, which are also impaired in some patients. Rare mutations have been identified in a growing list of genes: *NLGN3* and *NLGN4X* are involved in synaptogenesis (Jamain et al., 2003); *SHANK3* (*SH3* and multiple ankyrin repeat domains 3) is involved in synaptic scaffolding and interacts with the neuroligins (Durand et al., 2007); *SLC6A4* (serotonin transporter) mediates the reuptake of serotonin from the synapse and is the target of serotonin reuptake inhibitors, which are commonly used to treat the rigidity and ritualism of ASD (Sutcliffe et al., 2005). All of these findings provide valuable starting points in the brain to unravel the pathophysiology of these disorders.

Environmental Causes of Autism

A rather different body of work has been concerned with whether autism might be caused by environmental factors, such as obstetrical risk, immunizations, heavy metals, infectious agents, or pharmacological agents. This interest can be attributed in part to the common, although controversial and unproven, belief that we are in the midst of an autism epidemic (Fombonne, 2005a). Changes in both diagnostic criteria and public awareness (Fombonne, 2005b; Volkmar et al., 1994) have certainly contributed to the rise in the diagnosis of autism. Furthermore, the more common disorders of the autism spectrum (see Volkmar et al., Chapter 1, this volume) are often incorrectly equated with autism, in the strictly defined sense.

Early studies of pre-, peri-, and neonatal complications suggested increased rates of complications in children with autism. This early interest faded, however, as the strong role of genetic factors came to be appreciated—that is, that it is quite possible that apparent increased obstetrical risk comes as a result of genetic factors in the fetus. This would be compatible with the recent (and as yet unreplicated) observation of high rates of specific placental abnormalities (persistent trophoblast inclusions) in children with autism (Anderson et al., 2007). Recent work has been generally compatible with this notion. Glasson et al. (2004), for example, noted an increased risk for pre- and perinatal complications in a large series of children with autism as compared with a sizeable sample of unaffected siblings and a population based control. Furthermore, the nonaffected siblings were more like the control subjects in their profile of complications. Hultman and Sparen (2004) suggest that prenatal insults likely represent epiphenomena of a strongly genetic disorder. It must be noted that even for identical twins the concordance for autism, strictly defined, although high, is not 100%, leaving some potential for environmental factors (including intrauterine factors) to be involved in pathogenesis (Rutter, 2005a, 2005b).

Work on potential environmental factors in autism has been complicated by a number of issues, such as difficulties in diagnosis, overreliance on case reports (with a bias for producing positive but spurious correlations), and lack of developmental data. For example, early work on children with congenital rubella suggested that they were at high risk for autism, but the severity of these children's developmental difficulties compounded diagnosis and, as time went on, the more "autistic-like" features tended to diminish (Chess, 1977). Other viruses have also been examined for a putative role in the pathogenesis of autism, including measles (Singh, Lin, & Yang, 1998), herpes simplex virus (DeLong, Bean, & Brown, 1981), mumps (Ciaranello & Ciaranello, 1995), and cytomegalovirus (Stubbs, 1978). Common to all viruses, however, is the immune response they elicit in their hosts. Recent research has begun to examine the relationship between immune system irregularities and nervous system development—in particular, whether there is a critical developmental period during which an immune insult, such as a congenital viral infection, could lead to autism (Ashwood, Wills, & Van de Water, 2006). An excellent discussion of the relationship between viruses and autism can be found in Libbey, Sweeten, McMahon, and Fujinami (2005).

Similar problems complicate the interpretation of reports of autism associated with other infections or *in utero* exposure to toxins. Thalidomide, which received much attention because of a strong association with phocomelia, also has a well-documented association with autism. *In utero* exposure to the agent was associated with a 30% prevalence of autism (Stromland, Nordin, Miller, Akerstrom, & Gillberg, 1994). However, as a consequence of thalidomide's teratogenic properties, its current distribution is extremely limited, and it is of interest only because it highlights the fact that an *in utero* insult from a pharmacological agent may lead to autism. *In utero* exposure to valproic acid, an agent effective for stabilizing moods as well as for preventing seizures, has also been examined for its role in the pathogenesis of autism. Several lines of evidence, including case reports (Williams et al., 2001) and a theoretical mechanism (Narita et al., 2002) suggest the need for additional study of this relationship. Furthermore, although valproic acid is contraindicated in pregnancy, the fact that it is so widely used would most probably lead to cases of accidental *in utero* exposure. As noted in the review of Wing and Potter (2002), none of the data on environmental causes have, as yet, been convincing.

Undoubtedly the greatest interest in environmental factors in autism has arisen because of the now widespread public conviction that the measles, mumps, and rubella (MMR) vaccine has caused an increase in rates of autism. Clearly, not all children who are immunized with the MMR vaccine become autistic. Moreover, autism as a disorder predates both the introduction of vaccines in general and the advent of the measles vaccine in particular, which was introduced in 1963 (Kanner, 1943). Thus, the question becomes whether the members of a subgroup of autistic children were developing normally until they received the MMR vaccine. This issue caught the attention of the public after it was raised by Wakefield et al. in a study of a group of 12 children, all of whom had received the MMR, all of whom had an array of gastrointestinal symptoms, and all of whom had apparently quickly lost many of their developmental milestones (Wakefield et al., 1998).

In the February 1998 issue of *The Lancet*, Wakefield et al. suggested that the measles component of the MMR vaccine could cause an enterocolitis. This enterocolitis would disrupt gut absorption, leading, according to these authors, to the differential uptake of certain specific chemicals and thence to the anomalous neurological development characteristic of autism. On the basis of epidemiological and pathophysiological evidence, several researchers, including Wakefield, had already argued that the measles virus might play a role in the pathogenesis of various forms of enterocolitis, including Crohn's disease and ulcerative colitis (Daszak et al., 1997; Ekbom, Wakefield, Zack, & Adami, 1994; Feeney, Ciegg, Winwood, & Snook, 1997; Thompson, Montgomery, Pounder, & Wakefield, 1995; Wakefield et al., 1993). The suggestion of a link between enterocolitis and autism was not new (Asperger, 1961; Walker-Smith & Andrews, 1972). However, the causal chain described by Wakefield et al. (1993), as well as several of its components, and the resulting conclusion that measles immunization could cause autism, was surprising and electrified both the parent and medical communities. Although Wakefield and his coauthors allowed that more studies were needed, their positive claims were enough to generate an enormous amount of public interest.

In addition to the alleged links between measles and enterocolitis, and enterocolitis and autism suggested by Wakefield et al., at least two other factors helped to fuel the public's interest in the MMR theory after the publication of the *Lancet* article:

1. The onset of symptoms of autism in some children does occur shortly after they have been vaccinated with the MMR.
2. There has been an increase in the number of diagnoses of autism since the 1988 introduction of the MMR vaccine.

Shortly after the publication of the *Lancet* article, an industry grew up devoted to the sale of various dietary plans and supplements that were supposed to target the various parts of the causal chain proposed by Wakefield et al. and ultimately to cure autism, or at least to ameliorate its effects. In addition, many parents of normally developing children opted not to immunize them. Recent epidemiological studies indicate new and alarming trends in the direction of a resurgence of measles, mumps, and rubella, all potentially devastating diseases (English, Lang, Raleigh, Carroll, & Nicholls, 2006; Gupta, Best, & MacMahon, 2005; Savage et al., 2005). Smaller outbreaks of these diseases serve as striking reminders of the risks they carry. However, after very close scrutiny the entire pathophysiological mechanism proposed by Wakefield et al. has been rejected by responsible medical opinion (Afzal et al., 1998; Afzal, Armitage, Ghosh, Williams, & Minor, 2000; Black, Kaye, & Jick, 2002; Nielsen et al., 1998; Taylor et al., 2002).

Mechanisms other than the one proposed by Wakefield et al. have been suggested to account for the supposed association between MMR immunizations and autism. The most notable of these implicated thimerosal, the ethyl mercury-based preservative which, in the United States, was included until several years ago as a component of the MMR and other vaccinations (Bernard, Enayati, Redwood, Roger, & Binstock, 2001; Bernard, Enayati, Roger, Binstock, & Redwood, 2002; Blaxill, Redwood, & Bernard, 2004; D. A. Geier & Geier, 2003; M. R. Geier & Geier, 2003; Vojdani, Pangborn, Vojdani, & Cooper, 2003). There is some biological plausibility to this theory, in that neurodevelopmental abnormalities do occur subsequent to mercury exposure (Clarkson, 1997). As word of this possible association spread, a new industry appeared, claiming benefits to removing heavy metals directly from the body and from the diet. In particular, the drug therapy of chelation became common. However, a review of the current literature does not show any trials or reviews demonstrating the efficacy of chelation in the treatment of autism. On the contrary, chelation has been associated with adverse outcomes, including death (Brown, Willis, Omalu, & Leiker, 2006).

Population-level studies reject both the link between autism and thimerosal (Hviid, Stellfeld, Wohlfahrt, & Melbye, 2003; Madsen et al., 2003; Stehr-Green, Tull, Stellfeld, Mortenson, & Simpson, 2003) and the link between autism and the MMR vaccine (Chen, Landau, Sham, & Fombonne, 2004; Kaye, del Mar Melero-Montes, & Jick, 2001; Madsen et al., 2002; Taylor et al., 1999), suggesting that the observed temporal relationship between the MMR vaccine and the onset of autism can be attributed to chance. The important question raised by the history of the controversies about the MMR and thimerosol is whether a small subgroup of children might experience a regression subsequent to MMR immunization. This possible "regressive phenotype" has been examined by the Collaborative Program for Excellence in Autism (CPEA), both in general and with reference to the MMR. In a large sample it found "no evidence that onset of autistic symptoms or of regression was related to measles–mumps–rubella vaccination" (Richler et al., 2006). The staying power, however, of the claim of an association between vaccination and autism has been enormous. The American Academy of Pediatrics and the U.S. Institute of Medicine of the National Academies, among others, have found it necessary to issue statements that there is neither epidemiological nor pathophysiological evidence for the correlation between the MMR vaccine and autism.

MEDICAL CONDITIONS AND AUTISM

As the validity of autism as a distinct diagnostic category has come to be appreciated, various associations between autism and literally hundreds of medical conditions have been reported (e.g., see Gillberg & Coleman, 2002). However, there are many problems in interpreting such reports, including the bias for positive associations to be published over negative associations, duplicate publications, lack of rigor in diagnostic criteria, and so forth. As a result, the majority of studies fail to provide sufficient data to establish any association above levels expected by chance (Rutter, Bailey, Bolton, & LeCouteur, 1994). In his recent review, Fombonne (2005a) summarized the available literature on this topic, and based on epidemiological data, associations no greater than expected by chance were found for congenital rubella, phenylketonuria (PKU), neurofibromatosis, cerebral palsy, or Down syndrome. Although there is, of course, a possibility that any of these disorders and autism can coexist, the available epidemiological data do not support the idea that they occur more frequently than would be expected by chance. Similarly, although there has been great interest in gastrointestinal factors in autism, substantive data are lacking (see Erickson et al., 2006 for review).

Several medical conditions have documented associations with autism: fragile-X syndrome, tuberous sclerosis (Rutter, 2005a, 2005b), and epilepsy (Volkmar & Nelson, 1990); the latter likely arises as a result of the same factor or factors that cause autism (see Rutter et al., 1994, and Fombonne, 2005a, 2005b for discussions). Epilepsy appears to have bimodal peaks of onset in both early childhood and adolescence (Deykin & MacMahon, 1979; Volkmar & Nelson, 1990) (see Figure 10.1). In his recent review, Fombonne (2005a) reports that across available epidemiological studies the mean rate of epilepsy was 16.8%, although this is likely an underestimate, given the median age of available samples and the increased risk for onset of seizures throughout childhood and adolescence and in early adult life.

Genetic conditions associated with autism include fragile-X syndrome and tuberous sclerosis. It appears that approximately 1% of individuals with strictly diagnosed autism also exhibit the fragile-X abnormality (Rutter, 2005a). Similarly, the frequency of tuberous sclerosis in autism is 100 times higher than expected (Rutter, 2005a). It remains unclear whether this association is mediated by epilepsy, the presence of localized brain lesions, or direct genetic effects. There is some suggestion that an abnormality on chromosome 15 may also be associated with autism (Rutter, 2005a). Thus, although early reports suggested that almost 40% of cases of autism could be associated with specific medical conditions (Gillberg, 1992), more recent and stringent data have suggested that this rate is much lower—perhaps about 5% (Fombonne, 2005a). The available data on this issue are of variable quality, with studies ranging from questionnaires and retrospective parental reports to contemporaneous medical examinations.

MEDICAL EVALUATIONS OF THE INFANT AND YOUNG CHILD WITH AUTISM

Medical assessments should begin with a detailed history and examination, including developmental history and current presentation, course, family history, and relevant psychosocial issues. Diagnostic developmental information is typically derived from developmental assessment and speech–communication assessment, as well as observation of the child. As noted above, with the exception of a handful of conditions (seizure disorder, fragile-X syndrome, and tuberous sclerosis), the risk of associated medical conditions is relatively small, although for children with developmental delays that can be confused with autism, the list of potential organic etiologies is large (infective, endocrinological, metabolic, traumatic, or toxic). Medical assessments should be guided by the child's history and physical examination. Typically, these will include hearing screening and screening for fragile-X. There is some suggestion that individuals with autism may be at increased risk for hearing impairment (Jure, Rapin, & Tuchman, 1991; Rosenhall, Nordin, Sandstrom, Ahlsen, & Gillberg, 1999) and, as for autism, an early diagnosis of hearing impairment is central to early intervention. If suggested by history or examination, an electroencephalographic (EEG) study or neurological consultation should be obtained—for example, to rule out associated seizure disorder. It must be emphasized that in the absence of a specific indication, the likely positive yield of these procedures is relatively low.

There is general agreement that a genetics evaluation should be standard practice in the medical assessment of all individuals with ASD. A thorough physical examination, which includes assessment for dysmorphology, may identify a known syndrome, such as tuberous sclerosis or Angelman syndrome. In such cases, specific tests can be ordered to confirm the diagnosis. Otherwise, high-resolution karyotype should be obtained, given the greater frequency of chromosomal abnormalities in children with autism and ASD as compared with the general population. Fragile-X testing should also be routine, because there is a higher rate of this disorder—up to 2–5%, in ASD (Freitag, 2007). Detecting these anomalies can be important for the purposes of genetic counseling, as is clear for fragile-X.

Fluorescence *in situ* hybridization (FISH) is a technique that uses fluorescently labeled DNA probes to detect chromosomal abnormalities at individual loci. As mentioned above, the most common site of abnormalities in ASD is 15q11-13. Duplications of this segment, predominantly involving the maternal copy, have been reported numerous times in ASD (Veenstra-Vanderweele et al., 2004; Vorstman et al., 2006). Some researchers are advocating this single-locus FISH study in all patients with ASD (Abdul-Rahman & Hudgins, 2006) or in patients in whom intial karyotype and fragile-X testing are negative (Schaefer & Lutz, 2006).

The regions near the ends of chromosomes, known as subtelomeres, contain a high concentration of genes. There is an increased frequency of subtelomeric abnormalities in idiopathic intellectual disability, with an average rate of 4.6% across published studies (Xu & Chen, 2003). The more severe the intellectual disability, the higher the rate. Clinicians often question whether subtelomeric studies are also warranted in ASD. One study found that among 10 individuals with autism and moderate intellectual disability, one had a chromosome 2q37 subtelomeric deletion (Wolff, Clifton, Karr, & Charles, 2002). Two other studies found no subtelomeric abnormalities in 50 (Keller et al., 2003) and 71 (Battaglia & Bonaglia, 2006) patients with ASD. Therefore, there is not enough evidence presently to determine conclusively whether subtelomeric studies should be routine in ASD. They should still be considered for any individual who has moderate to severe developmental delay (Shevell et al., 2003).

As cytogenetic technologies advance, additional, higher-resolution chromosomal studies become available. For example, chromosomal microarray, also known as array comparative genomic hybridization (aCGH), can detect small chromosomal duplications and deletions that would be missed by standard high-resolution karyotypes. In a study of 29 patients with ASD and normal high-resolution karyotypes, aCGH detected chromosomal abnormalities in 8 (27.5%) patients (Jacquemont et al., 2006). This report shows that aCGH has the potential for high diagnostic yield. It should be followed up with additional studies of larger cohorts to determine whether aCGH should become a routine genetic investigation in ASD. Caution will be needed, however, in interpreting the results of such studies, because there are many instances of chromosomal deletions containing neuronally expressed genes in apparently normal individuals (Conrad, Andrews, Carter, Hurles, & Pritchard, 2006; Hinds,

Kloek, Jen, Chen, & Frazer, 2006; McCarroll et al., 2006). An advantage of aCGH is that it can simultaneously study duplications, deletions, subtelomeres, and individual loci of interest, such as 15q11-13 in one experiment, making it more cost-effective than several separate lab tests (Schaefer & Lutz, 2006). When genes for autism are clearly identified and replicated, the potential for genetic screening will significantly increase.

The majority of cases of Rett syndrome are caused by mutations in the gene *MECP2* (methyl-CpG-binding protein 2), which encodes a regulator of gene expression. Although mutations in *MECP2* do not appear to play a major role in autism (Beyer et al., 2002), they have been found in a few girls with autistic features who did not have or had not yet developed the full characteristics of Rett syndrome (Abdul-Rahman & Hudgins, 2006; Carney et al., 2003). Therefore, *MECP2* sequencing should be considered in young girls with developmental delay and/or autistic features if karyotype and fragile-X testing are negative.

Several metabolic disorders have been associated with autistic features, such as PKU (Schaefer & Lutz, 2006). However, a number of groups have concluded that the yield of metabolic testing is too low to justify routine screening in these patients (Abdul-Rahman & Hudgins, 2006; Battaglia & Carey, 2006; Schaefer & Lutz, 2006). Metabolic testing should certainly be pursued if there are suggestive findings from the history and examination, such as unclear newborn screening, dysmorphic or coarse features, lethargy, cyclic vomiting, early-onset seizures, and intellectual disability (Filipek et al., 2000).

By definition, there is much more phenotypic variability within the broader autism spectrum than in classical autism (and there is already considerable variability in the latter!) One might expect that there would be differences in the yield of genetics testing in the two populations. The broader spectrum includes individuals who have mild symptoms and are higher functioning, and who would not be suspected to have a high rate of genetic abnormalities, at least given the detection abilities of the current technology. The broader spectrum of patients can be considered comparable to the highly variable population of individuals with developmental delay/mental retardation (DD/MR). *Developmental delay* represents a delay in the attainment of developmental milestones and is used to describe deficits in children younger than 5 years of age. *Mental retardation* refers to cognitive disability in children older than 5 years, when IQ testing is considered reliable (Moeschler & Shevell, 2006).

A number of recent literature reviews have examined the diagnostic yield of genetics testing in individuals with DD/MR (Shevell et al., 2003; van Karnebeek, Jansweijer, Leenders, Offringa, & Hennekam, 2005; Moeschler & Shevell, 2006). The conclusions of these three reviews are largely similar to what has been recommended by groups specifically studying the ASD population. All three recommend routine karyotype analysis. Shevell et al.

(2003) and Moeschler and Shevell (2006) recommend routine Fragile X testing; van Karnebeek et al. (2005) recommend routine testing in boys with MR, and in girls if indicated, such as in the presence of a family history of MR. Although van Karnebeek et al. (2005) conclude that the yield of subtelomere analysis is relatively low and should be "selectively applied," other groups conclude that it should be pursued in all patients who have a normal karyotype (Moeschler & Shevell, 2006) or in those with moderate to severe developmental delay (Shevell et al., 2003; Schaefer & Lutz, 2006). Regarding *MECP2* screening, only Shevell et al. (2003) suggest that it should be investigated in girls with moderate to severe MR. There is general agreement that metabolic testing should not be routine, because of its low yield.

Challman, Barbaresi, Katusic, and Weaver (2003) specifically investigated whether there is a difference in the yield of genetic testing between autism and the broader spectrum. From a retrospective chart review, they found that 3.1% (2/65) of patients with autism had abnormal genetics test results, whereas 5.1% (6/117) of patients with PDD-NOS had abnormal test results. They recommended that karyotype and fragile-X testing be performed in all patients with ASD. Abdul-Rahman and Hudgins (2006) determined that 8.3% of their study population with ASD had positive genetics test results. Of their 7 patients (out of 84) with abnormalities, 5 had autistic features and 2 had Autistic Disorder. Three of the 5 patients with autistic features had Rett syndrome, which had not been diagnosed on examination alone. They, too, concluded that karyotype and fragile-X testing should be routine in all individuals with ASD. Based on their experience, they suggested that *MECP2* screening be performed in girls with autistic features, especially those under 4 years of age, inasmuch as the characteristics of Rett syndrome may not be apparent yet. They also recommended that FISH for 15q11-13 and 22q13 abnormalities be routine, as the associated phenotypes can be subtle.

Currently, most studies clearly favor routine karyotype and fragile-X testing in all patients with ASD, regardless of the specific diagnosis. Some groups recommend additional investigations, such as various FISH studies or *MECP2* screenings, based on their experience with their populations. Further studies are warranted to fine tune recommendations for genetics testing. They should have sufficient numbers of subjects representing the individual diagnoses in the spectrum. They should be prospective, so that standard measures are used to evaluate all of the participants. In addition, all patients, regardless of severity of symptoms, should undergo a uniform set of genetics tests. This can help to determine the yield of each test in patients across the spectrum. Clinical practice will continue to be shaped by diagnostic technology, which advances at a rapid pace. As more genetic information about each individual becomes accessible, it will be important to determine which pieces of data are clinically relevant and useful for genetic counseling.

EEG, Evoked Potentials, and Brain Size

Various EEG abnormalities are seen in autism; these include diffuse and focal spikes, paroxysmal spike and wave patterns, multifocal spike activity, and a mixed discharge. In the absence of a clinical seizure disorder, rates of EEG abnormalities in autism range from 10 to 83%, depending on the adequacy and length of the sample and the number of recordings obtained. However, in the absence of signs or symptoms suggestive of seizure disorder, the overall yield of EEG is relatively low. For individuals with a history of marked language regression, a sleep-deprived EEG may be helpful in ruling out the rare syndrome of acquired aphasia with epilepsy (Landau–Kleffner syndrome). In the latter condition, social skills are generally preserved and the clinical presentation is usually more that of an aphasia (Rapin, 1991).

Hearing testing should routinely be obtained. Deaf children may exhibit behaviors suggestive of autism. Studies of auditory brainstem-evoked potentials generally do not provide evidence of specific problems in auditory pathways if appropriate controls are used. Evoked potentials (e.g., the auditory P300) may be abnormal, suggesting problems in higher-level processing (Minshew et al., 2005).

In his original article, Kanner (1943) noted that children with autism had enlarged heads. The significance of this finding has been increasingly appreciated as magnetic resonance imaging (MRI) and postmortem studies have become available (Volkmar et al., 2004). The increased head size appears to reflect a basic shift in brain size, with recent studies suggesting that brain volume may be increased by as much as 10% in toddlers with autism (Courchesne et al., 2001; Sparks et al., 2002). Over time this effect diminishes, so that by adolescence and adulthood the effect is reduced (Aylward, Minshew, Field, Sparks, & Singh, 2002). Interestingly, head size does not appear to be enlarged at birth (Courchesne, Carper, & Akshoomoff, 2003). This finding is of interest because various factors may be responsible for early overgrowth. Longitudinal data are clearly needed for clarification, and the functional significance of this observation remains controversial (Volkmar et al., 2004). MRI is not routinely indicated in the absence of a specific concern.

ISSUES IN OBTAINING
AND PROVIDING HEALTH CARE

Various issues pose obstacles to provision of health care services to children included within the autism spectrum (Volkmar, Wiesner, & Westphal, 2006). These problems begin in infancy and persist into adult life. Some of these difficulties are a result of autism. Problems in social interaction and communication and limited tolerance for change pose substantial difficulties for providing high-quality, long-term health care. For example, an illness in a nonverbal child is more likely to present as behavior change. For individuals with autism, tolerating routine office visits can be problematic; when an individual is ill, this factor may be compounded. Physical examination can be difficult, and locating the source of pain or illness can be challenging. Other problems arise from the rather fragmented health care and insurance systems; for example, frequent changes in parental insurance may result in frequent changes of care providers, adding a further challenge for a child who has difficulty with change. Table 10.1 provides a list of frequent obstacles and some potential solutions for care providers.

Provision of regular well child care is particularly important to minimize difficulties associated with ASD. The pediatrician or other primary care provider often serves as the first point of contact for parents concerned about their child's development. As the American Academy of Pediatrics (2001) has noted, the pediatrician has a special role in diagnosis and management. Unfortunately, primary care providers' knowledge of autism is variable, with some of them still confusing autism with other forms of psychiatric illness, such as childhood schizophrenia (Heidgerken, Geffken, Modi, & Frakey, 2005). However, this situation appears to be changing. Guidelines for parents in choosing and working with care providers are available (Volkmar & Wiesner, 2004), as well as guidelines for pediatricians (Batshaw, 2002). Regular routine health care is particularly important, as are ancillary services such as dentistry.

TABLE 10.1. Challenges for Health Care Providers

Areas of difficulty	Possible solution
Marked social difficulties	Ensure familiarity with providers when possible (well child). Have family/familiar staff available. Slow down the pace, exaggerate social cues.
Problems with communication	Use visual supports (picture books, visual schedules). Keep instructions simple. Break procedures down into small steps. Provide ample wait time, talk before touching.
Difficulties with novelty	Familiarize child with office/setting when possible. Use picture books, visual supports, stories. As appropriate, allow child to manipulate materials.
Difficulties with organization/ attention	Minimize extraneous distractions. Use separate waiting area. Use picture schedules/visual aids.

Note. From Volkmar, Wiesner, and Westphal (2006). Copyright 2006 by Lippincott Williams & Wilkins. Reprinted by permission.

In summary, autism is associated with a variety of medical conditions, but is neither predominantly associated with nor the sole manifestation of any one condition. As such, the responsible health care provider working with this population must stay abreast of a large literature, both to provide educated answers to the variety of questions that parents will ask, and to guarantee a high standard of care for their patients. They must maintain some knowledge of the process and limitations of early diagnosis, keep up-to-date with the various etiologies being discussed in both the professional and popular literature, and above all, maintain vigilance for a variety of medical conditions. This is a population that communicates in unusual ways, and both the traditional signs and symptoms of a concurrent illness or disorder may be obscured by the autism itself. In addition, then, to helping parents obtain an initial diagnosis and services, the health care provider has an important and enduring role in ensuring the provision of high-quality care. For the very young child with (or at risk for) autism, the services of a knowledgeable health care provider are invaluable.

SUMMARY

In this chapter we examined various issues involved in the early diagnosis and screening of autism factors. We discussed some of the factors that have been linked to the etiology of autism, both in the popular press and in the literature. We described some of the challenges to health care providers working with children with autism, including the possible presence of a variety of associated conditions, while emphasizing the fact that symptoms of co-occurring conditions may manifest in atypical ways. Progress in defining the brain mechanisms underlying the symptoms of autism is being made in multiple disciplines, including genetics, neurobiology, pharmacology, and neuroimaging. Furthermore, the work of clinical researchers constantly refines the diagnostic process. As the genetics and neurobiology of the disorder are untangled and diagnostic tools are refined, we can expect to see interventions that are designed to target precisely the mechanisms that underlie the symptoms.

REFERENCES

Abdul-Rahman, O. A., & Hudgins, L. (2006). The diagnostic utility of a genetics evaluation in children with pervasive developmental disorders. *Genetics of Medicine, 8*, 50–54.

Afzal, M. A., Armitage, E., Begley, J., Bentley, M. L., Minor, P. D., Ghosh, S., et al. (1998). Absence of detectable measles virus genome sequence in inflammatory bowel disease tissues and peripheral blood lymphocytes. *Journal of Medical Virology, 55*(3), 243–249.

Afzal, M. A., Armitage, E., Ghosh, S., Williams, L. C., & Minor, P. D. (2000). Further evidence of the absence of measles virus genome sequence in full thickness intestinal specimens from patients with Crohn's disease. *Journal of Medical Virology, 62*(3), 377–382.

American Academy of Pediatrics, Committee on Children with Disabilities. (2001). The pediatrician's role in diagnosis and management of autistic spectrum disorders in children. *Pediatrics, 107*(5), 1221–1226.

American Psychiatric Association. (1994). *Diagnostic and statistical manual of mental disorders* (4th ed.). Washington, DC: Author.

Anderson, G. M., Jacobs-Stannard, A., Chawarska, K., Volkmar, F. R., & Kliman, H. J. (2007). Placental trophoblast inclusions in autism spectrum disorder. *Biological Psychiatry, 61*(4), 487–491.

Ashwood, P., Wills, S., & Van de Water, J. (2006). The immune response in autism: A new frontier for autism research. *Journal of Leukocyte Biology, 80*(1), 15.

Asperger, H. (1961). Die psychopathologie des coeliakakranken kindes. *Annales Paediatrici, 197*, 146–151.

Aylward, E. H., Minshew, N. J., Field, K., Sparks, B. F., & Singh, N. (2002). Effects of age on brain volume and head circumference in autism. *Neurology, 59*(2), 175–183.

Bailey, A., Le Couteur, A., Gottesman, I., & Bolton, P. (1995). Autism as a strongly genetic disorder: Evidence from a British twin study. *Psychological Medicine, 25*, 63–77.

Batshaw, M. L. (2002). *Children with disabilities.* Baltimore: Brookes.

Battaglia, A., & Bonaglia, M. C. (2006). The yield of subtelomeric FISH analysis in the evaluation of autistic spectrum disorders. *American Journal of Medical Genetics Part C: Medical Genetics, 142*, 8–12.

Battaglia, A., & Carey, J. C. (2006). Etiologic yield of autistic spectrum disorders: A prospective study. *American Journal of Medical Genetics Part C: Medical Genetics, 142*, 3–7.

Benayed, R., Gharani, N., Rossman, I., Mancuso, V., Lazar, G., Kamdar, S., et al. (2005). Support for the homeobox transcription factor gene ENGRAILED 2 as an autism spectrum disorder susceptibility locus. *American Journal of Human Genetics, 77*, 851–868.

Bernard, S., Enayati, A., Redwood, L., Roger, H., & Binstock, T. (2001). Autism: A novel form of mercury poisoning. *Medical Hypotheses, 56*(4), 462–471.

Bernard, S., Enayati, A., Roger, H., Binstock, T., & Redwood, L. (2002). The role of mercury in the pathogenesis of autism. *Molecular Psychiatry, 7*(Suppl. 2), S42–S43.

Beyer, K. S., Blasi, F., Bacchelli, E., Klauck, S. M., Maestrini, E., & Poustka, A. (2002). Mutation analysis of the coding sequence of the *MECP2* gene in infantile autism. *Human Genetics, 111*, 305–309.

Black, C., Kaye, J. A., & Jick, H. (2002). Relation of childhood gastrointestinal disorders to autism: Nested case-control study using data from the UK general practice research database. *British Medical Journal* (Clinical Research Ed.), *325*(7361), 419–421.

Blaxill, M. F., Redwood, L., & Bernard, S. (2004). Thimerosal and autism?: A plausible hypothesis that should not be dismissed. *Medical Hypotheses, 62*(5), 788–794.

Brown, M. J., Willis, T., Omalu, B., & Leiker, R. (2006). Deaths resulting from hypocalcemia after administration of edetate disodium: 2003–2005. *Pediatrics, 118*(2), e534–e536.

Campbell, D. B., Sutcliffe, J. S., Ebert, P. J., Militerni, R., Bravaccio, C., Trillo, S., et al. (2006). A genetic variant that disrupts MET transcription is associated with autism. *Proceedings of the National Academy of Sciences, 103*(45), 16834–16839.

Cantor, R. M., Kono, N., Duvall, J. A., Alvarez-Retuerto, A., Stone, J. L., Alarcon, M., et al. (2005). Replication of autism linkage: Fine-mapping peak at 17q21. *American Journal of Human Genetics, 76*, 1050–1056.

Carney, R. M., Wolpert, C. M., Ravan, S. A., Shahbazian, M., Ashley-Koch, A., Cuccaro, M. L., et al. (2003). Identification of *MECP2* mutations in a series of females with autistic disorder. *Pediatric Neurology, 28*(3), 205–211.

Casanova, M. F., van Kooten, I. A., Switala, A. E., vanEngland, H., Heinsen, H., Steinbusch, H. W. M., et al. (2006). Minicolumnar abnormalities in autism. *Acta Neuropathologica, 112*(3), 287–303.

Chakrabarti, S., & Fombonne, E. (2001). Pervasive developmental disorders in preschool children. *Journal of the American Medical Association, 285*, 3093–3099.

Challman, T. D., Barbaresi, W. J., Katusic, S. K., & Weaver, A. (2003). The yield of the medical evaluation of children with pervasive developmental disorders. *Journal of Autism and Developmental Disorders, 33*, 187–192.

Chawarska, K., & Volkmar, F. R. (2005). Autism in infancy and early childhood. In F. Volkmar, A. Klin, R. Paul, & D. J. Cohen (Eds.), *Handbook of autism and pervasive developmental disorders* (pp. 223–246). New York: Wiley.

Chen, W., Landau, S., Sham, P., & Fombonne, E. (2004). No evidence for links between autism, MMR and measles virus. *Psychological Medicine, 34*(3), 543–553.

Chess, S. (1977). Follow-up report on autism in congenital rubella. *Journal of Autism and Childhood Schizophrenia, 7*(1), 69–81.

Ciaranello, A. L., & Ciaranello, R. D. (1995). The neurobiology of infantile autism. *Annual Review of Neuroscience, 18*, 101–128.

Clarkson, T. W. (1997). The toxicology of mercury. *Critical Reviews in Clinical Laboratory Sciences, 34*(4), 369–403.

Conrad, D. F., Andrews, T. D., Carter, N. P., Hurles, M. E., & Pritchard, J. K. (2006). A high-resolution survey of deletion polymorphism in the human genome. *National Genetics, 38*, 75–81.

Coonrod, E. E., & Stone, W. L. (2005). Screening for autism in young children. In F. Volkmar, A. Klin, R. Paul, & D. J. Cohen (Eds.), *Handbook of autism and pervasive developmental disorders* (pp. 707–729). New York: Wiley.

Cooper, J. E. (1965). Epilepsy in a longitudinal survey of 5000 children. *British Medical Journal, 1*, 1020–1022.

Courchesne, E., Carper, R., & Akshoomoff, N. (2003). Evidence of brain overgrowth in the first year of life in autism [comment]. *Journal of the American Medical Association, 290*(3), 337–344.

Courchesne, E., Karns, C., Davis, H. R., Ziccardi, R., Carper, R. A., Tique, Z. D., et al. (2001). Unusual brain growth patterns in early life in patients with autistic disorder: An MRI study. *Neurology, 57*(2), 245–254.

Courchesne, E., Redcay, E., & Kennedy, D. P. (2004). The autistic brain: Birth through adulthood. *Current Opinion in Neurology, 17*, 489–496.

Daszak, P., Purcell, M., Lewin, J., Dhillon, A. P., Pounder, R. E., & Wakefield, A. J. (1997). Detection and comparative analysis of persistent measles virus infection in Crohn's disease by immunogold electron microscopy. *Journal of Clinical Pathology, 50*(4), 299–304.

DeLong, G. R., Bean, S. C., & Brown, F. R., III. (1981). Acquired reversible autistic syndrome in acute encephalopathic illness in children. *Archives of Neurology, 38*(3), 191–194.

Deykin, E. Y., & MacMahon, B. (1979). The incidence of seizures among children with autistic symptoms. *American Journal of Psychiatry, 126*, 1310–1312.

Durand, C. M., Betancur, C., Boeckers, T. M., Bockmann, J., Chaste, P., Fauchereau, F., et al. (2007). Mutations in the gene encoding the synaptic scaffolding protein *SHANK3* are associated with autism spectrum disorders. *National Genetics, 39*(1), 25–27.

Ekbom, A., Wakefield, A. J., Zack, M., & Adami, H. O. (1994). Perinatal measles infection and subsequent Crohn's disease. *Lancet, 344*(8921), 508–510.

English, P. M., Lang, N., Raleigh, A., Carroll, K., & Nicholls, M. (2006). Measles outbreak in surrey. *British Medical Journal (Clinical Research Ed.), 333*(7576), 1021–1022.

Erickson, C. A, Stigler, K. A., Corkins, M. R., Posey, D. J., Fitzgerald, J. F., & McDougle, C. J. (2006). Gastrointestinal factors in autistic disorders: A critical review. *Journal of Autism and Developmental Disorders, 35*(6), 713–727.

Feeney, M., Ciegg, A., Winwood, P., & Snook, J. (1997). A case-control study of measles vaccination and inflammatory bowel disease. *Lancet, 350*(9080), 764–766.

Filipek, P. A., Accardo, P. J., Ashwal, S., Baranek, G. T., Cook, E. H., Jr., Dawson, G., et al. (2000). Practice parameter: Screening and diagnosis of autism: Report of the Quality Standards Subcommittee of the American Academy of Neurology and the Child Neurology Society. *Neurology, 55*, 468–479.

Folstein, S., & Rutter, M. (1977). Infantile autism: A genetic study of 21 twin pairs. *Journal of Child Psychology and Psychiatry, 18*(4), 297–321.

Fombonne, E. (2005a). Epidemiological studies of pervasive developmental disorders. In F. Volkmar, A. Klin, R. Paul, & D. J. Cohen (Eds.), *Handbook of autism and pervasive developmental disorders* (pp. 1, 42–69). New York: Wiley.

Fombonne, E. (2005b). Epidemiology of autistic disorder and other pervasive developmental disorders. *Journal of Clinical Psychiatry, 66*(Suppl. 10), 3–8.

Freitag, C. M. (2007). The genetics of autistic disorders and its clinical relevance: A review of the literature. *Molecular Psychiatry, 12*, 2–22.

Geier, D. A., & Geier, M. R. (2003). An assessment of the impact of thimerosal on childhood neurodevelopmental disorders. *Pediatric Rehabilitation, 6*(2), 97–102.

Geier, M. R., & Geier, D. A. (2003). Thimerosal in childhood vaccines, neurodevelopment disorders and heart disease in the United States. *Journal of the American Physicians and Surgeons, 8*, 6–11.

Gharani, N., Benayed, R., Mancuso, V., Brzustowicz, L. M., & Millonig, J. H. (2004). Association of the homeobox transcription factor, ENGRAILED 2, 3, with autism spectrum disorder. *Molecular Psychiatry, 9*, 474–484.

Gillberg, C. L. (1992). The Emanuel Miller Memorial Lecture 1991. Autism and autistic-like conditions: Subclasses among disorders of empathy. *Journal of Child Psychology and Psychiatry, 33*(5), 813–842.

Gillberg, C., & Coleman, M. (2002). The biology of autistic syndromes. *Journal of the American Academy of Child and Adolescent Psychiatry, 41*(1), 104–105.

Glasson, E. J., Bower, C., Petterson, B., deKlerk, N., Charney, G., & Hallmayer, J. F. (2004). Perinatal factors and the development of autism: A population study. *Archives of General Psychiatry, 61*(6), 618–627.

Gupta, A. R., & State, M. W. (2006). Recent advances in the genetics of autism. *Biological Psychiatry, 61*(4), 429–437.

Gupta, R. K., Best, J., & MacMahon, E. (2005). Mumps and the UK epidemic 2005. *British Medical Journal (Clinical Research Ed.), 330*(7500), 1132–1135.

Heidegerken, A. D., Geffken, G., Modi, A., & Frakey, L. (2005). A survey of autism knowledge in a health care setting. *Journal of Autism and Developmental Disorders, 35*(3), 323–330.

Hinds, D. A., Kloek, A. P., Jen, M., Chen, X., & Frazer, K. A. (2006). Common deletions and SNPs are in linkage disequilibrium in the human genome. *National Genetics, 38*, 82–85.

Hultman, C. M., & Sparen, P. (2004). Autism—prenatal insults or an epiphenomenon of a strongly genetic disorder? *Lancet, 3654*, 485–487.

Hviid, A., Stellfeld, M., Wohlfahrt, J., & Melbye, M. (2003). Association between thimerosal-containing vaccine and autism. *Journal of the American Medical Association, 290*(13), 1763–1766.

Ido, A., Numata, M., Kodama, M., & Tsubouchi, H. (2005). Mucosal repair and growth factors: Recombinant human hepatocyte growth factor as an innovative therapy for inflammatory bowel disease. *Journal of Gastroenterology, 40*, 925–931.

Ieraci, A., Forni, P. E., & Ponzetto, C. (2002). Viable hypomorphic signaling mutant of the Met receptor reveals a role for hepatocyte growth factor in postnatal cerebellar development. *Proceedings of the National Academy of Sciences, 99*, 15200–15205.

Institute of Medicine, Committee on Immunization Safety. (2004). *Executive summary: Immunization safety review: Vaccines and autism*. Washington, DC: Author.

Jacquemont, M. L., Sanlaville, D., Redon, R., Raoul, O., Cormier-Daire, V., Lyonnet, S., et al. (2006). Array-based comparative genomic hybridisation identifies high frequency of cryptic chromosomal rearrangements in patients with syndromic autism spectrum disorders. *Journal of Medical Genetics, 43*, 843–849.

Jamain, S., Quach, H., Betancur, C., Rastam, M., Colineaux, C., Gillberg, I. C., et al. (2003). Mutations of the X-linked genes encoding neuroligins *NLGN3* and *NLGN4* are associated with autism. *National Genetics, 34*, 27–29.

Jure, R., Rapin, I., & Tuchman, R. F. (1991). Hearing-impaired autistic children. *Developmental Medicine in Child Neurology, 33*(12), 1062–1072.

Kanner, L. (1943). Autistic disturbances of affective contact. *The Nervous Child, 2*, 217–250.

Kaye, J. A., del Mar Melero-Montes, M., & Jick, H. (2001). Mumps, measles, and rubella vaccine and the incidence of autism recorded by general practitioners: A time trend analysis. *British Medical Journal (Clinical Research Ed.), 322*(7284), 460–463.

Keller, K., Williams, C., Wharton, P., Paulk, M., Bent-Williams, A., Gray, B., et al. (2003). Routine cytogenetic and FISH studies for 17p11/15q11 duplications and subtelomeric rearrangement studies in children with autism spectrum disorders. *American Journal of Medical Genetics, 117,* 105–111.

Klin, A., Chawarska, K., Paul, R., Rubin, E., Morgan, T., Weisner, L., et al. (2004). Autism in a 15-month-old child. *American Journal of Psychiatry, 161*(11), 1981–1988.

Klin, A., Jones, W., Schultz, R., & Volkmar, F. (2003). The enactive mind, or from actions to cognition: Lessons from autism. *Philosophical Transactions of the Royal Society of London. Series B: Biological Sciences, 358*(1430), 345–360.

Kolvin, I. (1971). Studies in the childhood psychoses: I. Diagnostic criteria and classification. *British Journal of Psychiatry, 118*(545), 381–384.

Kuemerle, B., Zanjani, H., Joyner, A., & Herrup, K. (1997). Pattern deformities and cell loss in Engrailed-2 mutant mice suggest two separate patterning events during cerebellar development. *Journal of Neuroscience, 17,* 7881–7889.

Lander, E., & Kruglyak, L. (1995). Genetic dissection of complex traits: Guidelines for interpreting and reporting linkage results. *National Genetics, 11,* 241–247.

Libbey, J. E., Sweeten, T. L., McMahon, W. M., & Fujinami, R. S. (2005). Autistic disorder and viral infections. *Journal of Neurovirology, 11*(1), 1–10.

Lord, C. (1995). Follow-up of two-year-olds referred for possible autism. *Journal of Child Psychology and Psychiatry, 36*(8), 1365–1382.

Madsen, K. M., Hviid, A., Vestergaard, M., Schendel, D., Wohlfahrt, J., Thorsen, P., et al. (2002). A population-based study of measles, mumps, and rubella vaccination and autism [comment]. *New England Journal of Medicine, 347*(19), 1477–1482.

Madsen, K. M., Lauritsen, M. B., Pedersen, C. B., Thorsen, P., Plesner, A. M., Andersen, P. H., et al. (2003). Thimerosal and the occurrence of autism: Negative ecological evidence from Danish population-based data. *Pediatrics, 112*(3, Pt. 1), 604–606.

McCarroll, S. A., Hadnott, T. N., Perry, G. H., Sabeti, P. C., Zody, M. C., Barrett, J. C., et al. (2006). Common deletion polymorphisms in the human genome. *National Genetics, 38,* 86–92.

Millen, K. J., Hui, C. C., & Joyner, A. L. (1995). A role for En-2 and other murine homologues of drosophila segment polarity genes in regulating positional information in the developing cerebellum. *Development, 121,* 3935–3945.

Millen, K. J., Wurst, W., Herrup, K., & Joyner, A. L. (1994). Abnormal embryonic cerebellar development and patterning of postnatal foliation in two mouse Engrailed-2 mutants. *Development, 120,* 695–706.

Minshew, N. J., Sweeney, J. A., Bauman, M. L., & Webb, S. J. (2005). Neurologic aspects of autism. In F. Volkmar, A. Klin, R. Paul, & D. J. Cohen (Eds.), *Handbook of autism and pervasive developmental disorders* (pp. 1, 453–472). New York: Wiley.

Moeschler, J. B., & Shevell, M. (2006). Clinical genetic evaluation of the child with mental retardation or developmental delays. *Pediatrics, 117,* 2304–2316.

Narita, N., Kato, M., Tazoe, M., Miyazaki, K., Narita, M., & Okado, N. (2002). Increased monoamine concentration in the brain and blood of fetal thalidomide- and valproic acid-exposed rat: Putative animal models for autism. *Pediatric Research, 52*(4), 576–579.

National Research Council. (2001). *Educating young children with autism.* Washington, DC: National Academy Press.

Nielsen, L. L., Nielsen, N. M., Melbye, M., Sodermann, M., Jacobsen, M., & Aaby, P. (1998). Exposure to measles *in utero* and Crohn's disease: Danish register study. *British Medical Journal (Clinical Research Ed.)*, *316*(7126), 196–197.

Okunishi, K., Dohi, M., Nakagome, K., Tanaka, R., Mizuno, S., Matsumoto, K., et al. (2005). A novel role of hepatocyte growth factor as an immune regulator through suppressing dendritic cell function. *Journal of Immunology*, *175*, 4745–4753.

Palmen, S. J., van Engeland, H., Hof, P. R., & Schmitz, C. (2004). Neuro-pathological findings in autism. *Brain*, *127*, 2572–2583.

Powell, E. M., Muhlfriedel, S., Bolz, J., & Levitt, P. (2003). Differential regulation of thalamic and cortical axonal growth by hepatocyte growth factor/scatter factor. *Developmental Neuroscience*, *25*, 197–206.

Rapin, I. (1991). Autistic children: Diagnosis and clinical features. *Pediatrics*, *87*(5, Pt. 2), 751–760.

Richler, J., Luyster, R., Risi, S., Hsu, W. L., Dawson, G., Bernier, R., et al. (2006). Is there a "regressive phenotype" of autism spectrum disorder associated with the measles-mumps-rubella vaccine?: A CPEA study. *Journal of Autism and Developmental Disorders*, *36*(3), 299–316.

Risch, N., Spiker, D., Lotspeich, L., Nouri, N., Hinds, D., Hallmayer, J., et al. (1999). A genomic screen of autism: Evidence for a multilocus etiology. *American Journal of Human Genetics*, *65*, 493–507.

Rosenhall, U., Nordin, V., Sandstrom, M., Ahlsen, G., & Gillberg, C. (1999). Autism and hearing loss. *Journal of Autism and Developmental Disorders*, *29*(5), 349–357.

Rutter, M. (1972). Childhood schizophrenia reconsidered. *Journal of Autism and Childhood Schizophrenia*, *2*(4), 315–337.

Rutter, M. (2005a). Environmentally mediated risks for psychopathology: Research strategies and findings [see comment]. *Journal of the American Academy of Child and Adolescent Psychiatry*, *44*(1), 3–18.

Rutter, M. (2005b). Genetic influences and autism. In F. R. Volkmar, A. Klin, R. Paul, & D. J. Cohen (Eds.), *Handbook of autism and pervasive developmental disorders* (pp. 1, 425–452). New York: Wiley.

Rutter, M. A., Bailey, A., Bolton, P., & LeCouteur, A. (1994). Autism and known medical conditions: Myth and substance. *Journal of Child Psychology and Psychiatry and Allied Disciplines*, *35*(2), 311–322.

Savage, E., Ramsay, M., White, J., Beard, S., Lawson, H., & Hunjan, R., et al. (2005). Mumps outbreaks across England and Wales in 2004: Observational study. *British Medical Journal (Clinical Research Ed.)*, *330*(7500), 1119–1120.

Schaefer, G. B., & Lutz, R. E. (2006). Diagnostic yield in the clinical genetic evaluation of autism spectrum disorders. *Genetic Medicine*, *8*, 549–556.

Schultz, R. T., Gauthier, I., Klin, A., Fulbright, R. K., Anderson, A., Volkmar, F., et al. (2000). Abnormal ventral temporal cortical activity during face discrimination among individuals with autism and Asperger syndrome. *Archives of General Psychiatry*, *57*(4), 331–340.

Shevell, M., Ashwal, S., Donley, D., Flint, J., Gingold, M., Hirtz, D., et al. (2003). Practice parameter: Evaluation of the child with global developmental delay: Report of the Quality Standards Subcommittee of the American Academy of Neurology and the Practice Committee of the Child Neurology Society. *Neurology*, *60*, 367–380.

Siegel, B., Pliner, C., Eschler, J., & Elliott, G. R. (1988). How children with autism are diagnosed: Difficulties in identification of children with multiple developmental delays. *Journal of Developmental and Behavioral Pediatrics, 9*(4), 199–204.

Singh, V. K., Lin, S. X., & Yang, V. C. (1998). Serological association of measles virus and human herpesvirus-6 with brain autoantibodies in autism. *Clinical Immunology and Immunopathology, 89*(1), 105–108.

Sparks, B. F., Friedman, S. D., Shaw, D. W., Aylward, E. H., Echelard, D., Artu, A. A., et al. (2002). Brain structural abnormalities in young children with autism spectrum disorder. *Neurology, 59*(2), 184–192.

Stehr-Green, P., Tull, P., Stellfeld, M., Mortenson, P. B., & Simpson, D. (2003). Autism and thimerosal-containing vaccines: Lack of consistent evidence for an association. *American Journal of Preventive Medicine, 25*(2), 101–106.

Stone, J. L., Merriman, B., Cantor, R. M., Yonan, A. L., Gilliam, T. C., Geschwind, D. H., et al. (2004). Evidence for sex-specific risk alleles in autism spectrum disorder. *American Journal of Human Genetics, 75*, 1117–1123.

Stone, W. L., Lee, E. B., Ashfor, L., Brissie, J., Hepburn, S. L., Coonrod, E. E., et al. (1999). Can autism be diagnosed accurately in children under 3 years? *Journal of Child Psychology and Psychiatry and Allied Disciplines, 40*(2), 219–226.

Stromland, K., Nordin, V., Miller, M., Akerstrom, B., & Gillberg, C. (1994). Autism in thalidomide embryopathy: A population study. *Developmental Medicine and Child Neurology, 36*(4), 351–356.

Stubbs, E. G. (1978). Autistic symptoms in a child with congenital cytomegalovirus infection. *Journal of Autism and Childhood Schizophrenia, 8*(1), 37–43.

Sutcliffe, J. S., Delahanty, R. J., Prasad, H. C., McCauley, J. L., Han, Q., Jiang, L., et al. (2005). Allelic heterogeneity at the serotonin transporter locus (SLC6A4) confers susceptibility to autism and rigid–compulsive behaviors. *American Journal of Human Genetics, 77*, 265–279.

Taylor, B., Miller, E., Farrington, C. P., Petropoulos, M. C., Favot-Mayaud, I., Li, J., et al. (1999). Autism and measles, mumps, and rubella vaccine: No epidemiological evidence for a causal association. *Lancet, 353*(9169), 2026–2029.

Taylor, B., Miller, E., Lingam, R., Andrews, N., Simmons, A., & Stowe, J. (2002). Measles, mumps, and rubella vaccination and bowel problems or developmental regression in children with autism: Population study. *British Medical Journal (Clinical Research Ed.), 324*(7334), 393–396.

Thomas, N. S., Sharp, A. J., Browne, C. E., Skuse, D., Hardie, C., & Dennis, N. R. (1999). Xp deletions associated with autism in three females. *Human Genetics, 104*, 43–48.

Thompson, N. P., Montgomery, S. M., Pounder, R. E., & Wakefield, A. J. (1995). Is measles vaccination a risk factor for inflammatory bowel disease? *Lancet, 345*(8957), 1071–1074.

van Karnebeek, C. D., Jansweijer, M. C., Leenders, A. G., Offringa, M., & Hennekam, R. C. (2005). Diagnostic investigations in individuals with mental retardation: A systematic literature review of their usefulness. *European Journal of Human Genetics, 13*, 6–25.

Veenstra-Vanderweele, J., Christian, S. L., & Cook, E. H., Jr. (2004). Autism as a paradigmatic complex genetic disorder. *Annual Review of Genomics and Human Genetics, 5*, 379–405.

Vojdani, A., Pangborn, J. B., Vojdani, E., & Cooper, E. L. (2003). Infections, toxic chemicals and dietary peptides binding to lymphocyte receptors and tissue enzymes are major instigators of autoimmunity in autism. *International Journal of Immunopathology and Pharmacology, 16*(3), 189–199.

Volkmar, F. R. & Klin, A. (2005). Issues in the classification of autism and related conditions. In F. R. Volkmar, A. Klin, R. Paul, & D. J. Cohen (Eds.), *Handbook of autism and pervasive developmental disorders* (pp. 1, 5–41). New York: Wiley.

Volkmar, F. R., Klin, A., Siegel, B., Szatmari, P., Lord, C., Campbell, M., et al. (1994). Field trial for autistic disorder in DSM-IV. *American Journal of Psychiatry, 151*(9), 1361–1367.

Volkmar, F. R., Lord, C., Bailey, A., Schultz, R. T., & Klin, A. (2004). Autism and pervasive developmental disorders. *Journal of Child Psychology and Psychiatry and Allied Disciplines, 45*(1), 135–170.

Volkmar, F. R., Lord, C., Klin, A., Schultz, R. T., & Cook, E., Jr. (2007). Autism and the pervasive developmental disorders. In A. Martin & F. R. Volkmar (Eds.), *Lewis's child and adolescent psychiatry: A comprehensive textbook* (4th ed., pp. 384–400). Philadelphia: Lippincott Williams & Wilkins.

Volkmar, F. R., & Nelson, D. S. (1990). Seizure disorders in autism. *Journal of the American Academy of Child and Adolescent Psychiatry, 29*(1), 127–129.

Volkmar, F. R., & Wiesner, E. (2004). *Health care for children on the autism spectrum.* Bethesda, MD: Woodbine.

Volkmar, F. R., Wiesner, E., & Westphal, A. (2006). Health care issues for children on the autism spectrum. *Current Opinion in Psychiatry, 19*, 351–366.

Vorstman, J. A., Staal, W. G., van Daalen, E., van Engeland, H., Hochstenbach, P. F., & Franke, L. (2006). Identification of novel autism candidate regions through analysis of reported cytogenetic abnormalities associated with autism. *Molecular Psychiatry, 11*(1), 18–28.

Wakefield, A. J., Murch, S. H., Anthony, A., Linnell, J., Casson, D. M., Malik, M., et al. (1998). Ileal-lymphoid-nodular hyperplasia, non-specific colitis, and pervasive developmental disorder in children. *Lancet, 351*(9103), 637–641.

Wakefield, A. J., Pittilo, R. M., Sim, R., Cosby, S. L., Stephenson, J. R., Dhillon, A. P., et al. (1993). Evidence of persistent measles virus infection in Crohn's disease. *Journal of Medical Virology, 39*(4), 345–353.

Walker-Smith, J., & Andrews, J. (1972). Alpha-1-antitrypsin, autism, and coeliac disease. *Lancet, 2*(7782), 883–884.

Wassink, T. H., Brzustowicz, L. M., Bartlett, C. W., & Szatmari, P. (2004). The search for autism disease genes. *Mental Retardation and Developmental Disabilities and Research Review, 10*, 272–283.

Williams, G., King, J., Cunningham, M., Stephan, M., Kerr, B., & Hersh, J. H. (2001). Fetal valproate syndrome and autism: Additional evidence of an association. *Developmental Medicine and Child Neurology, 43*(3), 202–206.

Wing, L., & Potter, D. (2002). The epidemiology of autistic spectrum disorders: Is prevalence rising? *Mental Retardation and Developmental Disabilities Research Reviews, 8*(3), 151–161.

Wolff, D. J., Clifton, K., Karr, C., & Charles, J. (2002). Pilot assessment of the subtelomeric regions of children with autism: Detection of a 2q deletion. *Genetic Medicine, 4*, 10–14.

Xu, J., & Chen, Z. (2003). Advances in molecular cytogenetics for the evaluation of mental retardation. *American Journal of Medical Genetics, Part C. Seminars in Medical Genetics, 117*, 15–24.

CHAPTER 11

Supporting Families

Karyn Bailey

The evaluation of a young child suspected of having autism spectrum disorder (ASD) effectively starts with the initial contact with the family. Although the primary goal of the clinicians is to gain a thorough understanding of the child's strengths and vulnerabilities, exploration of many other factors involved in the assessment process is essential for advancing positive outcomes for children and families living with ASD. This chapter summarizes a wide range of issues that need to be considered by clinicians and service providers that can potentially maximize adherence to this overarching mission. Such issues should both guide and anchor clinical efforts before, during, and after the evaluation.

SUPPORTING FAMILIES
THROUGH THE DIAGNOSTIC PROCESS

The Impact of Parental Early Concerns and Experiences

Many families that have young children with ASD bring a history of experience with professionals, family, and friends that often impacts their regard for the diagnostic assessment. More specifically, most of the parents have a sense that something is just not right from very early on (Howlin & Moore, 1997; Chawarska & Volkmar, 2005), sometimes as early as a child's birth (Wetherby, Prizant, & Schuler, 2000). In ideal circumstances, these concerns are shared with family, friends, and professionals who are sensitive and supportive and can assist the family in securing a comprehensive evaluation and warranted services. Such support does not necessarily eliminate the anxiety that families experience in anticipation of an evaluation that may confirm their worst fear for their child. In hindsight, however, families often express gratitude for such early assistance, as it serves as a springboard in the process of implementing early intervention services. Although the severity of their child's difficulties may bring sadness into their lives, parents who experience appropriate early support, especially from professionals, are able to act with greater confidence on their child's behalf. Careful attention to parental concerns may prevent a buildup of feelings of anger or guilt that parents may experience because of a prolonged lag between the onset of their concerns, the validation of their feelings by professionals, and the beginning of treatment.

Unfortunately, however, early parental concerns may be met with a dismissive attitude by professionals and family members. Comments such as "You're just an anxious parent" or "Boys talk later than girls" are not unusual. Although such comments may be heartfelt and well intentioned, they can potentially distract parents and derail efforts to pursue greater understanding of their child's challenges and may delay implementation of treatment. This is especially true when the comments come from professionals (DeGiacomo & Fombonne, 1998; Howlin & Asgharian 1999; Howlin & Moore, 1997). These comments may serve the parents' need to believe that all is well, yet the haunting sense that something is "not quite right" never fully abates.

Usually, by the time a child reaches the age of 2 or 3 years, professionals and other caretakers begin to share the parents' concerns. Although this is likely to happen earlier, as in the case of children who exhibit marked speech and/or cognitive delays, by the time the child is about 3 years old the concerns are likely to be corroborated even in the absence of significant delay in the development of language (Rapin, 2005). Even though there may be a sense of relief in having one's concerns finally validated and taken seriously, that same validation serves to exacerbate the ongoing anxiety about "what's wrong." Thus, many families come to an evaluation with mixed emotions (Randall & Parker, 1999), which are sometimes accompanied by a sense of mistrust of professionals.

It is very important to understand how and why this mix of emotions and the accompanying mistrust of professionals can impact the ultimate goal of advancing outcomes for children and families living with ASD. The emotional mix is a powerful and confusing combination of anxiety, sadness, fear, anger, guilt, and ambivalence that comes from both desiring and dreading to hear the "truth about my child." When parental concerns have been dismissed by professionals in the past and now those concerns are suddenly and finally confirmed, parents may feel a sense of ambivalence regarding professionals' competence. The risk is that the family may discount or dismiss the findings and recommendations of the evaluation and, consequently, may not pursue appropriate and necessary services for their child. In such cases, delays in implementation of appropriate treatment may impact the potential outcome, including the child's and the family's overall quality of life (Harris & Handleman, 2000). Thus, it is essential to establish trust and build a healthy working alliance with the family from the initial contact and to maintain this throughout the evaluation process and subsequent follow-up.

The Initial Intake Process

The first encounter with the clinical team can be crucial for the formation of an alliance between the parents and those involved in the assessment of the child. It often occurs in the context of collecting basic referral information necessary to determine the scope of the difficulties, as well as a basic developmental and medical history. It is important to keep in mind that this process should also be aimed at giving the parents an opportunity to express their concerns and ask questions about the upcoming evaluation. This has to be done in a clinically sensitive manner, as parents often feel compelled to give very detailed accounts about their child's medical and developmental history. In a way, the information may be more detailed than needed at this stage of the process. Yet the intake professional should listen attentively and with patience, because this will assuredly contribute to the establishment of trust and a working alliance with the parents.

In addition to attention to what parents have to say, awareness of what is not said, or more specifically, what is not asked, is quite useful. Most parents want to know what to expect during the evaluation, yet few will ask questions such as, "What instruments will be used, and what is their purpose?" "What happens, when, and how long will it take?" "Can I stay with my child and observe the assessment?" "Will I be able to discuss the results immediately with the assessment team?" "Can I bring along a family member or the child's therapist?" These are very important questions, the answers to which help to reduce uncertainty, and thus anxiety. Equally important, it will help parents prepare for the evaluation so that the conditions for maximal engagement of child and family are attained. Avoidable long waiting periods, indication of preferred waiting areas, even clear instructions for parking arrangements, all facilitate success or, alternatively their absence can exacerbate anxiety in all involved and can even exacerbate or trigger maladaptive behaviors in the child. Parents can also help the process by bringing a favorite toy or treat to entertain their child during transitions and waiting periods. Extended family members or family friends are often very helpful in supporting a parent and the child through the assessment process, which often extends for several hours at a time. Understanding the process of assessment and familiarity with its components helps parents face this potentially complex and stressful process.

Another clinical consideration for the intake process is the emotional state of the family. Understandably, most parents are greatly alarmed by the prospect of their child having a diagnosis of ASD, although many will work hard to mask their feelings. One way to explore their emotional state is to open with a statement aimed at normalizing the anxiety that naturally accompanies the evaluation, such as, "Most people are quite nervous about coming to the clinic. How are you doing with all of this?" This type of conversation often reveals key aspects of family coping strategies and informs the clinician about the most effective ways of communicating with the family about the assessment results and recommendations for treatment. For instance, the conversation during the intake process may reveal that one or both parents are struggling with such high levels of anxiety or depression that their ability to concentrate may be compromised. Such parents may benefit from recommendations from the assessment team that are clear, concise, and focused on two to three priorities. This subject is elaborated on in a subsequent section of this chapter.

Although gathering intake information alone may be technically sufficient, clinical sensitivity and exploration of the emotional states of the parent or parents lends an opportunity to normalize feelings, establish trust, build relationships, and discover how to tailor the evaluation process, especially the discussion of the results, to best meet the needs of the family. The essential point is that the aim of the assessment is not exclusively to learn about the child. A good assessment pursues and includes information about the family and uses that information to guide interactions. The hope is that the family will be better prepared and able to implement the recommendations and advocate effectively for appropriate services in a timely manner.

The Assessment Process

Ideally, a family arrives for a comprehensive assessment for the child already having a good understanding of the diagnostic procedures and the roles of the members of the assessment team. Nonetheless, it is often necessary and certainly helpful to recapitulate the main points, introduce the members of the team, and encourage the parents to seek clarification whenever they feel necessary.

Parents are often uncertain as to how they should behave during the assessment; therefore, it is important to facilitate a level of comfort by outlining the goals and course of each of the assessment procedures. Many parents are concerned that the standardized assessment conducted in an unfamiliar environment will skew the results and not reveal the child's true level of skills. Such concerns often stem from the fact that the child may only rarely or inconsistently display certain skills. It is often necessary to explain that it is necessary to sample the child's skills in unfamiliar contexts to gain a sense of the generalization of existing skills. Similarly, parents often need to be reassured that all measures will be taken (within reason) to obtain the child's optimal performance in such situations (see Chawarska & Bearss, Chapter 3, this volume). Consideration of how consistently a skill is displayed across people and across settings and specific situations is also helpful. One should assure parents that clinicians are not only measuring the child's skills but also learning about conditions that promote and support the child's learning. Moreover, an explanation as to the need to ascertain both strengths and deficits, and not simply reach a categorical diagnosis, is key in engaging parents about the ways in which the educational program should be designed and implemented. Responding to this type of parental concern affords the team members an opportunity to strengthen their credibility and alliance with the parents and helps parents to appreciate the complexity of the assessment process and their child's needs. The formation of such an alliance is likely to have significant implications for coping and the development of effective advocacy, as described in greater detail later.

Inviting a parent to join the young child in the assessment room and to observe the assessment process is essential for several reasons. First, it provides much needed comfort and a sense of familiarity for the child. Second, parental participation in the assessment process can greatly enhance subsequent discussions, when the meaning of specific behaviors that the parents and the clinicians observed can be elucidated. However, many parents can be quite uncertain as to how active they should be during the evaluation. A clear explanation of the goals of the procedures and the anticipated parental role (e.g., as an observer and supporter or as a play partner for the child) usually helps to alleviate this uncertainty and reinforce the parental sense of participation in the assessment process. Sometimes parents who are eager to bring out their child's best performance may take an active role in the assessment in ways that can be counterproductive, such as, for instance, by violating standard test administration conditions. Sensitive yet firm reminders by the professional may be warranted, along with an explanation of the degree of parental involvement that is typically helpful versus interfering.

Eliciting a parent's view of the child's functioning during the assessment, as compared with other, more natural settings, is also imperative (Klin, Saulnier, Tsatsanis, & Volkmar, 2005; see also Chawarska & Bearss, Chapter 3, this volume). As mentioned above, a discussion of differences in the child's presentation across contexts has implications for educational programming, as well as for parents' regard for the credibility of the evaluation and their motivation to follow through on recommendations.

Communicating Diagnostic Findings

Once the evaluation is completed, an immediate discussion with the parent or parents is preferable, as long delays may be difficult to tolerate. The discussion, often referred to as a parent conference or a feedback session, is essentially an opportunity to serve the family members and prepare them to serve their child (Klin et al., 2005). An effective feedback delivers details at the level of parental interest and probes for parents' questions.

Following a detailed discussion with the clinical team regarding the child's current level of functioning in various key areas and the diagnostic considerations, parents invariably feel compelled to project the current situation into the future by asking, "Will my child be 'high functioning,' " "Will her challenges be mild or severe?" "Will she be mainstreamed by the time of kindergarten?" and, at times, "What about college?" The questions relating to both short- and long-term outcomes are naturally very important for both parents and professionals. These are also questions very difficult to answer on a case-by-case basis, as our ability to predict long-term outcomes for very young children with ASD is still limited (Charman et al., 2003; Chawarska, 2007; Lord et al., 2006; see also Chawarska & Bearss, Chapter 3, this volume). Although some parents may find it reassuring that their child's future has not been "sealed," others find it difficult to accept, as they may be seeking guarantees that their child will eventually "outgrow" or "recover" from his or her social and cognitive disabilities. Providing parents with the most up-to-date information regarding the stability of the diagnosis and predictors of outcome (Howlin, Goode, Hutton, & Rutter, 2004; see also Bishop, Luyster, Richler, & Lord, Chapter 2, and Chawarska & Bearss, Chapter 3, this volume) may help them cope with the diagnosis and make decisions about treatment options. Early characteristics that bode well for more positive outcomes are the acquisition of speech, nonverbal cognitive strength, and a good rate of progress over time (Chawarska, 2007; Howlin et al., 2004). Highlighting the relative strengths of the child is critical, as this gives parents a sense of hope and provides a more complete picture of their child that extends beyond the identified delays and deficits. Hope inspires and energizes parents to take action (Marcus, Kunce, & Schopler, 2005), which, coupled with competent guidance, helps parents to pursue early, intensive, and appropriately focused interventions.

Another frequently asked question is, "What can we do to help our child now?" Effectively, this is a call for explicit guidance and instruction. Helping families to find answers to this question requires extensive training and familiarity with effective treatment approaches, as well as available resources. This question may need to be addressed on two levels. The first level involves recommendations on how to attain appropriate treatment and educational programming for the child, utilizing the community resources. The second level involves a question about what the parent or parents can do themselves to facilitate the child's development on a daily basis at home and in other settings, or ways in which they can extend their roles from parent to therapist. Both levels need to be addressed. It is typically the case that the more appropriate and structured the educational program is, the less stressed the parents are likely to be. Parents should also be encouraged to safeguard times in which they are unconditionally accepting and loving parents, not therapists, for their child. If every moment of the day is conceived as a moment for therapy, burnout can ensue. The child is unlikely to be able to please a parent in some situations of learning, which can lead to constant frustration. Thus, typical parent–child interactions, with periods of silly play and "winding down," can be very important to preserve the natural pleasures of parenting while also preserving the child's and the family's energy for the long periods of work and directed learning.

Although it is important to be aware of the general features of ASD, it is even more important to appreciate how ASD is manifesting in a particular child and to help parents understand and articulate their child's specific needs (Dunlap, 1999). This impacts the parents' efficacy as advocates when discussion on educational programming centers on identifying the child's needs (Volkmar, Cook, Pomeroy, Realmuto, & Tanguay, 1999). To simply report that the child has ASD is insufficient. Parents need to know how their child is functioning, as compared with same-age peers, in each area of development; therefore, it behooves professionals to identify and communicate this clearly to parents (Marcus, Flagler, & Robinson, 2001). Areas of intervention to consider for young children with ASD include safety; cognition; motor skills (both fine and gross); speech, language, and communication; social interaction skills; play and imagination; adaptive skills (e.g., toileting, dressing, bathing, feeding, sleeping, and coping); recreation; and the presence of interfering behaviors.

Undoubtedly, this list is extensive and reflects the wide range of needs that young children with ASD may have. It is also meant to highlight the fact that current law and the existing educational guidelines indicate that an appropriate program for children with ASD must address all areas of educational need that spring from the disability (20 U.S.C. § 1412 *et seq.*; National Research Council, 2001; Olley, 2005). Notably, educational need encompasses academic, developmental, and functional skills and abilities. It is essential that all of these areas be considered during the evaluation and that relevant recommendations be made for each area of need (Lord & Risi, 2000; Mandlawitz, 2005; Tager-Flusberg, Paul, & Lord, 2005; Klin et al., 2005). This effort should be explicit, as the current educational climate continues to focus primarily on academic instruction. Fortunately, this trend is shifting to include social and adaptive skill development, but the shift is slow and uneven across the country. Therefore, feedback discussions and written recommendations that clearly address all areas of need can give parents the awareness that these are key areas to target for services and the leverage to pursue them.

SUPPORTING PARENTS IN OBTAINING APPROPRIATE EDUCATIONAL SERVICES

Establishing Goals and Priorities

The needs of children with ASD can be so extensive and pervasive that it is essential to establish a hierarchy of priorities to be emphasized in a program. By law (20 U.S.C. § 1400 *et seq.*), each eligible child is entitled to an individually designed and implemented program. Professionals working with a child whose needs span many developmental areas should help the family develop a hierarchy of needs that the program should focus on systematically. Safety should always be at the pinnacle of this hierarchy. Common safety issues among young children with ASD include mouthing and/or ingesting nonfood items, darting, and climbing. Self-injurious behaviors such as head banging, or aggressive behaviors such as biting or hitting, are less frequent, but when they occur they must be treated immediately. Interfering behaviors may also occur, which essentially include anything that interferes with a child's ability to learn or use a skill functionally, including motor mannerisms, repetitive or restricted interests, distractibility, activity level, and so forth. Basic learning-to-learn skills also fall into the behavioral domain, and these include the ability to attend to speech, sit, monitor the therapist's behavior, follow directions, and engage in vocal and motor imitation. These skills prepare a child for the fundamental process of learning and are frequently and successfully addressed utilizing behaviorally based methods and techniques (Harris & Weiss, 1998; Hodgdon, 1995).

Any behavior that puts the welfare of self or others at risk should be systematically studied via a functional behavioral analysis (FBA) and addressed via positive behavioral supports (20 U.S.C. § 1415 *et seq.*; Powers, 2005). This is a dynamic process that involves a certain amount of trial and error. In order for the process to be successful, several elements need to be in place: (1) a competent professional to do the analysis and design the intervention, (2) ongoing monitoring of the intervention for effectiveness, (3) flexibility and change of the intervention as needed, and (4) collaboration among all team members, including parents, for consistency in the application of the intervention (Schopler & Mesibov, 2000). This effort should not be restricted to the school setting. If the difficulties exist outside the school—that is, at home or in the community—the child's needs should be addressed directly in those settings. The hierarchy of needs can vary from family to family and from child to child; however, a useful model puts safety first, interfering behaviors second, followed by a mix of efforts in the areas of communication, social interaction, adaptive skills, motor skills, and cognitive development as warranted.

The need for intervention in the areas of communication is self-evident, as impairments in this area are one of the defining features of ASD. However, it is important to help parents understand that teaching communication to young children is not equivalent to helping them to amass a large vocabulary. Intervention in this area needs to be focused on fostering an understanding of language: expressing needs, sharing interests, and commenting on experiences, as well as using nonverbal means such as gestures, facial expressions, and eye contact for communication (Wetherby et al., 2000; Prizant, Wetherby, & Rydell, 2000; Paul & Sutherland, 2005). For many children, the development of communication can be fostered with the use of pictures, signs, and assistive technology (Bondy & Frost, 1995). Parents need to advocate for intervention that targets the functional use of speech and language for the purpose of spontaneous and flexible communication, rather than simply the acquisition of verbal labels. Written reports should reflect this distinction in the "Recommendations" section.

Social impairments are another defining feature of ASD, which also warrant thoughtful intervention. Children who have some means for functional communication and imitation skills may benefit from adult instruction and facilitated support for peer interactions. Children who have not yet developed imitation skills in particular may be better served with individual adult instruction designed to develop these skills in preparation for peer interaction. The goal is to move the child toward independent and functional use of skills. The effort is informed by the child's present level of need and the pace, level of support, and context in which the child can benefit from intervention.

The typical repertoire of adaptive skills in young children includes feeding, toileting, dressing, sleeping, and personal hygiene skills. These areas can be quite challenging for children with ASD. The important point is that these are all legitimate and reasonable areas to target for intervention, by both early intervention providers and preschool settings. Self-reliance and independent living skills are essential long-term goals (Klin et al., 2007). The Vineland Adaptive Behavior Scales–II (VABS-II; Sparrow, Cicchetti, & Balla, 2005) is an example of a useful tool that can be used to formally identify specific adaptive needs. Common areas of adaptive need for young children with ASD include sleep (Didde & Sigafoos, 2001; Honomichi, Goodlin-Jones, Burnham, Gaylor, & Anders, 2002; Wiggs & Stores, 2004), feeding (Ahearn, Castine, Nault, & Green, 2001; Field, Garland, & Williams, 2003), and toileting (Volkmar & Wiesner, 2004; Wheeler, 2004). A feedback discussion, which includes identification of adaptive needs and guidance for setting treatment priorities, assists parents in making decisions and taking action to secure appropriate therapeutic and educational programming. Communication, social interaction, and adaptive skills often overlap. Although the specific teaching in each of these areas may be quite separate and different, the hope is that over time the skills will converge toward a higher level of functioning, especially in the context of peer interaction. For example, it is adaptive for a 4-year-old to be able to kick and throw a ball. Recreation is conducive to social interaction, which, in turn, is conducive to better communication.

Providing Information about Resources

One of the questions frequently asked by parents is, "Where can I find more information about ASD that I can trust?" This question is extremely relevant, considering the proliferation of both expert and nonexpert opinions about ASD, including its causes and treatment, via the Internet and various non-peer-reviewed publications. It is often helpful to provide parents with a reading list that can both give them more information about the disorder and provide them with suggestions on how to help their child in day-to-day situations. Books frequently cited as helpful by parents include *Healthcare for Children on the Autism Spectrum* (Volkmar & Wiesner, 2004), *Children with Autism and Their Families* (Powers, 2000), *Right from the Start* (Harris & Weiss, 1998), *More Than Words* (Sussman, 1999), *Visual Strategies for Improving Communication* (Hodgdon, 1995), and *Do–Watch–Listen–Say* (Quill, 2000). There is evidence suggesting that parents who are actively engaged in the delivery of intervention enjoy a greater sense of confidence and efficacy in the parenting role, and such involvement may contribute to greater progress for the child over time (Eyberg, Edwards, Boggs, & Foote, 1998; Schopler, 2001; Webster, Stratton, Reid, & Hammond, 2001). A word of caution is worth repeating: For a parent who is involved in helping the child, there is a risk that the role of therapist can supersede the role of parent. This speaks to the difficulty in maintaining appropriate roles and balance in a family living with ASD, which is discussed in greater detail subsequently.

Supporting Families in Accessing Services

To a large degree, helping a young child with ASD is a matter of securing appropriate services for an intervention program. Typically, services are available via a designated state agency. Early intervention services typically span the ages of birth to 3 years. At the age of 3, children are usually transitioned from the early intervention system to the public school system. The Special Education Law, formally known as the Individuals with Disabilities Education Improvement Act of 2004 (Public Law 108-446), and often referred to as IDEA-2004, mandates that these public systems provide appropriate intervention services and educational programming to those children who are deemed eligible. Specific eligibility criteria can vary from state to state, particularly in the early intervention system. Familiarity with the current governing regulations is critical in order to give good counsel to parents in their pursuit of services. Some states have published guidelines for educating children with ASD that help to frame and structure the content of a program (New York State Department of Health Early Intervention Program, 1999), which can be useful for professionals in making appropriate recommendations for programming and useful for parents in negotiating for services. If such state guidelines are not available locally, another good reference is *Educating Children with Autism* (National Research Council, 2001), which is written for both parents and professionals. It covers many topics, including guidelines for effective and appropriate programming for young children.

Why is it important to be aware of educational guidelines and special education law? Unfortunately, in some situations, guidelines and laws are not adhered to automatically or to their full extent. Thus, as Mayerson (2004) highlights, parents inherit the often unwelcome yet necessary responsibility to become effective advocates to secure services that their child needs and is entitled to by law.

Effective advocacy requires a knowledge of ASD in general, an understanding of how it is manifesting in a particular child, familiarity with educational guidelines (National Research Council, 2001; New York State Department of Health Early Intervention Program, 1999) and special education law, and utilization of negotiation and mediation skills (Volkmar et al., 1999). It may be daunting for parents to discover that they need to learn about and facilitate implementation of these guidelines while reeling from the news that their child has a developmental disorder. The task may at times be overwhelming, yet the need remains (Howlin & Moore, 1997). Parents who wish to become well versed in the educational guidelines and laws often find that it takes considerable time and effort to develop competence in this area, especially in the early years of adjusting to life with ASD. Professionals equipped with this knowledge are well positioned to give good counsel to families. Additional support often comes from various national and regional organizations and resource centers (Mandlawitz, 2005). These include such organizations as the Autism Society of America (ASA; *www.autismsociety.org*), Autism Speaks (*www. autismspeaks.org*) and local parent support groups. Such organizations can provide invaluable forums for connecting families with mentors (e.g., more experienced parents who have traveled a similar road), who may be able to help navigate the educational system and access resources in the community. Publications such as *From Emotions to Advocacy* (Wright & Wright, 2002) and *Wrightslaw* (*www.wrightslaw.com*) are informative and credible resources, which although not specific to ASD, are very relevant.

Supplementary Supports

Parents often pursue the option of supplementing the program offered by early intervention providers or school systems with additional services. Competent private practitioners, whether they are speech therapists, occupational therapists, physical therapists, ABA therapists, or individual or family therapists who are familiar with ASD in young children, are in high demand and short supply. An effective way to find such specialists is to network with other parents to explore who might be available in the community and how they may be helpful. The local chapter of the ASA may be a good place to network with other parents. There may also be other parent groups in the area, and some schools have special education parent–teacher associations. In addition, professionals who go to parent meetings have an opportunity to meet a broader array of families in the community, learn about their concerns and priorities, and learn more about recommended service providers. Taking time to meet providers and to gain an appreciation of their personal styles and working philosophies may also be helpful in matching them with particular families. A good fit is vital in sustaining a healthy and productive working alliance over time.

When a family starts creating an overall program that includes multiple providers, a word of caution is warranted. There is nothing inherently wrong with such a mix of professionals, and, in fact, it can be very effective, but it is imperative that all of the team members are communicating and coordinating their efforts with one another, with a view to reaching consensus about the child's level of need and how to address it (Schopler & Mesibov, 2000). Without such integration of efforts, there is a strong possibility that instruction and intervention across professionals will be fragmented and possibly at odds. When this occurs, the child is at risk of confusion, which impedes learning. The more service providers involved, the greater the need for clear communication, consensus regarding effort, frequent monitoring of efficacy, and flexibility to respond to changes as warranted.

Coordinating the schedules of multiple personnel can be quite challenging. Although the process can and probably will be fraught with frustration, striving for it is justified by the positive impact it will have on a child's opportunity for learning. Still, this can be more than some families can manage. If resources allow, having someone take on the role of service coordinator or education consultant to oversee the process can be very helpful. Even in cases where the child is receiving services from a single provider (e.g., public school), it is still valuable to hold regular meetings with teachers, therapists, and parents to ensure that everyone is working in ways that truly support learning. As generalization of skills is one of the most entrenched challenges in programming for children with ASD, a lack of integrated efforts across people and settings can significantly and deleteriously impact the eventual outcome of the program. In other words, it can undermine the entire effort.

LEGAL CONSIDERATIONS

Individuals with Disabilities Education Act

The Individuals with Disabilities Education Act (IDEA, 2004) mandates the provision of appropriate services for eligible children, yet the term *appropriate* is not defined in the statue (Wright & Wright, 2004). *Appropriate* has come to be understood as that which is effective in helping the child to make tangible and measurable progress. Progress that is apparent only in a particular context—that is, the testing environment or the classroom—does not constitute skill mastery. True progress, true skill mastery, is defined by spontaneous and flexible application of a given skill, with a variety of people and materials, across a variety of settings, and across time. Thus, each acquired skill needs to be further maintained and generalized (Klin et al., 2005).

Young children with ASD require intensive and explicit instruction and opportunities to practice their skills repeatedly in order to gain true mastery in natural and varied contexts. This process takes time, and there are differing opinions as to how much intervention time is necessary. The *Educating Children with Autism* report (National Research Council, 2001) has delved into this question extensively and determined that a reasonable and appropriate program for young children with ASD is full-time and full-year, meaning a minimum of 25–30 hours (15–20 hours for children under age 3) of instruction per week, running 12 months a year, and suplemented with additional hours of service provided for in-home and community support as warranted.

Early intervention programs are typically designed to run year-round, and services are delivered in the home and community. Public school programs are typically designed to run approximately 9 months of the year and are based at a school. Many public schools offer only half-day programs until the child enters first grade. Regardless of what educational programs are currently available, recommendations addressing the child's needs while following educational guidelines and federal law are needed. This gives parents leverage to negotiate and push for appropriate, reasonable, and individualized services, regardless of existing programming offerings. The complicating factor is that what is "appropriate" varies from child to child on the basis of his or her individualized profile of

needs and developmental assets, hence the importance of highly individualized assessments (see Bishop et al., Chapter 2; Chawarska & Bears,
Chapter 3; and Paul, Chapter 4, this volume).

It is reasonable for parents to request a full-time program even
though the school currently has only a half-day program for preschool
and kindergarten. It is reasonable to request programming through the
summer when the school typically closes during that time (Mandlawitz,
2005). It is also reasonable to request services for the family and the child
in the home and community that extend beyond the school day. Legal
statue (20 U.S.C. § 1400 *et seq.*) and educational guidelines (National
Research Council, 2001) support all such requests as required, given the
child's needs.

Just as parents benefit from a working knowledge of special education law, so too do professionals. The statue itself and *www.wrightslaw.com*
are useful resources. Familiarity with case law (Mandlawitz, 2002) quickly
reveals the power of language and the importance of choosing words carefully. This is true in meetings of record (e.g., school meetings), and it is
certainly true for written reports. It is essential for professionals to understand the implications of language and word choice in order to support
rather than undermine parents' efforts to secure *appropriate* services for
their child.

Free Appropriate Public Education

IDEA-2004 states that children deemed eligible for special education are
entitled to a free appropriate public education (FAPE) (20 U.S.C. § 1412
et seq.); however, as mentioned previously, "appropriate" education has
been left undefined. It is conventional to think of appropriate education
as that which is effective in supporting and moving a child toward progress in areas of need. The importance of word choice when making educational recommendations cannot be overstated. Public service providers
are not mandated to provide the "best" services possible, and their mission is not to maximize a child's potential (*Board of Education of Hendrick
Hudson Center School District v. Rowley*, 1982). Rather, they are responsible
for the provision of adequate services (Mandlawitz, 2005). Therefore,
when wording recommendations it is imperative that words such as *best,
excellent, optimal,* and *ideal* are excluded. These words can be counterproductive and in the worst cases can actually undermine the credibility of
the entire report. Surprisingly, the word *beneficial* is also problematic, as
any child could potentially "benefit from" the provision of practically any
intervention. Professional responsibility dictates an effort to identify the
child's needs and make reasonable and appropriate recommendations to
meet those needs with respect to one's particular area of expertise. Educational guidelines further help to frame what is reasonable.

Individualized Education Program

All eligible children with disabilities are entitled to an individualized education program (IEP) that is designed to address their specific and individual needs (20 U.S.C. § 1414 et seq.). This points again to the importance of delineating the child's specific needs and helping parents to articulate and prioritize these needs. It is inappropriate to place all children with ASD in the same classroom, targeting all the same goals, utilizing the same instructional methodology and the same supports. The key is that each child with ASD is an individual with specific needs that call for specific and individual attention. The potential benefits of early intervention and special education are compromised when instruction and intervention are not provided in ways and at levels from which a particular child can learn.

Common and worrisome experience shows that many children are offered the existing "autism program," which typically includes a standard and previously determined instructional approach, classroom designation, number of hours of instruction, intervention modalities, and goals. Such educational prepackaging should raise red flags for both parents and professionals. Instead, the designing of the intervention program should be collaborative and involve parents in the decision-making process. Decisions regarding the content and form of the program should be guided by the child's individual needs, including the child's profile of challenges and existing strengths.

Parents as Partners

The IEP process is designed to include parents as equal partners (20 U.S.C. § 1414 et seq.). An initial step in the process is to determine eligibility for special education. Once eligibility is established, the next step is to identify the child's present levels of functioning in all areas of development. This serves to highlight both the child's strengths and areas of need. Areas of need are further prioritized, and goals are established based on an understanding of those needs. The goals reflect the effort to help move the child toward progress in all areas of educational need with the understanding that these needs may span academic, social, emotional, motor, and adaptive skills that are generalized across contexts and maintained over time. The goals are typically thought to cover a 1-year period, with the expectation that progress can and will be measured objectively (20 U.S.C. § 1414 et seq.). Exactly how progress will be defined and measured is another factor to be discussed and agreed upon by the IEP team.

Once goals and measurement are agreed upon, the next step is to determine the logistics of the program. Which professional will be providing what service? Which methodology will be utilized, in what setting, how often, and for how long? Educational guidelines and special education law do not delineate specifics at this level. Although the guidelines suggest the total number of hours of programming that are generally considered appropriate, the specific number and duration of sessions of speech therapy, occupational therapy, physical therapy, applied behavior analysis (ABA), facilitated play, and so forth, are left to the IEP team to determine. Such determination can be daunting for both parents and professionals.

Professional Boundaries

Although a multidisciplinary approach to the evaluation of young children suspected of having ASD is typically recommended (Klin et al., 2005), practice limitations do not always allow for such an intensive process. In such situations, professional restraint is warranted to increase the credibility and usefulness of recommendations stemming from the evaluation. Specific recommendations limited to the parameters of one's particular professional discipline are necessary. Recommendations that span beyond the scope of a particular discipline can be problematic and counterproductive and can lead to questioning the credibility of the evaluation and subsequent recommendations. Although recommendations should highlight areas of identified need, professional restraint regarding the impulse to designate a specific number of hours or sessions or specific modality is encouraged. Instead, professionals in a given area of expertise may provide recommendations for a formal evaluation to be conducted by a professional in a different field, such as speech–language, occupational, or physical therapy, to assist in determining the frequency, duration, and specific approach of sessions warranted to adequately address the child's needs and help the child meet his or her IEP goals. Clearly, it is preferable when a group of professionals work together as a transdisciplinary team so that a single coherent view of the child can emerge from the evaluation process. When that is not possible, coordination of different expert opinions stemming from different areas of expertise is needed, particularly insofar as the operationalization and implementation of recommendations are concerned. Otherwise, parents may be left with the daunting task of having to integrate what might be, in some situations, a plethora of conflicted reports and recommendations.

Least Restrictive Environment

Another important consideration for the IEP team is placement. *Placement* refers to where the child goes to school: which school, which classroom, and with what level of support. IDEA-2004 (20 U.S.C. § 1412 *et seq.*) refers to the least restrictive environment (LRE), which is the environment closest to that of the mainstream classroom in which the particular child can benefit from instruction and make progress. The intent is to give children with disabilities opportunities to engage and associate with typically developing peers, rather than be automatically assigned to separate and more restricted environments. To automatically place all children with disabilities in a mainstream classroom is equally inappropriate. Placement decisions call for thoughtful consideration of the interaction of a given child's needs with the instructional environment and how that interaction can support versus undermine the child's learning. In many ways, the spirit of the law points to the placement of a child in an educational environment whereby the child can learn and profit from instruction with the fewest restrictions regarding access to typically developing peers.

The determination of appropriate placement hinges primarily on two factors: the child's ability to actually benefit from access to typically developing peers and access to the general curriculum (Handleman & Harris, 2001) and the level of competence and ready availability of professionals instructing the child (Simpson, 2004). In order to benefit from access to typically developing peers, a given child needs to have, at a minimum, a functional communication system, imitation skills, some degree of social interest, and an ability to at least briefly stay on task with or without adult support. Such a child, with appropriate levels of support, is more likely to be able to function, learn, and make progress in the mainstream setting and may be a good candidate for such a placement. A child manifesting behaviors that are aggressive, destructive, self-injurious, or highly distracting or who lacks the aforementioned basic skills is questionable if not inappropriate as a candidate for the mainstream setting until these problems are addressed in a more specialized educational setting. Placement is rarely an either–or decision, but instead is often a combination of mainstream and contained environments with varying degrees of adult support. Notably, few young children with ASD are able to function and learn in any school environment without at least some one-on-one adult instruction and support. Equally important, research has shown that a number of factors facilitate successful integration (Handleman & Harris, 2001) and that for many children, rather than a dichotomy of "fully mainstreamed" or "fully segregated" placement, it is a continuum of services that is needed.

Due Process

In the best of circumstances, families and service providers, be they early interventionists or school personnel, can easily and readily reach consensus regarding the child's needs and how to meet them appropriately. Rightly, legislators have anticipated that such an outcome will not always be the case, and therefore special education law includes a course of due process for those situations that call for legal intervention to resolve differences (20 U.S.C. § 1415 *et seq.*). The decision to pursue due process is a serious one, and consultation with an attorney who is well versed in special education law is advised. The decision should not be taken lightly as it will change the relationship between the family and the service providers, sometimes in ways that are irreparable (Mandlawitz, 2005).

Although due process is a valuable and sometimes necessary option, such a course of action warrants great care and much thought. Efforts to avoid due process are worthwhile and begin with a thorough understanding of the relevant information and access to resources. Professional responsibility encompasses highlighting the child's needs, making appropriate and comprehensive recommendations, and educating families about the disability, the guidelines, and the law in order for them to be effective advocates for their child. Resources that can assist parents' efforts at self-education include state guidelines (if available), *Educating Children with Autism* (National Research Council, 2001), as a national reference for educational guidelines, and *www.wrightslaw.com* for information regarding special education law and advocacy.

FAMILY IMPLICATIONS

In addition to issues related to diagnosis and treatment planning, there are a number of essential family-related issues that have a potential impact on the functioning of the entire family (Marcus et al., 2005). In many ways ASD is a family disability. Although a single child may be identified as affected with the disorder, the entire family, including extended family members, is affected by its emotional and financial fallout (Burack, Charman, Yirmiya, & Zelazo, 2001). How family members are affected, and to what degree, can vary significantly and can change over time. Here we focus on family implications that are typically seen in the young-child phase of family development and family functioning. As noted, it is quite common for parents of a child with ASD to have concerns early in the child's development. They often suppress these concerns, especially if this is their first child. By the time the child reaches the age of 2, professionals may concur with the parents' concern, especially when language development appears delayed. The parents often feel relief and confidence when their concerns are being validated; however, that same validation often stimulates anxiety. What will it mean if their child really does have a problem? Parents may also experience anger at having been dismissed previously. Anger and anxiety can further result from a sense that precious time for early intervention may have already been lost (Marcus et al., 2005), which is compounded by a complicated grief process surrounding the loss of the idealized child and family. The cumulative stress can be unbearable and depression often ensues (Siegel, 2003; Hastings & Johnson, 2001; Olsson & Hwang, 2002; Seltzer, Krauss, Orsmond, & Vestal, 2001; Tobing & Genwick, 2002).

Anecdotal evidence suggests that once a child is identified as having ASD, both parents typically experience an overwhelming sadness coupled with a sense of urgency that compels them to actively pursue intensive services for their child. The day-to-day details of this pursuit are often left to one parent. Both parents seem to struggle with depression and anxiety, and both typically take on a task-oriented approach to coping. One parent typically becomes immersed in his or her professional work, while the other parent takes on the responsibility for pursuing, organizing, and monitoring services for their child, to the extent that many such parents give up their professional careers (Gray, 2002; Seltzer et al., 2001). Both parents could probably benefit from some form of therapeutic support at this point, but the inclination is to be self-sacrificing—to ignore their own needs and focus almost exclusively on the work role that they have embraced. Some parents use medication to help them cope and keep up their energy, but they seem much less likely to engage in other pursuits that may offer therapeutic benefit. To do so is often regarded as selfish and frivolous when their child's needs are so grave and so immediate and the magnitude of financial responsibilities related to, for instance, supplementing the child's treatment, becomes apparent. Unfortunately, this dynamic has the potential to set down roots for unbalanced individual and family functioning in the future.

Imbalance

Imbalance is often the primary focal point in maladaptive or disrupted family functioning. It is also the most difficult area for therapeutic work. Regrettably, families often do not seek help until they are at the point of breakdown. Therefore, it behooves professionals to alert families to this inclination and help them to monitor for and identify signs that can essentially give them permission and impetus to help themselves. Interestingly, many parents are quite defensive about a direct recommendation for therapy for themselves. A typical response is, "You'd be going crazy too if you were going through what we are." Often a more helpful approach is to educate parents on the physical and cognitive signs that warrant clinical concern in general: change in appetite, weight, sleeping pattern, or sexual drive and presence of obsessive or persisting thoughts. Seemingly, parents find it more logical and more acceptable to think about these factors versus emotional factors as triggers for self-help. This may be especially true when the focus is on keeping themselves healthy so they can continue to have the energy and clear thinking necessary to help their child.

Not surprisingly, living with ASD and all of its ramifications puts enormous stress on families. Perhaps it is true of all disabilities, but it is certainly true that ASD is a family disability in that it impacts all family members (Powers, 2000), including extended family. The risks to the family include isolation, role imbalance, depression, anxiety, grief, guilt, blaming, and extreme self-sacrifice. Additional risks include financial hardship due to costs of supplementary services and/or due process expenses, and chronic sleep deprivation in cases involving children with disrupted or difficult sleeping patterns.

Some families experience isolation from their communities because of the child's behavior being idiosyncratic, unsafe, or disruptive to the extent that it becomes too difficult or too embarrassing to go out in public (Gray, 2002; Avdi, Griffin, & Brough, 2000). Isolation can also occur within the family. This tends to happen when parents are unable to agree on the needs of the child or how to meet those needs. In such instances communication between the parents diminishes along with emotional support, with one parent becoming overinvolved with professional work life, spending less and less time at home and being more withdrawn while at home. The other parent can become hyperfocused on the child with ASD, with the thought that everyone else in the family is able to function on his or her own. This seems to be driven by a parent's anxiety regarding the perceived ever-closing window for early intervention. It also seems to be driven by a deep-seated sense of guilt for somehow causing the ASD and/or a sense of guilt for not trusting his or her initial intuition of concern and not being more proactive in getting help for the child at the first moment of concern. Although these self-imposed pressures may seem irrational to an outside party, the stress is very real and can be quite debilitating for a family caught in this dynamic, all of which is further complicated in single-parent families.

The unrelenting effort, coupled with emotional weight, quickly becomes quite tiresome, and relations with spouse, other children, extended family members, and friends are easily strained if not neglected. The strains are particularly worrisome when the child with ASD makes limited progress. For, despite the best efforts of the family and service providers, some children unfortunately do not make much progress (Mundy, 2003). In such situations it is not unusual for the family to pursue less conventional therapies and practices (Marcus et al., 2005; Rapin, 2005; see also Smith & Wick, Chapter 9, this volume). Such is a time to help families think through options carefully and weigh hoped-for benefits against some very real risks that may have the potential to do harm.

Although many parents resist the idea of individual or family therapy, other families often choose to pursue this route. Families that cope well and manage life with ASD effectively appear to draw on their inherent strengths and various protective factors, which are discussed in a later section. They are also able to set priorities, stay focused, and pace their efforts effectively. The parents' goal is to support the needs of their child with ASD and still make room for the needs of the rest of the family, as well as themselves. Their goals are attainable and their expectations are reasonable. Families whose goal is to "erase" or "cure" autism often experience higher levels of frustration when their efforts do not meet expectations. At present, autism cannot be "cured," but children can make a great deal of progress toward independent, meaningful, and fulfilling lives.

Siblings and Extended Family

Siblings of a child with ASD often find their emotional needs somewhat neglected within their primary family (Harris & Glasberg, 1994). They tend to compensate for this experience by striving for excellence in all they do. Siblings are typically more mature than their same-aged peers and often take on responsibilities far beyond what would be expected from other children their age (Fishman, Wolf, Ellison, & Freeman, 2000; Konidaris, 2005). Typically, the most vulnerable sibling is the oldest female, who is most at risk for becoming quite parentified at a very early age. On the surface, siblings appear quite well adjusted and competent. Unfortunately, the heightened sense of responsibility and effort to excel may at times be driven by a very basic need for recognition, acceptance, and validation. Value as a person becomes associated with tasks and accomplishments versus simply being a child and a member of a family. External sources of validation (e.g., school) may become more reliable, and a sibling's natural sense of value within the family may be at risk for being diminished. The need for validation within the family remains a primary, yet in some instances an inadequately met, need. Typically, the sibling facing this situation can strive for years to be good enough, to be a great helper, to not be in the way, and to be content with a perceived secondary status in the family. Sadly, this effort becomes quite difficult for many to sustain over time. Preadolescence seems to be associated with emerging mental health concerns, particularly depression, which if left unchecked, may result in serious and potentially life-long challenges. Alerting families to the risks for siblings and guiding them to healthy family functioning can be invaluable. Lobato and Kao (2002) highlight evidence suggesting that participation in a sibling support group may also be beneficial.

Extended family members, especially grandparents, tend to follow one of several paths: (1) awareness of problems and supportive of needs,

(2) dismissal of problems, often stemming from a lack of understanding of ASD and/or an inability to accept its existence within their family, and (3) an attempt to "take over" the situation, pushing ahead with a plan without the full engagement of the child's actual parents. Dismissal of problems can undermine the parents' efforts to secure and maintain appropriate services for the child. It also serves to diminish and invalidate the stress that the family encounters. At its worst, dismissal breeds irreparable contention and conflict among family members and results in a cut-off of relations. Sharpley, Bitsika, and Ephrimidis (1997) point out that time and effort extended to educate and inform in such circumstances serves to increase understanding, which in turn can decrease stress on families. And if the actual parents are pushed aside at this critical juncture, this may lead to their dependence on others and lack of an active voice in a process that requires their decisive input. This often leads to a sense of powerlessness and ineffectual participation, thus delaying if not undermining altogether their becoming effective advocates for their children. From the standpoint of clinicians, this can be very confusing, as responsibility lies first with parents, and such confusion can lead to cross purposes.

Protective or Resilience Factors

There are many protective factors for family functioning that deserve to be cultivated and nurtured. A strong and committed partnership that supports the parental alliance as well as the marital bond is essential. A full understanding of the child's needs and a shared focus on how to meet those needs is also essential. Having practical knowledge of educational guidelines, special education law, and advocacy skills certainly assists in meeting the child's needs. Also, having an appreciation for the roles of the various family members and meeting their needs adequately can contribute to balanced and adaptive functioning of the entire family over time. A network of understanding and available friends can be protective, not only for emotional support but also for very practical needs such as child care and respite. Financial resources give families options regarding supplementary services and supports, which may contribute to a positive outcome for both child and family. The child's steady progress is also protective, as it gives parents assurance that their efforts are effective; thus, they are less distracted by the often tempting yet questionable alternative therapies. Finally, and perhaps most important, is a sense of hope. When family members perceive that they can be effective and that their child can make progress, they are energized by a strong sense of hope for the future, which fuels their motivation to continue their diligent work in service of the needs they face. Hope is powerful and necessary, and its cultivation is crucial.

CONCLUSIONS

When pondering the complexities of ASD, it is important to keep in mind that this essentially social disability can have a powerful and disturbing impact on the entire family. Restoring and maintaining balance within the family often becomes the focal point of therapeutic effort, which helps families get past feelings of blame and guilt, or the compulsion to erase all traces of ASD, thus enabling them to set healthy priorities for all family members while finding ways to accept and even embrace a life with ASD. Such work is very challenging, yet so worthy of effort.

An inspiring aspect of the work is the opportunity and privilege of witnessing families overcome very real and very difficult hurdles and come to view ASD as a "blessing in disguise" and an important factor in their sense of calling in life. Living with ASD opens many parents to self-discovery and personal growth that may not have happened otherwise. Countless numbers of families have noted that living with ASD has taught them to celebrate the little things in life, to not take anything for granted, to grow personally, to be brave, to be humble, and be grateful. Many have an intense appreciation of the value and strength of family and actively reach out and support the health and advancement of the wider community of families living with ASD. Professionals working in the field of ASD have an important mission to help families cultivate hope by highlighting their strengths and the strengths of their children, and by encouraging habits that further strengthen their efficacy as loving parents and advocates for their children. Good practice alerts families to the potential risks that may be inherent in living with ASD and serves as a pivotal element in facilitating positive outcomes for children and families living with autism spectrum disorder.

REFERENCES

Ahearn, W. H., Castine, T., Nault, K., & Green, G. (2001). An assessment of food acceptance in children with autism or pervasive developmental disorder-not otherwise specified. *Journal of Autism and Developmental Disorders, 31*(5), 505–511.

Avdi, E., Griffin, C., & Brough, S. (2000). Parents' constructions of professional knowledge, expertise and authority during assessment and diagnosis of their child for an autistic spectrum disorder. *British Journal of Medical Psychology, 73*, 327–338.

Board of Education of Henrick Hudson Center School District v. Rowley, 458, U.S. 176 (1982).

Bondy, A. S., & Frost, L. A. (1995). Educational approaches in preschool: Behavior techniques in a public school setting. In E. Schopler & G. B. Mesibov (Eds.), *Learning and cognition in autism* (pp. 311–333). New York: Plenum Press.

Burack, J. A., Charman, T., Yirmiya, N., & Zelazo, P. R. (Eds.). (2001). *The develop-ment of autism: Perspectives from theory and research.* Mahwah, NJ: Erlbaum.

Charman, T., Baron-Cohen, S., Swettenham, J., Baird, G., Drew, A., & Cox, A. (2003). Predicting language outcome in infants with autism and pervasive developmental disorder. *International Journal of Language and Communication Disorders, 38*(3), 265–285.

Chawarska, K. (2007). *Longitudinal study of syndrome expression: ASD from the second to the fourth year.* Paper presented at the Society for Child Development Conference, Boston.

Chawarska, K., & Volkmar, F. R. (2005). Autism in infancy and early childhood. In F. R. Volkmar, R. Paul, A Klin, & D. Cohen (Eds.), *Handbook of autism and per-vasive developmental disorders* (3rd ed., pp. 223–246). Hoboken, NJ: Wiley.

De Giacomo, A., & Fombonne, E. (1998). Parental recognition of developmental abnormalities in autism. *European Child and Adolescent Psychiatry, 7,* 131–136.

Didde, R., & Sigafoos, J. (2001). A review of the nature and treatment of sleep dis-orders in individuals with developmental disabilities. *Research in Developmen-tal Disabilities, 22*(4), 255–272.

Dunlap, G. (1999). Consensus, engagement, and family involvement for young children with autism. *Journal of the Association for Persons with Severe Handi-caps, 24,* 222–225.

Eyberg, S. M., Edwards, D., Boggs, S. R., & Foote, R. (1998). Maintaining the treat-ment effects of parent training: The role of booster sessions and other main-tenance strategies. *Clinical Psychology, 5,* 544–554.

Field, D., Garland, M., & Williams, K. (2003). Correlates of specific childhood feeding problems. *Journal of Pediatrics and Child Health, 39*(4), 299–304.

Fishman, S., Wolf, L., Ellison, D., & Freeman, T. (2000). A longitudinal study of siblings of children with chronic disabilities. *Canadian Journal of Psychiatry, 45,* 369–375.

Gray, D. E. (2002). Ten years on: A longitudinal study of families of children with autism. *Journal of Intellectual and Developmental Disability, 27,* 215–222.

Handleman, J. S., & Harris, L. D. (Eds.). (2001). *Preschool education programs for children with autism* (2nd ed.). Austin, TX: PRO-ED.

Harris, S. L., & Glasberg, B. A. (1994). *Siblings of children with autism: A guide for families* (2nd ed.). Bethesda, MD: Woodbine House.

Harris, S. L., & Handleman, J. S. (2000). Age and IQ at intake as predictors of placement for young children with autism: A four-to-six-year follow-up. *Jour-nal of Autism and Developmental Disorders, 30,* 137–142.

Harris, S. L., & Weiss, M. J. (1998). *Right from the start–behavioral intervention for young children with autism: A guide for parents and professionals.* Bethesda, MD: Woodbine House.

Hastings, R. P., & Johnson, E. (2001). Stress in UK families conducting home-based behavioral intervention for their young child with autism. *Journal of Autism and Development Disorders, 31,* 327–336.

Hodgdon, L. A. (1995). *Visual strategies for improving communication: Practical sup-ports for school and home.* Troy, MI: QuirkRoberts.

Honomichl, R. D., Goodlin-Jones, B. L., Burnham, M., Gaylor, E., & Anders, T. F. (2002). Sleep patterns of children with pervasive developmental disorders. *Journal of Autism and Developmental Disorders 32*(6), 553–561.

Howlin, P., & Asgharian, A. (1999). The diagnosis of autism and Asperger syndrome: Findings from a survey of 770 families. *Developmental Medicine and Child Neurology, 41,* 834–839.

Howlin, P., Goode, S., Hutton, J., & Rutter, M. (2004). Adult outcome for children with autism. *Journal of Child Psychology and Psychiatry,* 45, 212–229.

Howlin, P., & Moore, A. (1997). Diagnosis in autism: A survey of over 1200 patients in the UK. *Autism: Journal of Research and Practice, 1,* 135–162.

Individuals with Disabilities Education Improvement Act of 2004, 20 U.S.C. § 1400 *et seq.* (2004).

Klin, A., Saulnier, C. A., Sparrow, S. S., Cicchetti, D. V., Volkmar, F. R., & Lord, C. (2007). Social and communication abilities and disabilities in higher functioning individuals with autism spectrum disorders. *Journal of Autism and Developmental Disorders, 37*(4), 748–759.

Klin, A., Saulnier, C., Tsatsanis, K., & Volkmar, F. R. (2005). Clinical evaluation in autism spectrum disorders: Psychological assessment within a transdisciplinary framework. In F. R. Volkmar, R. Paul, A. Klin, & D. Cohen (Eds.), *Handbook of autism and pervasive developmental disorders* (3rd ed., pp. 772–798). Hoboken, NJ: Wiley.

Konidaris, J. B. (2005). A sibling's perspective on autism. In F. R. Volkmar, R. Paul, A. Klin, & D. Cohen (Eds.), *Handbook of autism and pervasive developmental disorders* (3rd ed., pp. 1265–1275). Hoboken, NJ: Wiley.

Lobato, D. J., & Kao, B. T. (2002). Integrated sibling–parent group intervention to improve sibling knowledge and adjustment to chronic illness and disability. *Journal of Pediatric Psychology, 27,* 711–716.

Lord, C., & Risi, S. (2000). Diagnosis of autism spectrum disorders in young children. In A. M. Wetherby & B. M. Prizant (Eds.), *Autism spectrum disorders: A transactional developmental perspective* (pp. 11–30). Baltimore: Brookes.

Lord, C., Risi, S., DiLavore, P. S., Shulman, C., Thurm, A., & Pickles, A. (2006). Autism from 2 to 9 years of age. *Archives of General Psychiatry, 63*(6), 694–701.

Mandlawitz, M. R. (2002). The impact of the legal system on educational programming for young children with autism spectrum disorder. *Journal of Autism and Developmental Disorders, 32*(5), 495–508.

Mandlawitz, M. R. (2005). Educating children with autism: Current legal issues. In F. R. Volkmar, R. Paul, A. Klin, & D. Cohen (Eds.), *Handbook of autism and pervasive developmental disorders* (3rd ed., pp. 1161–1173). Hoboken, NJ: Wiley.

Marcus, L. M., Flagler, S., & Robinson, S. (2001). Assessment of children with autism. In R. J. Simeonsson & S. L. Rosenthal (Eds.), *Psychological and developmental assessment* (pp. 267–291). New York: Guilford Press.

Marcus, L. M., Kunce, L. J., & Schopler, E. (2005). Working with families. In F. R. Volkmar, R. Paul, A. Klin, & D. Cohen (Eds.), *Handbook of autism and pervasive developmental disorders* (3rd ed., pp. 1055–1086). Hoboken, NJ: Wiley.

Mayerson, G. (2004). *How to compromise with your school district without compromising your child: A field guide for getting effective services for children with special needs.* New York: DRL Books.

Mundy, P. (2003). The neural basis of social impairments in autism: The role of the dorsal medial–frontal cortex and anterior cingulated system. *Journal of Psychology and Psychiatry. 47,* 793–809.

National Research Council. (2001). *Educating children with autism. Committee on Educational Interventions for Children with Autism. (Division of Behavioral and Social Sciences and Education).* Washington, DC: National Academy Press.

New York State Department of Health Early Intervention Program. (1999). *Clinical practice guideline: Report of the recommendations. Autism/pervasive developmental disorders, assessment and intervention for your children (age 0–3 years).* Retrieved August 2, 2003, from *www.health.state.ny.us/hysdoh/eip/menu.htm.*

Olley, J. G. (2005). Curriculum and classroom structure. In F. R. Volkmar, R. Paul, A. Klin, & D. Cohen (Eds.), *Handbook of autism and pervasive developmental disorders* (3rd ed., pp. 863–881). Hoboken, NJ: Wiley.

Olsson, M. B., & Hwang, C. P. (2002). Sense of coherence in parents of children with different developmental disabilities. *Journal of Intellectual Disability Research, 46,* 548–559.

Paul, R., & Sutherland, D. (2005). Enhancing early language in children with autism spectrum disorders. In F. R. Volkmar, R. Paul, A. Klin, & D. Cohen (Eds.), *Handbook of autism and pervasive developmental disorders* (3rd ed., pp. 946–976). Hoboken, NJ: Wiley.

Powers, M. D. (2000). Children with autism and their families. In M. D. Powers (Ed.) *Children with autism: A parents' guide* (2nd ed., pp. 119–254). Bethesda, MD: Woodbine House.

Powers, M. D. (2005). Behavioral assessment of individuals with autism: A functional ecological approach. In F. R. Volkmar, R. Paul, A. Klin, & D. Cohen (Eds.), *Handbook of autism and pervasive developmental disorders* (3rd ed., pp. 817–830). Hoboken, NJ: Wiley.

Prizant, B. M., Wetherby, A. M., & Rydell, P. J. (2000). Communication intervention issues for young children with autism spectrum disorders. In A. M. Wetherby & B. M. Prizant (Eds.), *Autism spectrum disorders: A transactional developmental perspective* (pp. 193–224). Baltimore: Brookes.

Quill, K. A. (2000). *Do-Watch-Listen-Say: Social and communication intervention for children with autism.* Baltimore: Brookes.

Randall, P., & Parker, J. (1999). *Supporting the families of children with autism.* Chichester, UK: Wiley.

Rapin, I. (2005). Autism: Where we have been, where we are going. In F. R. Volkmar, R. Paul, A. Klin, & D. Cohen (Eds.), *Handbook of autism and pervasive developmental disorders* (3rd ed., pp. 1305–1317). Hoboken, NJ: Wiley.

Schopler, E. (2001). Treatment for autism: From science to pseudo-science or anti-science. In E. Schopler, N. Yirmiya, C. Schulman, & L. M. Marcus (Eds.), *The research basis for autism intervention* (pp. 9–24). New York: Kluwer Academic/Plenum Press.

Schopler, E., & Mesibov, G. B. (2000). Cross-cultural priorities in developing autism services. *International Journal of Mental Health, 29,* 3–21.

Seltzer, M. M., Krauss, M. W., Orsmond, G. I., & Vestal, C. (2001). Families of adolescents and adults with autism: Uncharted territory. *International Review of Research in Mental Retardation, 23,* 267–294.

Sharpley, C. F., Bitsika, V., & Ephrimidis, B. (1997). Influence of gender, parental health, and perceived expertise of assistance upon stress, anxiety, and depression among parents of children with autism. *Journal of Intellectual and Developmental Disability, 22,* 19–28.

Siegel, B. (2003). *Helping children with autism learn: Treatment approaches for parents and professionals.* New York: Oxford University Press.

Simpson, R. L. (2004). Finding effective intervention and personnel preparation practices for students with autism spectrum disorders. *Exceptional Children, 70*, 135–144.

Sparrow, S. S., Cicchetti, D. V., & Balla, D. A. (2005). *Vineland Adaptive Behavior Scales–Second Edition (Vineland-II): Survey interview form/caregiver rating form.* Livonia, MN: Pearson Assessments.

Sussman, F. (1999). *More than words: Helping parents promote communication and social skills in children with autism spectrum disorder.* Toronto, ON: Hanen Centre.

Tager-Flusberg, H., Paul, R., & Lord, C. (2005). Language and communication in autism. In F. R. Volkmar, R. Paul, A. Klin, & D. Cohen (Eds.), *Handbook of autism and pervasive developmental disorders* (3rd ed., pp. 335–364). Hoboken, NJ: Wiley.

Tobing, L. E., & Glenwick, D. S. (2002). Relation of the Childhood Autism Rating Scale–Parent Version to diagnosis, stress, and age. *Research in Developmental Disabilities, 23,* 211–223.

Volkmar, F., Cook, E. H., Jr., Pomeroy, J., Realmuto, G., & Tanguay, P. (1999). Practice parameters for the assessment and treatment of children, adolescents, and adults with autism and other pervasive developmental disorders. *Journal of the American Academy of Child and Adolescent Psychiatry, 38*(12), 32S–54S.

Volkmar, F. R., & Wiesner, L. A. (2004). *Healthcare for children on the autism spectrum: A guide to medical, nutritional, and behavioral issues.* Bethesda, MD: Woodbine House.

Webster-Stratton, C., Reid, M. J., & Hammond, M. (2001). Preventing conduct problems, promoting social competence: A parent and teacher training partnership in Head Start. *Journal of Clinical Child Psychology, 30,* 283–302.

Wetherby, A. M., Prizant, M. B., & Schuler, A. L. (2000). Understanding the nature of communication and language impairments. In A. M. Wetherby & B. M. Prizant (Eds.), *Autism spectrum disorders: A transactional developmental perspective* (pp. 109–142). Baltimore: Brookes.

Wheeler, M. (2004). *Toilet training for individuals with autism and related disorders: A comprehensive guide for parents and teachers.* Arlington, TX: Future Horizons.

Wiggs, L., & Stores, G. (2004). Sleep patterns and sleep disorders in children with autistic spectrum disorders: Insights using parent report and actigraphy. *Developmental Medicine and Child Neurology, 46*(6), 372–380.

Wright, P. W. D., & Wright, P. D. (2002). *From emotions to advocacy: The special education survival guide.* Hartfield, VA: Harbor House Law Press.

Wright, P. W. D., & Wright, P. D. (2004). *Idea 2004.* Hartfield, VA: Harbor House Law Press.

CHAPTER 12

————•————

Opportunities for Research
Concepts and Future Directions

AMI KLIN
KATARZYNA CHAWARSKA
FRED R. VOLKMAR

The advent of prospective studies of infants at greater genetic risk for autism spectrum disorders (ASD)–the "baby siblings" studies, carries the promise of unveiling the mystery shrouding the first 2 years of life of these children (Zwaigenbaum et al., 2005). Until recently, models of the genetic, neural, and behavioral bases of autism were proposed and tested in the absence of solid knowledge of this critical period of development. Just as neuropsychological and brain imaging paradigms were combined in the past 15 years in order to generate levels of mutual constraint and synergy (Volkmar, Lord, Bailey, Schultz, & Klin, 2004), we predict that future genetic and neurocognitive hypotheses will be constrained by what we learn about the developmental profiles and trajectories of infants with ASD. This volume as a whole argues that the developmental nature of autism and its early onset need to take center stage in the process of discovery of causes and treatment of this complex family of conditions.

In fact, autism is the quintessential neurodevelopmental disorder. Disruptions occurring early in life lead to a cascade of pervasive clinical phenomena. This has critical implications for models of etiology and pathogenesis. By most accounts, the genetic liability involves an extremely variable genotype, whereby many susceptibility genes act in combinatorial fashion further complicated by variable activation timetables and other epigenetic factors (Gupta & State, 2007). In many ways, it is surprising that the ASD are expressed as a relative unitary syndrome, albeit vastly heterogeneous. What, in the face of so many "autisms," constrains syndrome expression? We propose that the answer to this question lies in the postnatal activities of infants and the experiences accrued from their attempts to "solve" fundamental, evolutionarily based adaptive tasks (Klin, Jones, & Schultz, 2003). Thus there is a need for charting what those experiences consist of, their timetable, and their trajectories.

Similarly, although a host of prenatal factors provide the blueprint for brain organization, both structure and function are sculpted by experiences, and the experiences of infants with ASD are atypical from very early on (Schultz, 2005). Sorting out causes of autism from the results of having autism is a critical, if vexing, issue in neuroimaging research, inasmuch as the determinism of brain growth and specialization is tempered by our knowledge that our brains also "become who we are" (LeDoux, 2002). The now prevailing "experience–expectant" framework of gene/brain and environment interaction posits that we are born with predispositions to respond to aspects of the world in certain ways so as to accomplish evolutionarily relevant tasks (Johnson & Karmiloff-Smith, 2004). The associated and equally prevailing framework of the activity-dependent nature of brain development signifies that brain specialization is the co-creation of genetic predispositions and experiences following the actions of infants in their world (Johnson, 2001). Both notions, therefore, prescribe the need for careful consideration of the experiences of infants in any attempt to understand the pattern of crystallization of brain structure and function.

The notion of multiple etiologies leading to a relatively singular and "boundable" or discrete syndrome has historically led to evocations of a "final common pathway." What might that be? Nature is replete with examples of animal shapes, forms, and behaviors that are not preprogrammed genetically (Thompson, 1942). Rather, they result from the interaction between biological and environmental forces that create regularities co-created as the result of this interaction. Understanding such regularities requires elucidation of both biological predispositions and the specific adaptive tasks that this specific biology is programmed to help the organism "solve." For human infants, one of the most fundamental evolutionary tasks is the engagement with their caregivers. Their fragility and utter dependence makes success in this task a question of survival (Tronick, 1980). It also provides a springboard for the acquisition of a wide range of communication and social-cognitive skills (Klin et al., 2003). We propose that variable etiologies associated with autism might result in similar phenotypes because they impact on the process of social engagement. After all, despite the impressive variability of various aspects of syndrome expression, the "constants," making the ASD a distinctive category in psychopathology, are both the impairments in socialization and their early onset (Volkmar et al., 2004). In this way, variable causes could lead to similar results.

But the process of social engagement is a recursive platform for ever more complex social-cognitive experiences. When, how much, and by which specific factors this process is disrupted would create fairly different results, corresponding to patterns of symptom onset and different levels of ability and disability. This is a well-known effect in developmental neurobiology. Activation or deactivation of the same gene at different embryological phases can result in extremely different phenotypes (DiCicco-Bloom et al., 2006). Though much less deterministic, there is enough knowledge of social-developmental processes to identify behavioral consequences of disruptions of social engagement at different stages in the first 2 years of life. Preferential orientation to auditory and visual social stimuli is online in the first weeks of life (Alegria & Noirot, 1978; Haith, Bergman, & Moore, 1979). Contingent and mutually reinforcing dyadic interaction is fairly advanced by 4 to 6 months of age (Trevarthen, 2005). With the emergence of joint-attention skills, triadic interaction is established in the first few months of the second year of life (Tomasello & Carpenter, 2007). Infants with autism whose engagement with others is disrupted at different stages of social development might all fail social-communicative tasks by the age of 2 years, but such a generalization would mask the possibly very meaningful differences resulting from differential timing of their symptom onset. And these different developmental pathways could represent significant mediators of outcome. To once again draw from embryology, the earlier the "lesion" the graver the outcome.

When seen in later development, children with ASD display baffling heterogeneity in syndrome expression and severity (Happé, Ronald, & Plomin, 2006). Because the onset of autism is almost always before 2 years of age (Chawarska, Paul, et al., 2007), and because until recently infants were never evaluated or studied, differences in onset patterns were not considered to be key factors in attempts to understand phenotypic heterogeneity. Though helpful, parental reports of syndrome recognition cannot be used with any degree of temporal precision as measures of symptom onset. Given the extraordinary rate of developmental change in infants, placing the onset of the disruption of socialization in the first month, or in the sixth, ninth, twelfth, or eighteenth month of life, would generate a respectable spectrum of syndrome manifestation. This hypothesis can now be tested because babies are carefully followed from birth, at least in some "baby sibling" studies. We suggest that this approach may greatly reduce phenotypic heterogeneity, which could otherwise introduce so much variability to group analyses to the point of diluting or masking key effects in research of older children. Although the concept of a "spectrum" of autism conditions is replacing more categorical definitions in research, it is important to remember that we know as yet very little as to what the dimensions generating this spectrum might be.

Another benefit of considering the social engagement task as the framework constraining phenotypic variability is that one may be able to go beyond symptom onset—when autistic behaviors are first evident, to studies of mechanisms of socialization—the reactions or skills underlying successful social adaptation. Note that this approach conceives of the possibility that there is no one-to-one relationship between etiologic factors and autistic symptoms, inasmuch as symptoms could be the result of disruptions of highly conserved social-adaptive mechanisms leading to a breakdown in socialization, that is, leading to autism (Klin et al., 2003). But there could be a one to-one causative connection between etiological factors and specific mechanisms of socialization, as these are robust features of the species. As such, they could be considered candidate "endophenotypes" (Dawson et al., 2002). In genetics, a fairly strong consensus is emerging as to the need to substantially increase the power of genetic analyses by focusing on meaningful mediating phenotypes rather than on complex symptom clusters (Geschwind et al., 2001; Gupta & State, 2007). What these might be is still a subject of speculation. What is not controversial is that such endophenotypes should correspond to developmental factors impacting on socialization in the first 2 years of life.

From a practical standpoint, this approach may also result in the earlier identification of vulnerabilities for autism. At present, the few existing studies have been focused primarily on the detection of the earliest symptoms of autism (Zwaigenbaum et al., 2005; Mitchell et al., 2006). If these are conceived as the result of failed mechanisms of social adaptation, then direct measurement of these mechanisms could provide an early benchmark for identification of vulnerabilities. For that goal to be achieved, there is a need for a much greater utilization of developmental science paradigms in the study of baby siblings. Experimental settings measuring typical social-cognitive accomplishments—from visual engagement to attentional mechanisms, to gaze cueing and face processing, to listening preferences—among other fields, have a history of several decades. Tentative but highly exciting findings are just emerging from such an effort in autism research (Chawarska & Volkmar, 2007; Chawarska, Klin, & Volkmar, 2003; Klin & Jones, 2007; Merin, Young, Ozonoff, & Rogers, 2007; Mitchell et al., 2006; Nadig et al., 2007; Paul et al., 2007). Thus, one should expect that quantification of social engagement processes, or other neurocognitive processes directly impacting on socialization, may elevate the early identification effort to a higher state of objectification of the diagnostic process. In this desired future, we may be able to identify vulnerabilities for autism even before the emergence of any autistic symptoms.

A consideration of the models of pathogenesis of autism has the potential of shedding light on several raging controversies in the field. Consider the phenomenon of regression in autism. Besides fueling unsubstantiated causative theories of autism such as vaccination and environmental toxins (Nature Neuroscience, 2005, 2007), it provides a substantially different guideline for neurobiological research. If autism represents a regressive phenomenon, our efforts should be focused on disease models that emphasize a cumulative effect of biological dysfunction resulting in the crossing of some threshold that unleashes the syndrome (such as in PKU or specific metabolic disorders). At present, the only irrefutable cases of regression are seen in the children with Childhood Disintegrative Disorder (CDD). These are extremely rare, their outcome is worse than in autism, and medical research has revealed as yet very little as to what factors are triggering such a dramatic developmental regression (Volkmar, Koenig, & State, 2005). Is CDD a good model for regressive autism?

There is a growing number of studies showing that some regression happens in a substantial number of cases, typically at about the first or second trimester of the second year of life (Brown & Prelock, 1995; Chawarska, Paul, et al., 2007; Christopher, Sears, Williams, Oliver, & Hersh, 2004; Davidovitch, Glick, Holtzman, Tirosh, & Safir, 2000; Goldberg et al., 2003; Lord, Shulman, & DiLavore, 2004; Siperstein & Volkmar, 2004; Tuchman & Rapin, 1997; Werner & Dawson, 2005; Wilson, Djukie, Shinnar, Dharmani, & Rapin, 2003). All of these studies, however, have relied on parental report or home movies of children prior to their regression. Although these represent a considerable improvement over the anecdotal notions of regression that preceded them, regression in autism has not as yet been the subject of more precise data collection—contemporaneous, direct, and quantified—which could in turn allow for more sophisticated conceptual scrutiny and analysis. For example, could the loss of a few words, one of the most discrete and measurable regressive symptoms, be the result of something other than a regressive process? By way of analogy, consider the case of babbling in congenitally deaf children (Lenneberg, 1967). They typically babble for several months before they cease to do so. Apparently this is so because of the absence of auditory feedback. This sound "gesture," which takes on communicative value with age, does not evolve in this fashion because it is not serving any function in the infant's efforts to respond adaptively to the approach of others. The congenitally deaf child cannot hear the sound that he or she is making and therefore cannot associate these sounds with the impact they have on their social interaction partners. Without an adaptive function, the babbling dies off. If infants with autism acquire words in echolalic fashion but these do not serve the purpose of social adaptation, there would be no function or use associated with them. So they may die off. If one were to be guided by the myriad behaviors displayed by older children with autism that mirror social or communicative behaviors, but when subjected to clinical scrutiny are found to be devoid of such content, it is plausible that parents, or professionals working on these clinical phenomena through the perspective of parents or only through indirect observations, may be unable to adequately assess the social intentionality of such behaviors in 12- to 18-month-old babies. After all, babies smile and vocalize in many ways, for many reasons, and in response to a wide range of stimuli (internal or external), and not only when they intend these to be acts of communication directed at their caregivers. In this light, we believe that this critical question can be elucidated only through direct prospective observation and quantification of these infants' development. This is likely to be one of the most significant contributions of baby sibling studies.

Finally, there are methodological advances of critical practical importance that need to result from the growing work with infants at risk for autism. Chief among these is the need for diagnostic criteria for children coming to clinical attention in their second year of life. Growing awareness of the importance of early intervention as a way of optimizing outcome (National Research Council, 2001) has generated an ever-increasing number of referrals for diagnostic evaluation and services. And yet there is still uncertainty as to what should be the defining criteria for infants and toddlers, and what instrumentation yields the greatest predictive power relative to subsequent confirmatory diagnosis (Zwaigenbaum et al., 2007). There is a substantial body of data for the diagnosis of 2-year-old children, and stability of diagnosis is quite strong (Lord, 1995; Lord et al., 2006), and the evidence regarding stability of the diagnosis in the second year of life is only beginning to emerge (Chawarska, Klin, Paul, & Volkmar, 2007). The field trials that led to the creation of research criteria for autism in the *Diagnostic and Statistical Manual of Mental Disorders*, fourth edition (DSM-IV) and the *International Classification of Diseases*, 10th edition (ICD-10) did not include a substantial number of children in this age group (Volkmar, Lord, Bailey, Schultz, & Klin, 2004). The use of these criteria by simple downward extension is therefore not warranted. Research on the sensitivity, specificity, and reliability of diagnostic criteria has been slow in coming because the gold standard is not only concurrent diagnosis made by experienced clinicians, but also confirmatory diagnosis obtained several years thereafter. Both research and services are negatively impacted by the absence of such criteria. It is therefore one of the greatest priorities in the field.

In the past 5 years, a confluence of findings in genetics and brain research generated the hope for a breakthrough in autism research. A number of genes were identified as being associated with a variable number of cases (see Gupta & State, 2007, for a review). These genes are primarily associated with factors impacting on brain growth and organization. These findings brought about hopes for pharmacological therapies targeting the proteins associated with these genes, possibly preventing autism before the onset of the pathological process.

At about the same time, evidence for atypically accelerated brain growth in the first 2 years of life of groups of children with autism began to mount, raising hopes for a biological marker of autism (e.g., Courchesne et al., 2001; Dawson et al., 2002; Hazlett et al., 2005). The association of these two lines of research strengthened the notions that fundamental brain architecture is altered in autism, and that further advances will link genes to brain growth factors and to anatomical and histological findings (through increasingly more sophisticated neuroimaging methods capable of mapping neural fiber structure and pathways, not only gross volumetric measures).

However, the impact of these gene–brain processes on behavior and development are not yet known. In the absence of such delineation, we are still left with sweeping generalizations. For years, research on the biology of autism had yielded little, whereas major strides were made in phenomenology and neuropsychology. In the context of studies on infants, it is now the latter, not the former, that is lagging behind. To narrow this gap and add meaning to the exciting new genetic and neuroimaging advances, there is a need to speed up the process of discovery related to behavioral development of infants with autism. As this volume signifies, the field is well poised to expedite these advances. In this sense, the next 5 years are likely to be even more exciting than the last 5.

REFERENCES

Alegria, J., & Noirot, E. (1978). Neonate orientation behavior towards human voice. *International Journal of Behavioral Development, 1,* 291–312.

Brown, J., & Prelock, P. A. (1995). The impact of regression on language development in autism. *Journal of Autism and Developmental Disorders, 25*(3), 305–309.

Chawarska, K., Klin, A., Paul, R., & Volkmar, F. R. (2007). Autism spectrum disorders in the second year: Stability and change in syndrome expression. *Journal of Child Psychology and Psychiatry, 48*(2), 128–138.

Chawarska, K., Klin, A., & Volkmar, F. (2003). Automatic attention cueing through eye movement in 2-year-old children with autism. *Child Development, 74*(4), 1108–1122.

Chawarska, K., Paul, R., Klin, A., Hannigen, S., Dichtel, L. E., & Volkmar, F. R. (2007). Parental recognition of developmental problems in toddlers with autism spectrum disorders. *Journal of Autism and Developmental Disorders, 37*(1), 62–72.

Chawarska, K., & Volkmar, F. (2007). Impairments in monkey and human face recognition in 2-year-old toddlers with autism spectrum disorder and developmental delay. *Developmental Science, 10*(2), 266–279.

Christopher, J. A., Sears, L. L., Williams, P. G., Oliver, J., & Hersh, J. (2004). Familial, medical and developmental patterns of children with autism and a history of language regression. *Journal of Developmental and Physical Disabilities, 16*(2), 163–170.

Courschene, E., Karns, C. M., Davis, H. R., Ziccardi, R., Carper, R. A., Tigue, Z. D., et al. (2001). Unusual brain growth patterns in early life in patients with autism disorder: An MRI study. *Neurology, 57,* 245–254.

Davidovitch, M., Glick, L., Holtzman, G., Tirosh, E., & Safir, M. P. (2000). Developmental regression in autism: Maternal perception. *Journal of Autism and Developmental Disorders, 30*(2), 113–119.

Dawson, G., Webb, S., Schellenberg, G. D., Dager, S., Friedman, S., Aylward, E., et al. (2002). Defining the broader phenotype of autism: Genetic, brain, and behavioral perspectives. *Development and Psychopathology, 14,* 581–611.

DiCicco-Bloom, E., Lord, C., Zwaigenbaum, L., Courchesne, E., Dager, S. R., Schmitz, C., et al. (2006). The developmental neurobiology of autism spectrum disorder. *Journal of Neuroscience, 26*(26), 6897–6906.

Geschwind, D. H., Sowinski, J., Lord, C., Iversen, P., Shestack, J., Jones, P., et al. (2001). The autism genetic resource exchange: A resource for the study of autism and related neuropsychiatric conditions. *American Journal of Human Genetics, 69*(2), 463–466.

Goldberg, W. A., Osann, K., Filipek, P. A., Laulhere, T., Jarvis, K., Modahl, C., et al. (2003). Language and other regression: Assessment and timing. *Journal of Autism and Developmental Disorders, 33*(6), 607–616.

Gupta, A. R., & State, M. W. (2007). Recent advances in the genetics of autism. *Biological Psychiatry, 61*(4), 429–437.

Haith, M. M., Bergman, T., & Moore, M. J. (1979). Eye contact and face scanning in early infancy. *Science, 198*(4319), 853–855.

Happé, F., Ronald, A., & Plomin, R. (2006). Time to give up on a single explanation for autism. *Nature Neuroscience, 9*(10), 1218–1220.

Hazlett, H. C., Poe, M. D., Gerig, G., Smith, R. G., Provenzale, J., Ross, A., et al. (2005). An MRI and head circumference study of brain size in autism: Birth through age two years. *Archives of General Psychiatry, 62,* 1366–1376.

Johnson, M. (2001). Functional brain development in humans. *Nature Reviews Neuroscience, 2,* 475–483.

Johnson, M. H., & Karmiloff-Smith, A. (2004). Neuroscience perspectives on infant development. In G. Bremner & A. Slater (Eds.), *Theories of infant development* (pp. 121–141). Malden, MA: Blackwell.

Klin, A., & Jones, W. (2007). Altered face scanning and impaired recognition of biological motion in a 15-month-old infant with autism. *Developmental Science.* Available online at: doi:10.1111/j.1467-7687.2007.00608.x

Klin, A., Jones, W., & Schultz, R. (2003). The enactive mind—from actions to cognition: Lessons from autism. *Philosophical Transactions of the Royal Society: Biological Sciences, 358,* 345–360.

LeDoux, J. (2002). *Synaptic self: How our brains become who we are.* New York: Viking Penguin Press.

Lenneberg, E. H. (1967). *Biological foundations of language.* New York: Wiley.

Lord, C. (1995). Follow-up of two-year-olds referred for possible autism. *Journal of Child Psychology and Psychiatry and Allied Disciplines, 36*(8), 1365–1382.

Lord, C., Risi, S., DiLavore, P. S., Shulman, C., Thurm, A., & Pickles, A. (2006). Autism from 2 to 9 years of age. *Archives of General Psychiatry, 63*(6), 694–701.

Lord, C., Shulman, C., & DiLavore, P. (2004). Regression and word loss in autistic spectrum disorders. *Journal of Child Psychology and Psychiatry, 45*(5), 936–955.

A mercurial debate over autism [Editorial]. (2005). *Nature Neuroscience, 10*(5), 531.

Merin, N., Young, G. S., Ozonoff, S., & Rogers, S. J. (2007). Visual fixation patterns during reciprocal social interaction distinguish a subgroup of 6-month-old infants at risk for autism from comparison infants. *Journal of Autism and Developmental Disorders, 37*(1), 108–121.

Mitchell, S., Brian, S., Zwaigenbaum, L., Roberts, W., Szatmari, P., Smith, I., et al. (2006). Early language and communication development of infants later diagnosed with autism spectrum disorder. *Journal of Developmental and Behavioral Pediatrics, 27*(Suppl. 2), S69–S78.

Nadig, A. S., Ozonoff, S., Young, G. S., Rozga, A., Sigman, M., & Rogers, S. J. (2007). A prospective study of response to name in infants at risk for autism. *Archives of Pediatric and Adolescent Medicine, 161*(4), 378–383.

National Research Council. (2001). *Educating children with autism.* Washington, DC: National Academy Press.

Paul, R., Chawarska, K., Fowler, C., Cicchetti, D., & Volkmar, F. (2007). "Listen my children and you shall hear": Auditory preferences in toddlers with autism spectrum disorders. *Journal of Speech, Language, and Hearing Research, 50,* 1350–1364.

Schultz, R. T. (2005). Developmental deficits in social perception in autism: The role of the amygdala and fusiform face area. *International Journal of Developmental Neuroscience, 23,* 125–141.

Silencing debate over autism. (2007). *Nature Neuroscience, 8*(9), 1123.

Siperstein, R., & Volkmar, F. (2004). Brief report: Parental reporting of regression in children with pervasive developmental disorders. *Journal of Autism and Developmental Disorders, 34*(6), 731–734.

Thompson, D. (1942). *On growth and form.* Cambridge, UK: Cambridge University Press.

Tomasello, M., & Carpenter, M. (2007). Shared intentionality. *Developmental Science, 10*(1), 121–125.

Trevarthen, C. (2005). Action and emotion in development of cultural intelligence: Why infants have feelings like ours. In J. Nadel & D. Muir (Eds.), *Emotional development: Recent research advances* (pp. 61–91). New York: Oxford University Press.

Tronick, E. (1980). The primacy of social skills in infancy. In D. B. Sawin, R. C. Hawkins II, L. Olszewski Waker, & J. H. Penticuff (Eds.), *Exceptional infant: Vol. 4. Psychosocial risks in infant–environment transactions* (pp. 144–158). New York: Brunner/Mazel.

Tuchman, R. F., & Rapin, I. (1997). Regression in pervasive developmental disorders: Seizures and epileptiform electroencephalogram correlates. *Pediatrics, 99*(4), 560–566.

Volkmar, F. R., Klin, A., Siegel, B., Szatmari, P., Lord, C., Campbell, M., et al. (1994). Field trial for autistic disorder in DSM-IV. *American Journal of Psychiatry, 151,* 1361–1367.

Volkmar, F. R., Koenig, K., & State, M. (2005). Childhood disintegrative disorder.

In F. R. Volkmar, R. Paul, A. Klin, & D. J. Cohen (Eds.), *Handbook of autism and pervasive developmental disorders* (3rd ed., pp. 70–87). New York: Wiley.

Volkmar, F., Lord, C., Bailey, A., Schultz, R. T., & Klin, A. (2004). Autism and pervasive developmental disorders. *Journal of Child Psychology and Psychiatry, 45*(1), 135–170.

Werner, E., & Dawson, G. (2005). Validation of the phenomenon of autistic regression using home videotapes. *Archives of General Psychiatry, 62*(8), 889–895.

Wilson, S., Djukie, A., Shinnar, S., Dharmani, C., & Rapin, I. (2003). Clinical characteristics of language regression in children. *Developmental Medicine and Child Neurology, 45*, 508–514.

Zwaigenbaum, L., Bryson, S., Rogers, T., Roberts, W., Brian, J., & Szatmari, P. (2005). Behavioral manifestations of autism in the first year of life. *International Journal of Developmental Neuroscience, 23*(2–3), 143–152.

Zwaigenbaum, L., Thurm, A., Stone, W., Baranek, G., Bryson, S., Iverson, J., et al. (2007). Studying the emergence of autism spectrum disorders in high-risk infants: Methodological and practical issues. *Journal of Autism and Developmental Disorders, 37*(3), 466–480.

Index